Eros *and* Illness

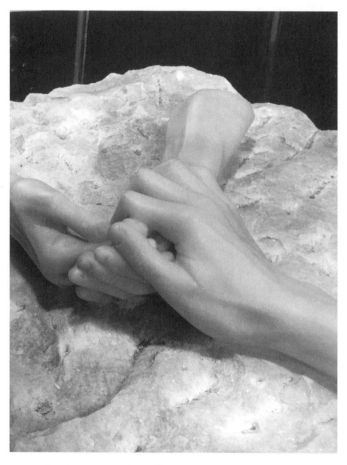

Louise Bourgeois. *Cell: You Better Grow Up*. 1993.
Detail. Installation. © The Easton Foundation.
Licensed by VAGA, New York, NY.

Eros

and

Illness

David B. Morris

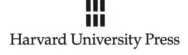

Harvard University Press

Cambridge, Massachusetts
London, England
2017

First printing

Library of Congress Cataloging-in-Publication Data

Names: Morris, David B., author.

Title: Eros and illness / David B. Morris.

Description: Cambridge, Massachusetts : Harvard University Press, 2017. |
Includes bibliographical references and index.

Identifiers: LCCN 2016038760 | ISBN 9780674659711 (cloth)

Subjects: LCSH: Sick—Psychology. | Medicine and psychology. |
Desire (Philosophy) | Personalized medicine.

Classification: LCC R726.5 .M666 2017 | DDC 610—dc23

LC record available at https://lccn.loc.gov/2016038760

For Ruth

Contents

Eros *and* Illness

INTRODUCTION

What Is Eros?

Eros is everywhere. It is what binds.

JOHN UPDIKE, QUOTED IN *NEW YORK TIMES* (1998)

*E*ROS IS CENTRAL not only to love, its traditional domain, but also to illness. This crucial relationship, however, goes mostly unrecognized and unaddressed, with incalculable harm to patients, to doctors, and to loved ones. The importance of eros in illness proved an unavoidable, unwelcome fact in my own experience as I gradually came to recognize that I was living in a condition of conflict—almost like a civilian in a war zone—caught between two mighty forces that, lacking an established vocabulary, I came to call *medical logos* and *medical eros*. The conflict turned weirder than any ordinary combat because, although medical logos is highly visible and almost inescapable, medical eros remains largely unseen, living in the shadows, as if its distinctive superpowers included a cloak of invisibility. The conflict and the terms that I invented in order to describe it are both unfamiliar enough to require a brief, preliminary account.

Eros is the ancient Greek god of desire. Desire, under the rule of Eros, usually brushes directly or indirectly against sexual passion, so some classical authorities describe Eros as the god of love or as the god of

1

fertility, a powerful figure depicted on a fifth-century BCE Greek vase as a dark-haired muscular young archer, with an athlete's washboard abdomen and a wingspan massive enough to suggest Andean condors. In later Roman art, as if forgetting his former godlike powers, Eros mostly dwindles into the mischievous, wanton, and sometimes downright cruel boy Cupid: ancestor of the chubby putto with vestigial wings who shows up on Valentine's Day bearing a box of chocolates and a heart-shaped card full of amorous pieties. Eros includes all these figures and more, far more, from Cleopatra to *The Rocky Horror Picture Show* and onward into the gender-questioning future, as desire circulates, pulses, and overflows beyond images and words, beyond thought and music, beyond flirtation, romantic dalliance, one-night stands, or shocking lustful abandon.

Why should we bother with a defunct classical god? Even if we think of Eros merely as a figure who represents love—and no one seriously disputes the importance or complexities of love—Eros is much more than an ancient fictitious deity. As a classical god, Eros gives visible shape to the lowercase internal psychic force (eros) that has forged both a complex social history and far-reaching connections with other human forces, from lust and compassion to violence. The classical god Eros, in this sense, bears some resemblance to fire. Fire in the ancient world has its designated gods—Hephaestus in Greece, Vulcan in Rome—but fire can assume many different shapes, from the blacksmith's civilizing flame (associated with Hephaestus) to the volcanic eruptions that derive their name from Vulcan. We no longer believe in Vulcan or Hephaestus, but it would be a serious miscalculation to doubt the reality of fire. Like fire, eros can do great harm—burn, injure, devastate—but it also holds a primal power for good, much as the mythic flame that Prometheus stole from Mount Olympus and delivered to humankind could warn sailors with a coastal light or warm a cold hearth. Reconfigured as an internal human force, eros today would not resemble a classical archer but might instead assume the charisma and plasticity of contemporary shape-shifters from androgynous rock stars to the wizarding world of J. K. Rowling.

Eros in its continual changes and ceaseless circulation, especially in what John Updike rightly calls its power *to bind*, once held absolute preeminence as the original cosmic creative force. The early Greek poet Hesiod (ca. 800 BCE) depicts Eros as the oldest of the gods, who brings about the fruitful union of earth (Gaia) and sky (Uranus). Several centuries later Eros—still celebrated as a god, or at least godlike in its power—remains so important as to constitute the single topic of discussion in Plato's *Symposium*. Socrates, a foundational figure in Western philosophy and a key participant in the Platonic dramatic dialogue on love, claims that eros is the only subject he knows anything about. His contribution, however, is to retell a story or myth once told to him by an obscure prophetess. This secondhand tale—about a ladder that leads from the love of beautiful bodies to the love of ideal form—carries an implicit caution from the master ironist: that whatever we say about eros (even reconfigured as a modern, lowercase, internal power) will fall short of absolute truth and occupy only the secondary, indirect status of a myth, narrative, or symbolic approximation.

Eros, in short, cannot be reduced to a concept. It is not accessible through propositions or argument. It is rather a primal force that, in its typical motion, sweeps us away, depriving us of reason, logic, and even coherent speech. As it turns out in Plato's *Symposium*, no one gets the last word on eros, where the one truly inexhaustible erotic pleasure seems to be *talking* about love. The philosophical talk, really a competitive form of oratorical display, occurs on a high plane of discourse, while erotic desire (on the lower plane of libido) circulates invisibly among the talkers: Socrates, we learn, wants to seduce Agathon, Agathon is already the boyfriend of Pausanias, and (toward the inconclusive conclusion of the speeches) Alcibiades breaks in, very drunk and uninvited, to describe at length his sexual longing for Socrates. Plato depicts a semicomic scene, then, in which reason, logic, rhetoric, and philosophy pay extended homage to Eros as a god, while eros as a human power (in conjunction, as so often, with wine) sweeps away both rationality and consciousness as all the participants finally slip off into inebriated slumber, leaving Socrates—the ironic philosophical storyteller—to walk away, alone, into the dawn.

Socrates offers a distinguished pedigree for the claim that eros, even when configured as a secular human force, cannot be adequately represented in concepts, arguments, or definitions. Eros embraces desire in all its colorful and passionate varieties up to and including delirium. Its inherent excess or surplus—what reason cannot explain or contain—puts it in conflict with the widely shared belief (a founding principle of natural philosophy or early science) that the implicit duty of words is to match up with clear and distinct ideas. Eros is more amenable to description than to definition, and its descriptive history includes the ancient recognition that the erotic signified a "way of being": for Homer, a way of being that emphasized participation in a sacred dimension of life overseen by the goddess Aphrodite.[1]

Today the view of eros as a primal or sacred force finds at best minority expression among scattered writers, scholars, post-Freudians, and eco-spiritualists. Ceaseless news of celebrity hookups, however, along with online dating sites, porn flicks, and sexualized ads suggest that eros, in shape-shifting mode, secretly dominates popular culture.[2] Popular culture no doubt constitutes a distinctive way of being, at least for individuals fully immersed within it, and eros through sheer omnipresence might stake a viable claim as the patron saint of late consumer capitalism. The circulation of capital, as we endlessly consume new films, new music, and all manner of shiny new digital objects, is inseparable from the circulation of erotic impulses and from ad-driven or peer-driven manipulations of desire.

The absence of a consensus-sanctioned definition, if regrettable, luckily does not constitute a fatal flaw, but it creates an implicit obligation to sketch out, early on, the rough boundaries of my usage (Figure 0.1).

Eros, as the diagram suggests, is not a fully knowable quantity—something we can pin down, define, measure, and reconstitute as an object of knowledge; it inhabits shifting relationships, spontaneous actions, and hidden states that desire (often without our knowledge or even against our better judgment) draws us into. Eros and desire are finally far less about knowledge than about altered states of being, unruly impulses, hidden biological and psychic forces, charismatic bodies, everyday selves at risk, and a vertigo of lost control. It is almost inseparable from the exhilarating, dangerous feel of letting go.

My diagrammatic figure of proliferating erotic relations includes a deliberate measure of self-parody in its stable geometric patterns used to clarify a shifting, uncontainable force. A better diagram would be three-dimensional, spinning nonstop like a pinwheel, and embedded with a kill switch to self-destruct when the formula approaches hazardous clarity. A

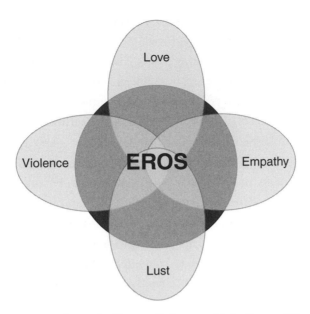

FIGURE 0.1. Logos in (Doomed) Quest to Make Sense of Eros.
David B. Morris.

simplified bird's-eye view, like weather maps, cannot avoid error; however, it remains useful here in representing eros as a libidinal energy that suffuses a wide variety of disparate states from empathy to lust. The diagram also recognizes that eros always implies a potential to make contact with energies that circulate entirely *outside* eros. Mindless brutality, for example, is as unerotic as a butcher shop. Can we fully account for the history of war, human sacrifice, ritualized cruelty, and rape, however, without positing an erotic dimension concealed *somewhere* within even extreme violence? In their violent sexuality, the Marquis de Sade's novels and the high-opera *Liebestod* offer a glimpse into the dark ranges of eros: Tosca, the innocent object of Baron Scarpia's evil lust, hurling herself over the parapet. Such troubling glimpses suggest again that reason will never fully comprehend eros. Eros is at home with chaos and the anarchic. It embraces the *in-definite*, the *a-logical*, the *in-comprehensible*. By definition, it resists definition. My overly geometrical, clockface diagram at least allows for fifty-six additional un-named shades of erotic practice, not all of them pleasant. One key assertion about eros, however, seems to me as reliable as bedrock. Eros, whatever it is, is *not* identical with sexual activity.

Sexuality, sexual activity, and lust are all central to eros, of course, but when it comes to human beings, these basic forms of desire often lead to and become entangled with other forms. "Sexual reproductive activity is common to sexual animals and men," writes French polymath Georges Bataille in *L'érotisme* (1957), "but only men appear to have turned their sexual activity into erotic activity."[3] Bataille, still the modern Continental thinker most at home with eros, does not shy away from exploring dark, perverse, or grotesque episodes when erotic pleasure, sexual passion, and carnal delirium make contact with violence, pain, torture, and death.[4] Its darkest excesses confirm for Bataille that eros cannot be confined to sexuality. Eros certainly shares common ground with sexual activity, but human erotic life extends to distant and indirect psychological inflections of desire played out within the arena of experience that Bataille calls "the inner life" (*la vie intérieure*). A sonnet sequence can prove erotic, or e-mail innuendos, or a certain smile, the sway of bodies, a hint of perfume, or even (under the right circumstances) a lullaby. The inner life matters for eros as much as do erogenous zones, while the free play of mind can provide a self-sufficient erotic pleasure. Sexual activity is a trait widely shared within the animal kingdom. "Human eroticism," as Bataille nails down the crucial distinction, "differs from animal sexuality precisely in this, that it calls inner life into play."[5]

Inner life is what makes eros both irresistible and dangerous. Its danger and its dark side were evident long before Bataille collected and celebrated examples of what he called *the tears of eros*. Cupid's arrows can turn lethal as lovers' quarrels slide recklessly toward violence. Every neighborhood seems to house its convicted sex offenders. Eros is not only not identical with love but also regularly shatters settled romantic relations with spontaneous flings and disastrous betrayals. It persists as heartbreak in love's absence. From classical lyric to modern tragedy, eros disrupts and torments the inner life that it calls into play. It rips apart marriages and plunges alliances into disarray, justifying the frequent references to love as an addiction, torment, plague, and disease. Anne Carson, classicist, philosopher, and gifted contemporary writer, explains that ancient Greek lyric poets simply assumed as a matter of self-evident fact that eros is "hostile in intention and detrimental in effect." "Alongside melting," she remarks, adding up the classical epithets attributed to eros, "we might cite metaphors of piercing, crushing, bridling, roasting, stinging, biting, grating, cropping, poisoning, singeing, and grinding to a powder."[6] Eros regularly extends the range of romantic afflictions from mild obsession to disease. Lovesickness in the Middle Ages was a standard medical diagnosis: a famous English bishop supposedly died from it.[7]

"The whole business of eroticism," Bataille asserts, "is to destroy the self-contained character of the participators as they are in their normal lives."[8] Normal lives, as Bataille believed, may well benefit from the destruction of spirit-crushing bourgeois routines and from the demolition of capitalist self-denials. Illness too destroys (or threatens to destroy) the patterns of our normal lives, but the complex underground associations that link illness with eros and desire—including possible benefits that might arise from the ashes—simply did not register during the prolonged period when medical eros and medical logos trapped me within their unseen, incessant crossfire in my role as sudden caregiver for my wife, Ruth.

Here is how I came to see the conflict. Medical eros, which I would describe—too simply, but for practical purposes—as the operations of desire within the context of health and illness, is engaged in a massive and mostly concealed struggle with the reigning power in Western health care, usually called biomedicine. *Biomedicine*, under the alias medical logos, views illness as calling for scientific knowledge, for evidence-based treatments, and for public policies governed by statistical, cost-benefit analysis. It encloses the patient within concentric systems of logos or reason that affect every aspect of medical care, from electronic records and computerized diagnoses to research agendas, training modules, state-of-the-art hospitals, and automated reimbursement programs. Every procedure must have its designated billing code.

Despite its ancient roots, biomedicine gathered its modern strength and scope in the early 1870s with the advent of new science-based medical schools. Physician and medical historian Kenneth M. Ludmerer describes how the new university-based agenda extended medical study to three years, added new scientific subjects to the curriculum, required laboratory work of each student, and added full-time medical scientists to the faculty. The new Johns Hopkins Medical School (opened in 1893) became the model by which other medical schools were measured.[9] Soon thereafter the influential Flexner Report (1910), financed by the Carnegie Foundation, sealed the future of American medicine with its recommendation (based on the Hopkins model) that all medical schools should engage medical faculty in research and train physicians to practice in a scientific manner.[10] With its electron microscopes, genetic therapies, stem-cell research, and molecular nanotechnology, to name only a few modern advances, biomedicine ranks among the most impressive by-products of Enlightenment reason: a lifesaving enterprise that extends the breakthrough nineteenth-century clinical gaze not only far within the opaque surface of the body but also, as medical logos probes our DNA and peers into the remotest molecular units of our individual heredity, far inside *the inside* of the body.

Medical logos in its Flexnerized genealogy gives biomedicine the knowledge and prestige that allow it to rule supreme in its standard institutional settings from hospitals, laboratories, and health-care systems to grant agencies, insurance programs, clinics, and doctors' offices. Today it augments its power through the support of such equally massive, overlapping, inescapable systems as the worldwide pharmaceutical industry, philanthropic foundations, and multilayered government-sponsored agencies, from first-responder teams to the World Health Organization. The genius of biomedicine, its detractors might say, lies in the prodigious science-based power that allows it to defang and absorb—often under the rubric of experimental trials—all but its most rigidly antagonistic opponents. Medical logos, no matter how alien the term, is familiar to almost everyone who lives under the health-care umbrella of modern Western democracies. By contrast, medical eros often passes wholly unrecognized. It is a daunting challenge to provide a cogent description of a power so unfamiliar, elusive, and hard to recognize, but it is an important challenge to take on, even if the highest possible goal is likely no more than modest clarification.

Medical eros, in its focus on the large but limited arena of human health and illness, encompasses all the various emotional, psychological, and personal implications of desire. Medicine today, of course, carries out its business (and medicine *is* big business) in a space remote from erotic experience. But not entirely. Surgeons regularly get asked how soon after surgery it's safe to resume sex, and sexually transmitted diseases get their own medical specialty, but such exceptions hardly constitute an institutional embrace of medical eros. The professional space of medicine bears very little resemblance to its eros-rich simulation in televised hospital dramas and soap operas, which are indistinguishable (except for a few tense code blues) from other sexualized television fantasylands such as coffee houses and police departments. Off camera, patients and doctors understand illness as calling for scientific rationality, evidence-based decisions, antiseptic sterility, and cool digital technologies so that illness seems not just remote from eros but actually *opposed* to the erotic.[11] Serious illness, of course, can drain people of vigor, including erotic energies; even common colds can leave us limp and cranky, from the German *krank* (ill)—or, in the euphemism for no-sex-tonight, *indisposed*. At a polar remove from the common cold, dying patients may drift off in a near-comatose state where eros appears only as the negative space opened up as life slips away: what is missing, not present, gone. Such limit-case instances, however, cannot undo the bond between eros and illness. Illness, despite the prominence of medical reason, often also unfolds in an unseen, unlikely erotic dimension. This erotic dimension, where inner life is always in play, proves as basic to illness as drugs, surgeries, and doctors. It is also where illness makes direct contact with the state of not-knowing.

Medical eros operates in a realm given over to uncertainty, fluidity, and profound lack of knowledge, and its intimate relation with not-knowing makes medical eros both resistant to a succinct definition and also in continual need of piecemeal clarifications. The best procedure, in my view, is a slow, open-ended accumulation of specific instances. The cultural history of *eros* is already far more complicated than a single concept can encompass, and theorists abound. A thousand years after Plato's *Symposium* depicted Eros as a divine, cosmic ruling force, mediating between gods and humankind, Freud came to regard *eros* as the life force engaged in perpetual struggle with *thanatos*, or the death wish. Jung, rarely in sync with Freud, sees *eros* as a feminine principle opposed to the masculine and rational force of *logos*, while Lacan, in his creative revisions of Freud, writes about desire as desire for the desire of the other, where the other may be another person or an almost impersonal nonconscious force such as language or ideology. Too simply: we desire expensive cars not merely for transportation but, in part, because we desire whatever (we imagine) might increase our desirability, even if the desire of the other that we desire is our own displaced or unacknowledged narcissistic self-love.

I prefer thinkers such as Georges Bataille and Ann Carson to theorists who construct elaborate systems, and my preference is not to ally *eros* with one particular thinker but rather to layer up a thick collage of specific instances and insights, which avoids confining the erotic to a system or restricting its range to sexual passion and to romantic love. Illness invokes multiple varieties of desire. The urgent task, which I undertake here in an exploratory spirit suitable to a realm where not-knowing far outstrips knowledge, is to recognize and begin to address the various, multidimensional roles of *eros* in illness.

An example here might add welcome concreteness. "The Use of Force" (1938)—a classic short story by poet and pediatrician William Carlos Williams—so powerfully describes an encounter with medical eros that some readers view it as a default warning *against* contaminating medicine with erotic impulses. A routine digital throat examination goes terribly wrong as an ordinary house call careens out of control. The overworked doctor and his patient, a young girl who fiercely resists his exam, lock wills in a struggle that slides, ominously, toward violence. The doctor confesses to an impassioned, irrational drive that reflects how eros, as Bataille claimed, can destroy the self-containment of the participants as they are in their normal lives. Nothing remains normal. "I could have torn the child apart in my own fury and enjoyed it," the doctor admits. "It was a pleasure to attack her. My face was burning with it."[12]

Interpretations of Williams's story often focus on ethics, rightly calling attention to its undercurrent of sublimated rape. Rape is about power, however, and sexual power does not describe the other forces also at stake—specifically, contagious erotic impulses that carry a competent physician far beyond the bounds of medical logos. "But the worst of it was that I too had got beyond reason," says the doctor. The girl's passion, in its fierceness, contains a truth that rings even truer as it exposes a double dose of adult falsity. "I smiled in my best professional manner," says the doctor as he begins his exam—perhaps following the manual written by medical logos. The girl's parents compound his falseness with abjection.

"Such a nice man," coos the mother. The doctor, however, soon passes beyond banalities. Force begets force, as the story insists, and the girl now is frantic. Her ferocious struggle elevates her in the doctor's eyes as the opposite of false or abject, and her passionate authenticity is what seems to draw him, not primarily her attractiveness (which he notes) or a sexualized male drive for power. Their struggle becomes an impure, impassioned contest of conflicting values—her childlike authenticity against his adult medical responsibility—and ultimately the physical strength of the doctor prevails "in a final unreasoning assault." Medical logos has won, but not by virtue of reason. Eros, writes Anne Carson as she describes the thrilling, dangerous, authentic, fiery sense of aliveness that it evokes in her, is like an *electrification*.[13]

An interpretation less focused on ethics or on cautionary lessons and more attentive to the electrifications of eros need not harden the doctor into an icon of professional misconduct. His "fury" represents unprofessional conduct, no doubt, but he also ultimately establishes a diagnosis of diphtheria—a highly contagious, fatal disease—and in obtaining the diagnosis he protects both the girl and the community. His conduct is culpable, then, but he merits some sympathy not only for a life-saving diagnosis but also for his sudden amoral free fall into erotic not-knowing. Eros takes vertigo as a defining state, and it always implies a tendency to move beyond benign release toward a loss of self-control so radical that it threatens even the self. This terrifying, exhilarating breakthrough opens onto terrain suitable for poets but not for pediatricians. (Williams as poet celebrated the amoral lure of the senses and even addressed a poem—with the command-like title "Smell!"—to his nose.) In his erotic free fall, however, Williams's doctor at least meets the girl's truth-in-passion with his own passionate truth, very human if unprofessional, and powerful enough in its truth to demystify the false and sanitized portraits of saintly rural doctors currently circulating in popular magazines and irrelevant to the normal life of an overworked, exhausted urban physician on a three-dollar house call in a poor neighborhood where a child whom he suspects of carrying the diphtheria bacterium refuses to open her mouth for a digital throat examination. "I have seen at least two children lying dead in bed of neglect in such cases," says the doctor as he exchanges a splintered wooden tongue depressor for a smooth-handled metal spoon. The stakes were high. According to figures from the Centers for Disease Control and Prevention, the United States reported 100,000 to 200,000 cases of diphtheria during the 1920s, with 13,000 to 15,000 deaths annually, largely among children.[14]

The stakes are equally high today when it comes to medical interventions and decisions. As the son of a physician, brother of a psychiatrist, husband of a medical librarian, and friend to talented, generous physicians whom I would trust with my life, I am not about to bash individual doctors. Medical logos, however, at least in the United States where its power approaches absolute, has a lot to answer for. The Commonwealth Fund is a private U.S. foundation devoted to improving health care, and it issues regular reports that compare different national systems across various measures. "The United States health care system is the most expensive in the world," its most recent report observes, "but comparative analyses consistently show the U.S. underperforms relative to other countries on most dimensions of performance." Compared with Australia, Canada, France, Germany, the Netherlands, New Zealand, Norway, Sweden, Switzerland, and the United Kingdom, as the Commonwealth Fund report concludes, the United States "ranks last."[15]

Biomedicine in the United States produces not only the most expensive (and, arguably, the least efficient) health-care *system* in the developed world but also a system marked by immense and proliferating complication. It is a system in which, according to recent studies, U.S. doctors prescribe over 14,000 different drugs; a system in which 82 percent of American adults take at least one medication and 29 percent of adults take over four; a system in which the United States spends $3.5 billion annually on adverse drug events, which is a bureaucratic euphemism for illnesses and deaths *caused* by drugs. In addition, about 1.5 million Americans are injured each year because of preventable errors in medication. *Nosocomial* infections (in plain English, infections acquired from the environment or staff of a health-care facility) kill some 99,000 Americans each year—twice the number of Americans killed in traffic accidents. Medical logos cannot rule out or control every harm. In the United States, however, some 225,000 deaths annually are attributed to *iatrogenic* causes. (The Greek noun *iatros* means physician.) Its own statistical tools thus provide solid evidence that something is amiss in the evidence-based world of biomedicine. Statistical studies are always open to debate, but it is reason for concern when a 2016 study of medical error in the United States finds that doctors are the third-leading cause of death.[16]

Medical eros implies a sideways critique of biomedicine as focused too exclusively on reason, science, evidence, statistics, and data, but medical eros too includes its dangers. Eros, in its most worrisome implications for good conduct and norm-keeping, appears at times both unavoidable and uncontrollable. Like fate or the uncanny return of the repressed, eros finds us and grips us even as we seek to elude or contain it. It casts us back into a primal space that we cannot avoid because we carry it within us: it is part of our psychic apparatus. In Williams's story, eros as sideways critique exposes not only a professional artifice built into the medical encounter but also wider and less visible medical applications of force. The *cordon sanitaire* of material barriers and of forced confinement once designed to halt contagious disease now extends to various invisible applications of state biopower that, in the name of public health or professional decorum, tend to isolate patients and to rope off eros. Doctors, however, cannot exclude eros from their lives any more than priests, teachers, or politicians can, and sex scandals seem to tarnish every profession. (The term *doctors*, I should add, will sometimes here refer to MDs and otherwise serve as an all-purpose reference to health professionals.) If no professional discipline seems able to quarantine eros, perhaps the greater harm lies less in eros (since eros includes benefits, too) than in rigid practices, policies, and ideologies that seek to deny or exclude eros, as if to expunge it from the medical encounter, which is like seeking to expunge your own pancreas. Far better, when lives are at stake, to recognize eros and to deal with it—the good and the ill—mindfully.

It will be easier to deal with the erotics of illness if we recognize one key point: medical eros and medical logos are not binary opposites (fixed adversaries or polar opposites) but rather contraries. The difference is crucial. As contraries, medical eros and medical logos share many areas of harmonious overlap, alignment, and collaboration.

The key distinction between contraries and binary opposites merits clarification. Binary opposites follow a closed artificial logic wherein a switch, say, is either on *or* off. Binaries—zero *or* one—make perfect sense in computer codes; a switch cannot be both off and on simultaneously.

Contraries, in contrast, do not exist within a closed, logical, artificial, either/or relation where they designate an unchanging and mutually exclusive opposition. Rather, they are fluid, changeable elements within a heterogeneous and often open-ended field where they may enter into new and surprising alliances. Binaries never overcome their fixed polar opposition, that is, but contraries can join forces and even produce unexpected unities. For example, biologist Donna Haraway rejects the usual binary opposition between *nature* and *culture*, arguing that humans and animals inhabit a heterogeneous realm of "naturecultures"; anthropologist Bruno Latour agrees, proposing the hyphenated concept "nature-cultures."[17] The ancient concept of *concordia discors* offers a similar vision in which cosmic order emerges only from ceaseless conflict among the four separate elements of classical physics: earth, air, fire, and water. Music too, for Renaissance theorists, offered an emblem of the harmony emerging from the contrary relations among differing instruments, rhythms, melodies, and sounds. Not surprisingly, they associated this creative, musical *concordia discors* with the classical god Eros.

Medical logos and medical eros as contraries will likely remain to some degree in opposition and potentially antagonistic—if only because the difference in social power between them is so vast. Medical logos rules the health-care system; medical eros slips into the bedside shadows. Individual patients, however, may decide to construct their own personal *concordia discors*, adjusting the proportionate power of logos and of eros as their particular illness changes or as their personal goals and purposes change. For patients and families facing serious illness, such individual adjustments are far too important to dismiss simply because they fall short of a perfect or collective system-wide solution to disease. What matters most here is to clarify the conflicts between medical logos and medical eros as the necessary prelude to any personal or systemic remedies.

Contraries certainly do not guarantee harmony. Unredeemed discord pretty well sums up my experience. Unaware, with no safe house or elevation from which to gain an understanding, I was simply caught between two mighty forces, clueless, swept up in the fog of a bulletless, surreal civil war. Medical eros in its limits and in its possibilities thus raised urgent questions for me in my new role as caregiver navigating the day-to-day encounters with doctors, insurance companies, lawyers, banks, hospitals, assisted-living facilities, and faceless bureaucracies, while of course also trying to keep house, job, and marriage from caving in around us. It became an occasion for guilt as I recognized how deft I had become, in public, at covering up the social slips and verbal miscues that Ruth's illness entailed. Stories that she launched into with friends would often get lost in midcourse, and (with an artificial smile) I would catch the flapping, loose end, weaving it neatly into a finished tale. Were my spousal cover-ups an act of love or love's betrayal? My frustrations grew daily as I tried to manage my slippery emotions, a full teaching schedule, the medical establishment, and a shifting patchwork of daytime helpers. I couldn't get angry at everyone, but sometimes I wanted to. Isolation, suppressed anger, and continual irritation ultimately led me to question the larger, hidden conflict that I felt trapped in. I ultimately discovered that the unseen conflict between medical logos and medical eros reached far beyond my own private distress. The fatigue and confusion I felt were not mine alone. Illness often transports patients and family and caregivers into an unreasonable, uncanny, inverse realm where knowledge is far less common than not-knowing. It is a desire-haunted space of the inner life (given over equally to terrors, guilt, and fantasies) that Susan Sontag, in an accurate metaphor, calls "the night-side of life."[18]

We urgently need to explore the place of desire in illness because illness is no longer *simply* the nightside of life: a quasi-natural feature of the human condition. Most people fall ill, but illness now falls under the supervision of biomedicine, and biomedicine is a gigantic state-run, state-regulated, and state-supported system dominated, as we will see, by the new *molecular gaze*. The molecular gaze extends throughout the international pharmaceutical industry, which provides the first line of biomedical treatment, and it also governs the standards that apply both within huge government agencies (such as the U.S. Federal Drug Administration or Veterans Health Administration). This new biomedical giant with its cell-piercing panopticon eyesight certainly brings unprecedented advances, much as the new "personalized medicine" employs our distinctive genetic data to guide treatment and to forestall disease. The biomedical, molecular gaze continues to produce astonishing discoveries. Researchers announced in 2015, for example, that the brain is connected to the immune system by vessels previously unknown. "I really did not believe there were structures in the body that we were not aware of," said neuroscientist Jonathan Kipnis, whose laboratory made the breakthrough discovery with its profound implications for immunotherapy treatments. "I thought the body was mapped."[19]

But what does this indispensable, deep-seeing biomedical giant miss? What does its astonishing molecular vision neglect, overlook, or disregard as wholly irrelevant? Simply put: biomedicine, both in clinical practice and in bench science, ignores the role of desire in illness. Desire, legitimized as medical eros, offers a power that can help make the passage through illness far less onerous, a power that offers a more truly "personalized" medicine than genetic profiles alone can promise. An exploration of desire in illness depends on looking beyond (but not ignoring) randomized double-blind experiments; it means looking beyond (but not ignoring) telephone surveys and check-the-box questionnaires. It means especially focusing on such nonstandard biomedical data as memoirs, essays, paintings, performances, experiences, and images—from the nudes of Modigliani to my own stumbling efforts as caregiver—which in their own way offer firsthand testaments to the place of desire in illness. They, too, count as evidence. The goal is to cross restrictive boundaries and to open perspectives that can alter what happens when you or someone you love enters into the nightside of life and falls under supervision of the molecular gaze.

An e-mail (a fragmentary illness narrative) just arrived from an old friend who has recently faced sudden, unexpected surgery for breast cancer. "I won't know for a while what treatment, if any, I'll need next," she writes from within the immense vistas of not-knowing: "Another period of waiting to find out. Well, it's a good lesson, to live with the unknown, because actually the next moment is always an unknown, we just like to think we have it under control."[20] I couldn't match her wisdom and her courage; in my role as caregiver, mostly I just muddled on. I discovered, however, that medical eros tends to pick up and desire tends to intensify exactly where the reasonableness of medical logos leaves off, leaves us unattended, in need of hope, companionship, consolation, affection, wisdom, and healing. My aim here, in sorting out my confusions, is not to undertake an exhaustive or even orderly analysis but rather to begin a wide-ranging exploration among the fertile possibilities that an understanding of medical eros opens up: possibilities for scholarly study, for professional development, and, most important, for individual change, healing, and solace. Eros and illness together—in their endless, surprising, personal permutations—touch us all: there is no refuge, no asylum, no escape.

Medical eros is far less a concept than a lens that offers an inside view of illness as a lived experience. It is experience so diverse that it can range from a doomed sense of fatal entrapment to a liberating burst of life-transforming gratitude and insight. My excursions through literature, philosophy, art, film, memoir, and the environment—as discourses that mediate the immediacy of inner life and outer life—constitute merely an exploratory sample. It is an exploration in which illness appears less as a diagnostic category than as a lived experience embracing not only body, mind, and spirit but also relevant biological and cultural contexts, including the all-pervasive culture of medicine. On any such headfirst exploratory journey, of course, it's best to expect a fairly wild ride.

We need medical eros, by whatever name, because serious illness so often arrives like a sudden blow, plunging us into a twilight of not-knowing where everything looks strange, where nothing feels under control, including our own bodies with their sudden odd aches and ominous spasms, or thoughts as feverish as dreams, reminding us that, despite all our science and statistics and medical knowledge, we have no idea, not a clue, what may be circling overhead like a drone or hidden around the next corner, waiting . . .

Part One

The Contraries

CHAPTER ONE

The Ambush: An Erotics of Illness

"The right art," cried the Master, "is purposeless, aimless! The more obstinately you try to learn how to shoot the arrow for the sake of hitting the goal, the less you will succeed. . . . What stands in your way is that you have a much too willful will. You think that what you do not do yourself does not happen."

EUGEN HERRIGEL, *ZEN IN THE ART OF ARCHERY* (1953)

*E*VERYTHING CHANGED with the blessing of the candles. Something awful was going on. After months of untethered suspicion, as dishes turned up in random cabinets and a mislaid exercise rope triggered meltdown rages, I couldn't any longer take refuge in excuses. The secular Jewish family I married into blessed the candles only on Passover, and the traditional prayer always fell to Ruth. With the grace of a natural-born dancer fully blossomed into her fifties, flanked by family and by our closest friends, she stretched her hands above the lighted candles—eyes closed, palms down, elbows raised—ready to intone the customary Hebrew words, softy, slowly, as she had done since childhood. *Barukh Ata Adonai, Eloheinu Melekh Ha-olam* . . . Ruth's almost trancelike state as she re-enters this ritual space visibly softens the edge that served her well as a mid-level administrator and corporate crisis manager, as if the ancient

21

blessing draws her into a deeper order of time and being. After twenty-five *Sedarim* together, I know the sounds and rhythms (in a language I don't understand) almost as well as the hymns from my childhood. I always feel a reassuring warmth as Ruth sings the blessing. It seems to affirm a preverbal bond that connects us in a closeness that friends marvel at, much as touches, sighs, and glances count for more, among lovers, than words and meanings.

On this night, now forever different from all other nights, with Ruth's hands floating palms down above the white tapers, her face serene and her skin glowing in the candlelight, I turn stone cold as she stumbles over the opening phrases. *Impossible! She can't remember?* I'm repeating the familiar Hebrew syllables in my head as if to help her, to jog her memory. But this, I sense, is no normal forgetting. I've read enough popular neuroscience to suspect that you don't ordinarily forget patterns so deep, but I still don't understand what's going on. All at once I'm knee-deep in the not-known. There must be severe damage, a powerful synaptic disorder. Ruth's halting and peculiarly unmelodic contralto accent only adds to my well-mannered, unnoticed dinner-table panic. I have no idea about the hidden nightmare ahead.

Ruth—impossible to intimidate under any circumstances—does not appear to feel embarrassed or upset by her sudden memory lapse. I feel confused and blindsided, as if masked, black-clad troops are sliding down ropes to land on our roof in a surprise assault.

Losing Control

I want to explore—beginning with that awful night and with the journey it initiated—what, from a medical point of view, is an unreasonable and entirely counterintuitive position: that doctors and patients might do well to consider and even embrace the role of eros. As the ancient Greek god of sexuality and desire, Eros would seem to have no place in contemporary evidence-based medicine, where rationality, employed like a scalpel in the service of health care, governs the entire modern medical enterprise, from laboratory science and randomized, double-blind clinical trials to the commonsense expectation of patient compliance. Medicine tends to flee the erotic, with good reason. Eros, as an ancient representative of passion and irrational desire, is the sworn enemy of instrumental reason and thus an unwelcome figure at the bedside. *Noncompliant* is the pejorative, technical term for patients who elude rational control. This preference for rationality and control helps explain why medicine, when it doesn't openly reject the erotic as unruly, which it is, simply ignores it as irrelevant. In its affirmations of desire and of excess, eros opposes key values that medicine has endorsed to advance a firm knowledge of disease and to promote patient safety ever since the scientific heirs of Hippocrates ousted his powerful archaic predecessor, the dream god Asklepios.

Serious illness, from the patient's point of view, is all about losing control, a crash course in the insufficiency or radical limits of reason. As I discovered, patients and families routinely enter into a territory hostile to medicine and native to eros. The irrationalities of illness, which do not exclude a comic side or even gallows humor, might be well represented in *A Midsummer Night's Dream*, where the eros-figure Puck deploys a potent drug to upend control and to disorder social hierarchies so thoroughly that the beautiful fairy queen Titania instantly falls in love with the buffoon-like tradesman Bottom the Weaver. Puck, whose impish humor runs toward cruelty, had deployed his magic drug to endow Bottom with the long ears and high-octave rasp of the likeable jackass he more or less is, but Titania (love blinded) dotes on him all the more. Illness and eros can also abruptly transport us into an eerie dreamscape where everything changes and intensifies. "Bless thee, Bottom! bless thee!" cries a companion on seeing his jackass-headed friend: "Thou art translated."[1]

Translational medicine refers to a discipline within biomedicine and public health research designed to bring the findings of laboratory or bench science to the practical aid of patients and communities.[2] It seeks to "translate" relatively abstract rational discoveries into new diagnostic tools and policies. The unofficial "translations" of eros often, in practice, bring only confusion and disorder, even nightmarish hallucinations, as in Henry Fuseli's erotic / demonic illustration (Figure 1.1) that depicts Bottom—oblivious to the embrace of Titania—stuck in an Ovidian metamorphosis somewhere between animal and human form.

Bottom bears the signature of eros as trickster, the unruly antagonist of reason, introducing the civilized world to its uncivil, undomesticated dark side, as Fuseli suggests by including two unscripted eighteenth-century

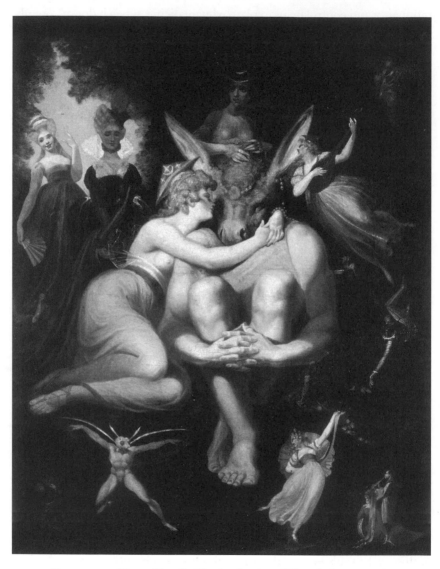

FIGURE 1.1. Henry Fuseli. *The Awakening of Titania* (1793–1794).
Photo credit: Album / Art Resource.

society belles (their charms tastefully on display) framed by a small clearing in the thick, dark, wooded canopy. The jackass head, however appropriate for Bottom, also gestures toward the dark woods: unlike its tame cousin the donkey, the jackass since biblical times has a reputation for wildness, much as eros maintains contact with primordial forces that underlie our civilized facades. Serious illness also can initiate a Bottom-like nightmare regression, in which the sensuous body reclaims its original (wild) precedence over reason and thought. Eros and serious illness both center us in the body with its often inexplicable feelings and wayward desires. Illness translates *us*: it carries us into an unfamiliar, even malign, humpty-dumpty realm where, without our consent and against our wishes, we change and our lives change. As cancer survivor and sociologist Arthur W. Frank writes, "When the body breaks down, so does the life. Even when medicine can fix the body, that doesn't always put the life back together again."[3]

Eros, in short, far from irrelevant to medicine, regularly suffuses the experience of illness, marking it with damage, deficit, forfeit, and loss: loss of health, loss of function, loss of future. It punctuates the medical encounter with its invisible interruptions and even its telltale nonappearances, as when serious illness interrupts or terminates former intimacies. "No more fucking!" insists poet Jane Kenyon when her poet-husband, tactlessly, reminds her of their thousands of afternoon erotic "assignations" on the same bed where she now lies stricken with end-stage leukemia.[4] Eros at such times makes its presence known obliquely through passionate refusals, grief, or anger. It produces gaps as palpable as the vacant space in a once-shared marriage bed. Eros is at work even in such apparent absences, but its more intrusive presences also tend to remain invisible because biomedicine has schooled us not to recognize eros or (if we sense its unseen ghostly presence) to disregard and to unsense it.

Ruth's struggle to bless the candles in a voice eerily flat and unmusical—at the will of the body—hid a stark truth: the catastrophic death of brain cells and wrecked neural paths. It was my nonstatistical introduction to Alzheimer's disease, the incurable, fatal, degenerative illness afflicting over 5 million Americans, including 200,000 under age 65 who, like Ruth, suffer younger-onset Alzheimer's. Alzheimer's disease (the sixth leading cause of death in the United States, if we ignore medical error) kills over half a million seniors each year; nationwide, it is the single most expensive medical condition, with annual costs in 2016 estimated at $236 billion—projected at $1.2 trillion by 2050.[5]

Numbers so massive quickly pass through my mind, disappearing like abstractions, but I cannot omit two brief and crucial personal notes. First, on ethics: Ruth's story belongs to Ruth, and I need to respect her privacy as far as our joint experience allows. Second, on method: as caregiver, I am a paramedical figure, with rights and responsibilities at the bedside, but my role is more complex than duties and privileges suggest. Family caregivers cannot put aside the interlaced social and emotional filaments that bind them to the patient, which infiltrate my account in ways that prevent me from dividing subjective experience and critical inquiry into separate compartments.

Susan Sontag wrote brilliantly about metaphors of illness and the dilemmas that they create without once mentioning her own breast cancer. (Her son, David Rieff, calls Sontag's *Illness as Metaphor* "almost *anti-autobiographical*.")[6] "What I write about," Sontag says of her nonfiction works, "is other than me." She grants, however, a sizeable concession to her writing as a novelist: "Needless to say, I lend bits of myself to all my characters."[7] The shards of my experience that I "lend" here, sparingly, fall outside the memoirs of illness that scholar Ann Jurecic describes as "a thriving genre in the late twentieth and early twenty-first centuries."[8] My own fragments contribute, I trust, to an emerging composite portrait of the caregiver.[9] The commonness of my experience taps into what makes the caregiver both a representative figure of our time and also, compounding the dilemmas that caregivers face, an uncannily invisible figure.

The general claims that follow—less logical propositions than a loose network of positions supported through a makeshift ensemble of evidence, argument, and illustration—begin with the observation that eros is often an unseen and unacknowledged presence at the sickbed. A focus on caregivers helps expose some of the varied manifestations of medical eros, especially its contact with lost control and with the not-known. It raises practical and ethical questions about what to do—not only when medicine reaches its limits or outright fails but also when eros, too, leads us into losses, failures, and dead-ends. Caregiving, finally, calls attention to a major change within the understanding of illness that holds important implications for biomedicine as well as for those who fall seriously ill and for their companions in illness. It helps demythologize the outdated, nostalgic health-care dyad of doctor and patient. Caregivers represent the far fuller opening up of the dyad.

The doctor/patient dyad, almost like a traditional romantic couple, offers a useful image for the contractions of focus that eros (in its contemporary shapes) disrupts, shatters, and expands. Medical eros in its multiplier effect turns the caregiver into a figure with resonance for patients, doctors, and a wide range of health-care professionals, as well as for family, friends, lovers, and bystanders who are caught up in the circumference of illness. The caregiver is an in-person metaphor. We are all in some sense caregivers, or potential caregivers, even as patients (surrounded by medical professionals and by significant others) engage in their own visible or invisible acts of self-care. They are caregivers enlisted in the service of their own porous patienthood. Physicians, of course, will not confuse their legitimate role—as the designated resource for primary and specialized care—with the position of informal or formal caregivers, but an opening up of the doctor/patient dyad allows us also to recognize the larger personal, social, and professional affiliations that doctors cannot always shed or set aside at the patient's bed. Is the doctor going through a divorce, concerned about a sick child at home, a closeted gay, or desperate with guilt over a medical error? Medical eros is crucial to an expansion of focus that opens up the doctor/patient dyad and moves individual illness beyond traditions that, even in the era of biomedicine and of managed care, no longer apply.

Supra-dyads: Eros at the Bedside

Eros and illness both usually send us under the bedcovers, and beds remain so basic to the vocabulary and practice of medicine that hospital supply firms manufacture them in truckloads. The bedside, then, serves both as a real-world place and as a metaphor: the actual site of privileged medical exchanges and a theoretical space where patients encounter the representatives of medical logos. In its metaphoric sense, the bedside functions as an edge, a boundary or borderland where two adjacent worlds touch and sometimes collide. This edge, however, always in practice acquires thick historical real-world particularities that locate it in specific times and cultures, much as the Victorian bedside (enfolded within the home) differed significantly from the modern hospital cubicle. Eros, then, at *whose* actual bedside? When? Where? Who is officially or unofficially licensed to be there? *Enter the caregiver.*

The caregiver, at least under that name, may be a fairly recent invention. The famed *Oxford English Dictionary* lists the first appearance of the noun *caregiver* in 1966, when it emerges into language as a role distinct from the mostly female figures (grandmothers, aunts, mothers, daughters, sisters, spinsters, nuns) who for centuries assumed a caregiving function. The work, if devalued previously, is often unpaid or reimbursed with obscenely low wages, perhaps partly because gender stereotypes still associate caregiving with women and with unskilled labor. There are 2.5 times more women than men providing intensive "on duty" twenty-four-hour-a-day at-home care for Alzheimer's patients. In my experience most of the daily hands-on staff in nursing care facilities are women, often minority women. In 2015, unpaid caregivers—I'd guess, disproportionately female—provided an estimated 18.1 billion hours of care to people with Alzheimer's and with other dementias, work valued at $221.1 billion (or eight times the total revenue of McDonald's).[10]

Equity, economics, and gender raise serious issues, but here a focus on the underpaid, overworked, and largely invisible caregiver helps add a touch of reality to archaic fantasies of medical attention. Today teams of rotating specialists mostly replace the single family doctor; even family practice offices are often staffed with multiple doctors, who trade off as needed. Meanwhile, patienthood has expanded far beyond the image of a single person who occupies the sickbed. Alzheimer's, I came to see, is at least a two-person disease. The intrinsic doubleness of Alzheimer's disease is in truth more like a polygon, a many-sided figure, in which it resembles much serious illness, wherein one of the many persons is not the doctor and also not the patient.

The caregiver emerges as a representative of our changing conceptions of health and illness. It is a change that also includes patients. In 2008, medical sociologists Kirsten Smith and Nicholas Christakis described a new health-related pattern that they call "supra-dyadic effects."[11] Supra-dyadic effects extend in networks beyond a single patient to include not only spouses or parents but also children, relatives, neighbors, paramedical help, and others, from the playmates of children and the neighbors of neighbors to far-flung friends of friends of friends. Christakis and Smith argue that obesity spreads through supra-dyadic networks, but patterns of illness also change as emerging technologies alter both the networks to which we belong and our relations to other people. Eating disorders, for example, are now a semicontagious global phenomenon as new media, from cell phones to Internet video clips, expand social networks. In the remote island of Fiji, girls were free of eating disorders prior to the introduction of television in 1995, but after several years of television 11.3 percent of adolescent girls in Fiji reported purging at least once to lose weight.[12] Even divorce tends to "cluster" within social networks.[13] Susan Sontag's short story "How We Live Now" (1986) perfectly captures the operation of a supra-dyadic social network, as readers encounter a nameless HIV/AIDS patient exclusively through conversations among his acquaintances, with each speaker offering tidbits of advice: "Meat and potatoes is what I'd be happy to see him eating, Ursula said wistfully. And spaghetti and clam sauce, Greg added. And thick cholesterol-rich omelets with smoked mozzarella, suggested Yvonne, who had flown from London for the weekend to see him. Chocolate cake, said Frank. Maybe not chocolate cake, Ursula said, he's already eating so much chocolate."[14] It is a perfect polygon of quasi-medical advice.

The supra-dyadic bedside, with its disruption of the patient/doctor dyad, finds its typical contemporary figure, I would argue, in the family caregiver. I would learn as Ruth's unofficial primary caregiver that doctors tended to disappear, and her illness became a condition that wrapped us up together, both in its sometimes ragged, ever-expanding outward circles as friends and family stopped by, but especially in its centripetal contractions, when for long periods we were like castaways adrift on a single raft. Caregiver spouses, for example, are bound to the patient not only by complex emotional entanglements but also by semiofficial paramedical duties; almost inescapably they become the communications center for far-flung family members, friends, coworkers, and acquaintances.

Mass e-mail updates shoot out like duplicate Christmas letters. Emotional entanglements range from romantic love to anger and schadenfreude. Is the old boyfriend welcome? The horrible in-laws? Rotating teams of health-care providers come and go, along with waves of semiprofessional investigators—*good*-nurse, *bad*-nurse—sent to enforce insurance company protocols, but the figure who stays, day in, day out, and who absorbs the costliest toll on spirit, mind, and body is of course the family caregiver. The caregiver experiences the supra-dyadic bedside edge as a highly permeable membrane where to be fully present is almost inescapably to be wounded.

All family caregivers face a significant risk of serious illness and even death.[15] A few bullet points help blow holes in any suspicion that I am talking here mainly about myself:

- The United States has an estimated 36 to 38 million caregivers according to a 2004 survey by the American Association of Retired Persons (AARP) and the National Alliance for Caregivers.
- The AARP estimates that the total unpaid value of labor by caregivers is at least $350 billion per year.
- Caregivers are at increased risk for heart disease, arthritis, cancer, diabetes, and other stress-related diseases.
- Caregivers suffer depression at twice the rate of noncaregivers.[16]

The illnesses that caregivers contract or stand at much increased risk of contracting point to a significant additional problem: wounded caregivers not only continue to care for patients but also affect others in the social network. Illness spreads across the network of support even as practical help recedes. I quickly came to realize, as Ruth's disease worsened, that medical logos had no effective treatments to offer her. She grew weary of appointments in which her neurologist posed questions designed to track her cognitive losses and to map the brain damage. Author and neurologist Oliver Sacks objected to what he calls a "mechanistic neurology," which focuses on deficits.[17] Ruth quickly came to dislike such medical visits that focused on what she *couldn't* do. How many times do you need to fail to know what day it is today or what the doctor's lapel is called? As doctors receded and Ruth's deficits increased, I slowly emerged

as the lone figure in charge, a position for which I was both wholly un-
qualified and totally unprepared.

Family caregivers in general are overtasked, underprepared, and thoroughly worn down as they struggle on with little more than good intentions as a guide. Medical eros is their native turf, but nobody tells us about
eros. Instead, stressed-out exhaustion serves as a powerful antiaphrodi-
siac, which I failed to recognize as illness opened fissures in our once rock-
solid marriage. My frustration mounted each time Ruth screwed up
ordinary household exchanges. *Please close the front door.* A blank stare
simply intensifies my frustration. *The cat got out!* Ruth panics. *Now what?*
Spent, I climb the stairs only to discover a bathroom faucet running full
blast. My outbursts, no longer rare, cause Ruth physical distress, like the
stereo volume suddenly turned up ultra-loud; so I school myself to
(a hair-trigger) calm. I can't leave Ruth alone to shop, but shopping with
Ruth turns a quick ten-minute errand into a maddening, hour-long chore.

Every day brings the same tearful plea: "I want a *dog.*" Of course, I'm
the bad guy who keeps saying no. *Who'll feed the dog, walk it, clean up
the mess? Me, that's who.* Reluctantly, worn down, I get a dog—a cute
rescue mongrel with heart disease, a huge disaster. But Ruth pays it
almost no notice. Was "dog" a metaphor? I understand next to nothing
about how her mind works. One hot August day, preparing my syllabus
for fall courses at the university, I suddenly know (as if a disembodied
hand scrawls the warning in blood on my study wall) that one more semester teaching full time and also organizing Ruth's care when I'm not
caring for her, morning, nights, and weekends, will flat out kill me. I put
down the syllabus, turn on the word processor, and compose my letter of
resignation.

Nothing here will surprise family caregivers. Our standard guidebook—
accurately titled *The 36-Hour Day*—details the surreal Beckett-like contradictions: "I can't go on, I'll go on."[18] Through it all, I feel the old, abiding
deep love for Ruth, enhanced with the extra concern that a parent might
feel for an injured child, but mingled with suppressed resentment that my
own life has shrunk to the pleasureless round of kitchen, stairs, and bedroom. I have been "translated" into a mechanical man, a zombie, a dead
man walking. In robbing Ruth of her health, Alzheimer's disease has worn
me down to the nub, robbed me of a loving daily companion, and left me

little but deadlines, meetings, and useless biweekly pill containers. I didn't recognize myself in the person who kept missing appointments and forgetting plans. I began to wonder if dementia could be contagious. Isn't this the weak point (the heart as dazed and crazed as the head) where the failures of eros—the everyday losses and erosions that it entails— begin to raise questions of ethics? Pose basic questions about how to live and what to do?

Medical logos has good reason to control the free play of eros. Codes of conduct, however, control mainly the disruptive powers of eros, while failing to maximize its positive contributions, which include the widening, postdyadic circles of empathy.[19] Empathy is a topic of increasing interest in medicine, and an empathetic stance toward patients represents a major advance beyond the "detached concern" that doctors once (wrongly) thought they should cultivate. Empathy in medicine has no more persuasive advocate than Danielle Ofri, a physician whose challenging patients at Bellevue Hospital in New York City at times gave even Ofri pause; however, her book *What Doctors Feel* (2013) has emphasized, with vivid accounts, how the "final outcomes can be strongly influenced by a doctor's emotional state."[20] Medical educators disagree about whether empathy can be taught, but it certainly can be modeled and encouraged as a positive value, with a shaping influence on outcomes.

Empathy nonetheless has its limits. I can't empathize with serial killers, rapists, and mass-murderers; their victims and families have my concern. Moreover, so-called empathetic *behaviors*—sometimes recommended by medical authorities—strike me as bogus, no more than a clinical charade if practiced merely to improve patient-satisfaction scores or to forestall lawsuits. A colleague once interviewed Pueblo elders in New Mexico for a report on Native American attitudes toward end-of-life care. She had no interest in eros but rather asked (one question among many) if the elders would like their Anglo doctors to show greater "empathy." *No*, the elders replied. *They did not want empathy. They wanted respect.* Empathy is a force for good: it radiates kindness, understanding, and connection. Eros, however, is not always a force for good, and empathy (if cheapened into a behaviorist charade) can quickly transform patients into objects of manipulation. Objectification, even with good motives, eventually poisons a relationship, much as pity can turn the other person into an object of charitable condescension. Empathy, respect, and even self-respect all seemed, in my case, dire casualties of Alzheimer's disease.

Medical Eros and Patient-side Transformations

Eros, despite the casualties that illness inflicts, can also hold benefits equally helpful for patients, doctors, caregivers, and the entire supra-dyadic network of the ill. Illness, even through the fires of its sometimes inescapable destructiveness, can bring advantageous as well as harmful changes, and the helpful changes need not follow the scripts laid out by tenderheartedness. "The kindest thing anyone could have done for me, once I'd finished five weeks' radiation," writes American novelist Reynolds Price after spinal cord cancer left him a wheelchair-bound paraplegic, "would have been to look me square in the eye and say this clearly, *'Reynolds Price is dead. Who will you be now?'* "[21]

Price's unlikely description of the kindness he desired, far from drill-sergeant, suck-it-up tough love, expresses a recognition that serious illness, like eros, puts not only lives at risk but also selves. Life as a biological state—*bare life*, as philosopher Giorgio Agamben calls it—involves signaling and self-sustaining properties absent in organisms that are dead. In mammals, it is almost equivalent with breath. King Lear, holding the corpse of his daughter Cordelia, cries out, "Why should a dog, a horse, a rat, have life, / And thou no breath at all?"[22] Selves, as distinct from bare life, are social, cultural, emotional, psychological, and often spiritual beings. Spinal cancer—compounded by the radiation damage caused by medical treatment—had left Reynolds Price in a position to know how catastrophic illness can destroy not just the ability to walk but the lineaments of a former self. Illness, like eros, may include episodes of violence and destruction that coincide with dark failures of personal identity: *"Reynolds Price is dead."* Reason is not the power most likely to produce a new self, unless perhaps you are a philosopher. Desire, however, provides the thrust toward change necessary for almost anyone; for Price, self-transformation and recovery both included an erotic push.

Eros played into recovery and self-transformation for Price in the specific sense that his personal inflection of Christian belief drew him toward

the biblical injunction to "choose life." Life for Price means—at a far remove from breath or bare life—chiefly love and work. *Love and Work*
(1987) is, in fact, the title of a book he wrote about a writer recovering from
despair. Eros and its sustaining powers also play a significant, almost spiritual role in his poetry. Christ and Eros, according to literary scholar
Victor Strandberg, are the two major figures interwoven "across his whole
poetic oeuvre."[23] Price leaves no doubt about the importance of eros to
both his creative work and his personal relations, and eros remains basic
to his own return to health. *Health*, in its etymology, refers to wholeness,
but no medical cure could reverse his paralysis and return his body to a
precancerous wholeness. The title of Price's autobiographical illness narrative, *A Whole New Life* (1994), embraces a punning doubleness: its colloquial meaning suggests simple renewal, while the adjective "whole" also
suggests a transformation or redefinition of what we understand by health
and wholeness. Health, in Price's creative movement through illness to
recovery, does not mean the restoration of prior function. It means the
emergence of a new self, full and unimpaired in its altered wholeness, for
whom eros provides indispensable thrust: *Who will you be now?*

Recovery for Reynolds Price holds significance beyond his personal
story because it also challenges the assumptions of theorists who tend to
ignore, discount, or deny the erotic movement through loss and damage
to self-transformation. Like Bataille, they celebrate eros for its power to
destroy bourgeois illusions and to burn away or demystify repressive social structures and obsolete belief systems, including what some theorists—
at the crossroads where Marxist critique meets radical psychoanalysis—
regard as the bourgeois illusion of a stable or coherent self. Price certainly
sees a possible move from an older stable self to a new stable self that
emerges from the fires of trauma, but he does not experience the new,
hard-won, coherent ("whole") selfhood as illusory or as a bad-faith ca-
pitulation to dominant bourgeois ideologies.

Biological anthropologist Helen Fisher, melding neuroscience with
field data, identifies three distinct stages of erotic life: lust, romantic love,
and attachment.[24] *Attachment* (if the least familiar aspect of eros) merits
special attention here as vitally important in its personal, social, and spiritual dimensions, and everyday experience confirms that erotic experience contains the power to promote affective bonds reaching far beyond

mere sexual pleasure. Recovery, as Price understands it, depends on erotic attachments that extend to life itself. Choosing life means feeling grateful even for breath. "Grieve for a decent limited time over whatever parts of your old self you know you'll miss," he advises. "Then stanch the grief, by whatever legal means. Next find your way to be somebody else, the next viable you—a stripped-down whole other clear-eyed person, realistic as a sawed-off shotgun and thankful for air."[25]

Caregivers, no less than the patients they care for, pass through the fires. They stand no less in need of attachment, emergence, and self-transformation. After thirty years of marriage and a decade as caregiver, I needed plenty of help. Mostly, given my solitary habits, help was absent. I was left alone to decide—the hardest day of my life—when it was time for Ruth to leave the home we had built together. She could no longer make decisions: it was all left to me. When I asked for help from her all-star medical center team, her neurologist replied coolly (from the far-side of logos): "Not a medical issue."

Many caregivers know the unthinkable bitterness of leaving a loved one behind. The distress is almost mythic, evoking, for me, memories of Eurydice disappearing into the underworld. A miraculous recovery and reunion was what I longed for—Ruth's return to health and the restoration of our life together—so I set out on a literary journey to find my own consoling myth. What I discovered, instead, was the inescapability of loss and failure.

Psyche is a young princess so beautiful that even Venus, goddess of love, envies her. Fired with resentment toward a mere human rival, Venus sends her wayward son Cupid to afflict Psyche. Cupid, famous for mischief and malice, enjoys undermining marriages and defiling public morality, but not even Cupid, as it turns out, is safe from eros. The beauty of Psyche proves so enchanting that Cupid too falls helplessly, hopelessly, in love. After numerous improbable twists, many engineered by Psyche's two wicked sisters, they marry. Their fairy-tale marriage, however, includes an ironclad proviso: Psyche as mortal is not allowed to gaze upon her winged-god husband. Hence they meet only after dark. Psyche, alas, whose innocence tends toward naïveté, falls for a plot devised by her evil sisters. One evening she lights an oil lamp to gaze secretly at her sleeping husband, and the vision of her golden-ambrosial husband so dazzles her that, unluckily, a drop of lamp oil falls on Cupid's shoulder. He wakes, sees that she has broken the marriage provision, and without a word flies off on powerful wings, with poor Psyche hanging on to one leg until, exhausted, she slips down to earth. As the years pass, she wastes away, tormented in ordeals devised by the still-vengeful Venus, wandering the earth in futile search for her lost lover and lost husband.

The myth of Cupid and Psyche has an equally improbable happy ending—a reunion and remarriage ordered by Jupiter—but the deus-ex-machina happy ending gets less happy the more I think about it. In one version, Jupiter gives Psyche a cup of ambrosia to drink that transforms her from mortal to immortal. In the more common version, she lies worn out and near death from years of futile searching when Cupid, out of nowhere or prompted by the god of comedy, suddenly reappears. He revives Psyche with a famous kiss that both saves her life and confers immortality. It is this moment of erotic transformation that neoclassical sculptor Antonio Canova captures in a marble embrace so fluid it seems lifelike (Figure 1.2).

As if its eroticism were too dangerous to accept outside the sanitizing process of allegory, various Neoplatonic writers interpreted the passion that Canova celebrates as expressing the soul's desire for union with the divine. I interpret it differently through my decade as worn-down caregiver. Eros is both poison and antidote, as signified in the Greek term *pharmikon*, and the same formula holds for medical eros. While Cupid's kiss reflects the power of eros to redeem the loss and failure always implicit in eros, certain experiences of loss and failure can also be unfixable and irredeemable. The erotic antidote does not work; the creative self-transformations do not occur. Cupid, outside myth, fails to show up just in the nick of time.

Loss and failure—not amyloid plaques and neurofibrillary tangles—may be what Alzheimer's disease is all about for the entangled caregiver. Mere statistics that rank Alzheimer's among the leading causes of death serve to hide the unnumbered thousands of caregivers exhausted and distraught as a spouse or parent slowly slides into a protracted, unresponsive death-in-life. Such caregivers, wedded to loss and failure, are not the sixth leading cause of anything. Some disasters, over which we have no control, may be slightly easier to accept than *preventable* losses and failures. My failures as caregiver were sometimes, frankly, very preventable.

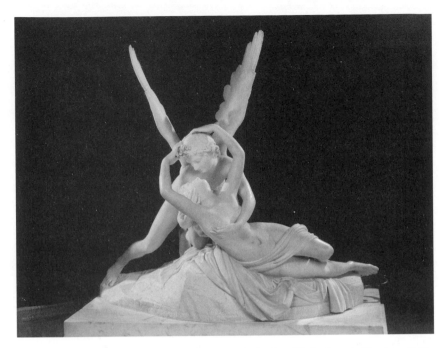

FIGURE 1.2. Antonio Canova. *Psyche brought back to life by Amor's Kiss* (ca. 1818).
Photo Credit: Bridgeman-Giraudon / Art Resource, NY.

I once confided my failures in an e-mail to religious friends of high moral character: "I know that what I'm describing may offend your principles," I wrote. "It offends my principles too. I just couldn't survive on principles." Sheer survival as a caregiver may require such violation of principles and failures of best intentions that you cannot but emerge (in your own eyes) *less*. Eros, too, as Anne Carson writes, can reduce the lover to a state of *less-ness*. This is not the self-criticism of a crank perfectionist. At times I just plain failed.

Failure is preordained for caregivers of Alzheimer's patients. This note-to-self, which applies in other desperate medical conditions, might at least offer solace to fellow caregivers distressed or tormented by their deficiencies. Caregiving is like a game that you cannot win and cannot refuse to play, but it is also no game. It belongs to the awful paradox that caregiver Carol Levine calls "accepting the unacceptable."[26] A wise physician advised me, in reference to my struggles as caregiver, that the first rule for lifeguards is *don't drown*. I was drowning. Failure here is not an error to be excused with a heartfelt mea culpa or with a Hamlet-like nod to human frailty: it constitutes the caregiver's daily experience. We can't help but fail. Such unavoidable spirit-eroding failure and loss, as your strength runs down, is the immersion in a hyperflawed state of being: an experience of indelible mistakes that you cannot expunge and cannot repair, what Reynolds Price once called *permanent errors*. If you set high expectations for yourself, you will fall short. You will fall short anyway. Period. I was ambushed, a second time, less by Alzheimer's disease than by my inescapable, irreparable failures.

Caregiving, according to Arthur Kleinman, a physician, medical anthropologist, and family caregiver, is a "defining moral practice." He adds, "It is a practice of empathetic imagination, responsibility, witnessing, and solidarity with those in great need."[27] A moral practice must take account of its own failures, including failures of empathic imagination. One Alzheimer's caregiver described himself as chained to a corpse—worse, a corpse that "complains all the time."[28] Empathy? In nonstop thirty-six-hour days, caregivers cannot discharge all their duties with honor and distinction. Respite is so desperately needed that medical insurance (even Medicare) regularly covers it, although many caregivers—thanks to eros again—can't or won't accept relief. I wouldn't. My empathetic imagination hit bottom one day when Ruth put my car keys in her purse . . . and forgot. *Cue the frantic two-hour key search.* An everyday nuisance? How often do you find ice cream puddled in a kitchen cabinet? I'm patient, but caregivers run out of patience. Ruth didn't know which of the three doors in our bedroom led to the toilet. (The toilet, as one caregiver told me, was where her husband washed his hands.) Every nighttime bathroom trip for Ruth requires supervision, as I wearily roll back the covers. My frustration, long held in check, at times spills out wildly.

A serious ethical question for Alzheimer's caregivers is not how to avoid failure, because failure is inescapable, but how to understand and to deal with the self-diminishments it entails, especially for people who are competent, loving, and desperate to help. Alzheimer's disease, unlike many medical conditions, ramps up the likelihood of moral, physical, and emotional failures because it enlists caregivers without their knowledge in a distinctive and damaging erotic economy. *Erotic economy* is an unusual concept in medicine. If the moral practice typical of caregivers, however, is carried out amid inescapable failures and loss, it cannot be fully understood apart from the idea of an erotic economy and, in my case, apart from understanding which specific erotic economy it is that typifies Alzheimer's disease.

An Erotic Economy of Illness

This is how the erotic economy worked: as Ruth's condition deteriorated, my concern for her intensified. Love and affection can't be quantified, of course, but they can change, even measurably. People fall in and out of love, divorce happens, and our degrees of concern ratchet up and down. Ruth's deterioration kicked my attention, concern, love, and a variety of related feelings into overdrive. My hyperintense emotional investment occurred at the exact moment when Alzheimer's disease was shutting down not only Ruth's cognitive functions but also, disastrously for me as well as for Ruth, her emotional responses. In effect, she was fading away emotionally, just when I felt in greatest need of her ordinarily loving expressiveness. Oddly, I could deal with her failures of memory and household lapses. What was hardest for me was her unusual absence of emotion. The subtly modulated flow of mutual affection established over thirty years of marriage suddenly went haywire. Ruth gave back less and less just as I was giving more and needing more. I began to feel something like emotional impoverishment. What would happen when my own heart registered as wholly bankrupt?

Historians employ the concept of "moral economy" to identify the complex flow of competing interests and obligations among diverse groups in a society, such as eighteenth-century street mobs, cottagers, and landowning aristocrats.[29] My coinage of an *erotic* economy refers to the complex flow of affections within a household, within a relationship, or within the extended supra-dyadic social networks created by illness. In Alzheimer's disease, the usual flow of reciprocal affections between patient and caregiver swerves crazily out of balance. It also alters in inverse patterns that threaten breakdown, with consequences often less dire for the unknowing patient (progressively unaware or possibly already lost in dementia) than for the knowing, anxious, increasingly distraught caregiver.

Economics, which Thomas Carlyle famously described as *the dismal science*, seems a bleak metaphor applied to love, but literal money is often a real source of anxiety for caregivers, with the power to undermine affection and to trump eros. Fortunately, Ruth and I had bought long-term care policies, doubtless a white upper-middle-class privilege, but still I worried about money, and now I worried about work, too. Work, according to some major thinkers, stands in direct opposition to eros. Economic activities and erotic activities, they argue, are linked only through a weird misalliance. Bataille, for example, associates eros with the concept of *dépense*, and *dépense* in his specialized usage refers not merely to expense but to specific irrational and excessive expenditures: not only unproductive but also deliberately *wasteful*. From ritual gifts to blood sacrifice, eros for Bataille belongs to the profligate, wasteful expenditures of *dépense*—which differ fundamentally from capitalist values that focus on production and profit. As he writes of *dépense*, "the accent is placed on a *loss* that must be as great as possible in order for that activity to take on its true meaning."[30] My loss seemed as great as possible but—perhaps because it was unchosen or because I was simply unable to recognize the extent of my own wasteful erotic expenditures as caregiver—I felt little beyond meaningless fatigue and emotional numbness. Eros, for me, had just gone missing.

The erotic economy of Alzheimer's disease, in short, had transformed an intimate and loving act—caring for a disabled spouse—into almost the opposite of intimacy. Days became a to-do list of never-ending chores. Our social life dried up in direct correlation with Ruth's increasing inability to communicate. Naively, I had imagined that sexual intimacy would survive Ruth's increasing loss of speech—isn't sex supposed to be the secret language of love?—but I discovered that sexual communication depends on a continuous mutual relay of subtle signals, unspoken to be sure; the signals failed with the failures of language. The sex life of an Alzheimer's couple, often nonexistent, is at best a study in asymmetries: in one study, only 27 percent of the Alzheimer's couples were sexually active.[31] The erotic economy of Alzheimer's disease, then, stripped away sex, too, just when I most needed its unspoken intimacies.

Numb, I was hanging on for dear life, and eros had disappeared in a plodding execution of only the most unavoidable tasks. "One goes on to the end," says William Carlos Williams's doctor as he pursues his digital examination in a spirit of grinding, impersonal labor.[32] He and I might have benefited from a glimpse at sociologist Jean Baudrillard's theory of *séduction*. *Séduction*, for Baudrillard, sheds its libertine aura and refers instead to purposeless, unproductive erotic play. Erotic play, much like *dépense* for Bataille, stands as a positive alternative to the prevailing bourgeois, capitalist work ethic centered on a profit-and-loss mind-set. "Seduction," he sums up, "is, at all times and in all places, opposed to production."[33] I was in no mood for francophone theory. I fretted that I could barely read or write. It was not that I opposed either production or play—I like them both. Writing for me, I learned, is directly connected with pleasure and desire, but I was unable to feel pleasure, was drained of desire, and was without a spark of creative juice. It was all loss and failure all the time, and the seductions of play were, frankly, the last thing on my mind.

The erotic economy of Alzheimer's disease has a specific time signature that no doubt differs from the tempo of other illnesses. While *dépense* and *séduction* take place in an archaic or fantasy world without clocks, the Alzheimer's caregiver lives in a paradoxical world in which there is never enough time for the tasks left undone, and meanwhile we know that one day soon (the disease-clock is ticking) radical changes will occur. At a moment of intense distress, I contacted the local Alzheimer's Association office and arranged to meet with a volunteer. My advisor turned out to be a white-haired, elderly widow, flawlessly attired in a skirt and matching cashmere sweater as if just arrived from the country club. I doubted she could help—my prejudice against country clubs had somehow survived the emotional insolvency—but nonetheless I poured out my distress as she sat and listened. Only later did I realize that widowhood meant she had probably nursed her own spouse through Alzheimer's disease. When I at last finished, she said quietly, "It will get worse."

Maybe I just needed to lighten up—not a likely scenario—but eros certainly failed to carry me as caregiver into a lighthearted zone where time is measured in happiness. What does time feel like, I wonder, in the erotic economy of children pressed into service as de facto caregivers for a mother shut down in depression, say, or for an alcoholic father? Such

children must not only give affection without return but also likely
receive, for their trouble, mainly indifference and abuse. What if as a
teenager I'd had to raise my younger sister and three younger brothers?
Dépense and *séduction* belong to worlds far different from the strange
nightside territory into which Alzheimer's disease pulls the unwitting
caregiver—a realm all the more uncanny because everyday surroundings
tend to remain unchanged while the clocks whir madly backward and
forward, or just stop. The time signature that defined my life in the erotic
economy of Alzheimer's disease was split into either nonstop busyness
and constant fatigue or (as Ruth edged ever further into unresponsive,
emotion-stripped need) what seemed like interminable and purposeless
waiting.

Standing-By: Medical Eros and Waiting

Waiting is such a common experience in medicine—waiting for laboratory results, for a hospital bed, for an appointment—that it even receives
its designated space: the waiting room. As scenes of waiting, hospitals and
clinics are so similar to airports and motor vehicle departments that we
might be tempted to dismiss waiting as simply an unavoidable modern
inconvenience, like temporary gridlock. Samuel Beckett, in a more philosophical vein, represented waiting as an image of the modern condition.
In *Waiting for Godot* (1953) the main characters spend their time
talking, with no clear purpose other than passing time. Waiting is just
what they do, almost a vocation or a state of being. The postmodern era
adds its own twist to inaction. Waiting, in a popular culture that praises
agency, self-actualization, and empowerment, is automatic disempowerment; it implies timidity, nonassertiveness, diminished selfhood, and
loss of control. It signifies almost culpable or shameful failures of will. If
you were truly self-actualized, empowered, and in control, you wouldn't
be waiting. Your oil would already be changed, your plane forever at
the gate, the doctor always in.

Caregivers, in their encounter with waiting, are not likely to benefit
from philosophical distinctions between time and duration, however fascinating.[34] My experience brought a rough-hewn, pragmatic recognition
of two *kinds* of waiting. These alternate modes might be called—to borrow

an old-fashioned distinction from grammar—transitive and intransitive waiting.

Transitive waiting implies waiting *for* something. An anticipated event would complete the action of waiting, the verb will eventually find its object, and the practical questions that then arise mainly concern timing: how *long* to wait for the anticipated closure. For example, I silently waited for the dreaded day that I knew would arrive when Ruth would have to leave home. Most family caregivers know this dread, and in my case I waited—a serious mistake—far too long. I felt that Ruth was better off at home. I couldn't bear the thought of losing her, and I didn't know that there are now some truly remarkable facilities designed and staffed for dementia patients. Instead, as I arranged for daytime home care during the workweek, I also failed to understand two important facts.

First, Ruth was growing dismayed at her unwilling transformation into the one household member who was forever making mistakes. She liked to say, laughing, that she was only "dinged." We both knew it was no joke, but we kept up the subterfuge. It shocked me, when she finally left home for a residential facility, that she thrived in the company of patients equally (or far worse) *dinged*.

Second, I worried that when I brought her home for brief visits that Ruth would be choked up with nostalgia. I was shocked again to find that she was wholly indifferent to her old home surroundings. Now—*idiot*—I get it. Her brain no longer worked like my brain, so I had no inner compass to estimate her thoughts and feelings. We were out of sync. What I might experience as nostalgia, she didn't, especially as Alzheimer's gradually blocked the neural pathways linking recognition, memory, and emotion. On entering the house, Ruth would barely glance around before setting out to find Pounce the cat. Unfortunately, her cognitive loss included losing the sense that warns us to watch out when cats pin back their ears, so her visits home often ended in blood and tears as Pounce, each time, whacked the hand that stroked her.

The dreaded day had eventually arrived, of course, when my transitive waiting was at an end. It had occurred to me that, in my state of continual exhaustion, it was very possible—and I cautioned myself against self-dramatizing worst-case scenarios—that Ruth might one day wake up beside a corpse. It could happen. The thought spurred me to visit a few local residential Alzheimer's facilities. In bed one morning, I timidly worked up the nerve to tell Ruth that I had visited a live-in facility. She shocked me once more. Without emotion or spark of curiosity, she replied in an even voice, "*Can we go see it?*"

Intransitive waiting implies waiting *without* an object, and I became an expert at intransitive waiting. You didn't wait *for* something, not even for an imaginary or real Godot who never comes; you just wait. The elderly residents at Ruth's Alzheimer's facility seem to me absorbed in an intransitive waiting, with no object and no purpose as they slump in a ragged semicircle of overstuffed chairs. Is *waiting* even the right term for their motionless state? Or have they entered an almost timeless condition? I don't know—their demeanor seems so alien. A few residents will say that they are waiting for a visitor, or waiting to go home. I'll find them days later lingering by the locked door, overcoat on. The staff knows better than to correct them. Then I reflect that I, too, am waiting, intransitively. There's no one to correct *me* either. I am not waiting *for* anything—for Ruth to get better (which won't happen) or to get worse (which will).

I am on the go, like Psyche, busy visiting the facility every day, taking Ruth on hour-long walks, but this busyness has no real object, like the unending tasks I perform, from scheduling Ruth's hairdresser and taking her out for (necessary) pedicures—nail salons an uncharted terrain—to accompanying her through the emergency room, orthopedic ward, and rehabilitation facility after unwisely prescribed antipsychotic drugs caused a fall that broke her leg at the hip. (Dementia patients cannot follow directions. Within days of surgery, she regularly escaped her wheelchair and paced the halls on a newly pinned femur in danger of splintering.) My waiting may be disguised as busyness, but I am as powerless as the elderly resident endlessly waiting by the locked door with her overcoat on.

Waiting enfolds family caregivers in an almost invisible ethical dilemma basic to medical eros. Eros is what drives us, expressed in affection for the patient and in our deep desire to help, but eros is also what makes our lives so confusing as, driven, we wait and wait. Is intransitive waiting, paradoxically, our action? Or is it the *absence* of action? Such questions tangled my intestines in knots, which is why I felt pleased later to find theologians W. H. Vanstone and Henri Nouwen.[35] In their writings, both respond to the devaluations that depict waiting as passivity and lost control: action delayed, deferred, or abandoned. Both writers, surprisingly, offer an unequivocal affirmation of waiting. They regard inaction (and especially objectless, unproductive waiting) as endowed with moral value. Jesus is their model of intransitive waiting. In particular, they point to the period, after Gethsemane, when his active ministry concludes and Jesus almost passively hands himself over to the political world. Thereafter, his ministry complete, he simply . . . waits. Vanstone and Nouwen view the passiveness after Jesus has *completed* his ministry not as disempowerment but rather as the relinquishment or abandonment of an active, productive, purposeful role.

Medical eros might discover in waiting a hidden erotic affirmation of life: life as affirmed and valued *despite* the absence of production, despite the loss of activity. Such a revaluation of waiting would provide at least a counterweight to the burden of self-reproach that so easily accompanies the caregiver's personal sense of loss and failure. An erotic revaluation of waiting, however, faces stiff resistance. Inaction has a bad name, and idleness, if no longer a deadly sin, is now regarded as a prime capitalist blunder in a world where time is money. It evokes the vaguely sinister image of guys just hanging out on a street corner. Ad campaigns depict even retirees as golfing, hiking, sailing, and partying (good consumers of recreational activities) until the golden sun goes down. No one, of course, wants to see ads that feature pale, ailing, decrepit old folks slumped in an arc just, as it may be, waiting.

Just waiting, however, is exactly what Vanstone and Nouwen revalue. Their concern with well-being across the *entire* life span—including times of sickness, retirement, and very old age, when significant action may be physically impossible—imparts to waiting the same positive value that Bataille sees in deliberate and excessive loss, as if the sheer objectless-ness of intransitive waiting gives meaning to an otherwise pointless or dismal state, time not just slipping away but disregarded or even squandered. Ethics concerns not only right actions but also right values.[36] Medical eros might well insist that there is ethical value in simple waiting: not *failure* to act but rather the gentle *acceptance* of unwilled inaction.

A gentle acceptance of passive inaction and of intransitive waiting goes against the American grain, and I still struggle with it. Shouldn't I be *doing* something for Ruth? Isn't acceptance another name for resignation, despair, and surrender? Why should I accept the unacceptable? Medical eros can help us address such questions, which fall outside the expertise or even the purview of medical logos, even if eros can't answer them in every instance. In any case, whatever value medical eros might assign to the intransitive waiting typical of Alzheimer's disease must focus, as Lisa Diedrich recommends, on failure and loss, especially the moral or psychic state of *being at a loss*.[37] Of not-knowing. Such a focus includes more than the patient's lost health, failed abilities, or incomprehension. It implicitly acknowledges the *two-person, plural*, or *polygon* structure of certain illnesses—in which caregivers too so often enter into a twilight state of *being* at a loss: a condition of free-fall, vertigo, and not-knowing. Caregivers are new residents of an *at-loss* state. Their radical helplessness, despite nonstop caregiving, links them with another set of cultural figures who famously wait: lovers.

Lovers wait *for* the beloved, in at least a semitransitive state, but often the objects of romantic love recede out of reach, desired but unattainable: the bright stars of Keatsian longing, the return home or the return to health for an Alzheimer's patient. Eros and illness both tend to plunge the person who waits—lover, caregiver, patient—into a passiveness where loss is the only steady state, where wished-for objects recede endlessly in a hopeless, imposed, intransitive waiting. Did Ruth truly want a dog? I, too, want something, and I don't know how to name it. Is it nameless? So what else can caregivers do? I wait.

A gospel song that I heard after Ruth left home poses a question that caregivers in particular will recognize: "What do you do when you've done all you can?" I often found myself at this impasse, out of options, out of strength, empty. *What do you do when you've done all you can?* The three-word gospel response: "You just stand."[38] Just standing doesn't sound impressive, but in the world of gospel music it cannot occur without God's help. It also embraces a radical acceptance that medical eros would associate with divine love. The at-loss state of standing and waiting constitutes a similar state of radical acceptance for the seventeenth-century dissenting Protestant poet John Milton. In the famous sonnet on his blindness, he asks how a poet without eyesight can still serve God. The response: "They also serve who only stand and wait."[39] Standing and waiting, nothing more, nothing less, signify for Milton an ethical state entangled in loss—in failures beyond lost eyesight—which he regularly represents in images of falling. Falling, for Milton, almost always contains an implicit theological reference to The Fall. In Miltonic theology, to stand thus also means to remain upright, to do your duty. To stand and wait means—crucially—*not to fall*. More secular caregivers, such as I am, can substitute their own highest values to be served in the paradoxical act of inactive, objectless, upright, and no less devoted intransitive waiting.

"If you are uncomfortable with the implication of the erotic attraction of a woman at eighty," E. S. Goldman reports, "—eighty-five as I write this—suffer more: the sagging breasts, iconic of the destiny of an aged woman, draw the surface of globes taut so that in the midst of physical degradation the breast is as smooth as a bride's. I did not abdicate the nightly privilege of helping her undress until a year or so ago, in her fourth year of Alz, when an aide took over. I stand by."[40] Goldman's account as octogenarian caregiver belongs to an erotics of illness, and medical eros might especially value in Goldman's sweetly loving account its distinctive concern with *presence*. Presence needs to be distinguished, as a moral state, from witnessing. Witnessing—an important concept in trauma studies and in palliative care—is an action: rational, teachable, even measurable as true or false (as in the concept of bearing *false* witness). *Presence*, in its erotic inflections, differs from the act of witnessing. It is not quite, either, the opposite of absence. It signifies *being there*, in the moral sense of standing by in a fully embodied, deeply attentive waiting. Presence implies an ethical state beyond reason, rules, or duties—an acceptance of the often unspoken bonds that draw people together. It evokes various meanings of not-to-fall: standing firm, taking a stand, standing by, ready as needed. Presence means *being there* as distinct from *doing something* or *knowing something*. It means, in its full moral implications, a stance of nonabandonment.

Medical eros might regard presence or standing by as among the highest goods in a new ethics befitting the flawed, depleted, failed, at-loss caregivers who have run out of hope, run out of options, done all they can, and now just wait. "Presence," Goldman says, "is what counts."[41]

It has been twelve years now since the blessing of the candles. So much has changed. The cost that dementia incurs worldwide currently equals over 1 percent of global gross domestic product.[42] Such figures mean little to the caregiver. Ruth no longer recognizes me. Waiting is now a strictly one-sided expression of desire with no response possible: a situation where there is nothing more, almost nothing, to lose. Still waiting. Medical eros, in providing the basis for an ethics of loss and failure, can offer help to caregivers for whom simply waiting, waiting without an object, with no expectation, no purpose, just being there, has to be barely enough, an upright (if brokenhearted) place to stand. Medical eros, too, can remind caregivers and all who enter the kingdom of illness that their dilemmas come with a silent history, and we are standing on the site of an invisible conflict that defines us and the ground we stand on, much as a Civil War battlefield recalls the unseen wounds that still define and divide Americans. The individual experience of illness today, including the hidden conflicts and confusions that grip both patients and caregivers, owes much to a forgotten antagonism between medical eros and medical logos, so any personal understanding to dispel confusion or any future resolution of conflict requires a step back into the history of this ancient, effortless forgetting.

CHAPTER TWO

Unforgetting Asklepios:
Medical Eros and Its Lineage

Without Contraries is no progression.

WILLIAM BLAKE, *THE MARRIAGE OF HEAVEN AND HELL* (1789–1790)

"*H*E RUINS MORTALS and causes them every kind of disaster." So Euripides writes of Eros.[1] Eros as depicted by the ancient Greeks embodies fearsome destructive powers that, simply put, can rip your life apart. A late Latin romance, *The Golden Ass* (ca. 170–180 CE), offers a seriocomic version of the same wanton, deceitful, destructive power, as the author, Apuleius, describes Eros (now Romanized as the mischievous boy Cupid) "rampaging through people's houses at night armed with his torch and arrows, undermining the marriages of all."[2] Roman and Greek lyric poets agree about the betrayals and agonies coiled with the blandishments of love. The lover, it appears, is almost set up not only for suffering but also for diminishment and self-attrition. "Eros is expropriation," as classicist Anne Carson sums up the ancient lyric consensus. "He robs the body of limbs, substance, integrity and leaves the lover, essentially, less."[3]

Why then would anyone take a chance on eros? Puck, as an immortal spirit, offers one solid answer in *A Midsummer Night's Dream*: "Lord, what fools these mortals be!"[4] Eros, however, is far more than a sign of human folly or even a dubious consolation prize for our death-haunted mortality. Something else must be at stake. Eros, that is, regularly encodes an inherent doubleness. "Bittersweet" (*glukopikron*) is the poet Sappho's preferred epithet for eros, as Anne Carson emphasizes, and the bittersweet mix of sensations perfectly captures an erotic duality that includes the power not only to ruin lives but also to fill them with delight and exalt the lover to inexpressible, transcendent, and even (as in Sappho's famous ode 31) "godlike" heights. Eros, then, encompasses the dual possibilities of total abjection and utter exhilaration, sometimes compacted into a single night. "Use me but as your spaniel" (II.i.205), Helena implores her turncoat lover, Demetrius, in *A Midsummer Night's Dream*; but once they have passed through the erotic chaos of the dark forest night, it is the same inconstant Demetrius who suddenly announces that all his faith, virtue, and pleasure is "only Helena" (IV.i.171). So it goes, red hot and ice cold, with eros. The doubleness within eros, where eros embraces a roller-coaster range of contrary experience, offers at least a useful model for thinking about the early history and contemporary relevance of medical pluralism. It is a pluralism lived out in ancient times through a simultaneous allegiance to the figures of Asklepios and Hippocrates.

The god Asklepios and the mortal Hippocrates can stand here as iconic contraries in the conflict between medical eros and medical logos. The ultimate victory of Hippocrates and the triumph of so-called rational medicine, for which he is so often cited as founder, make sense within a positivist history of medicine. In this familiar narrative of scientific progress, medical knowledge advances (leaving behind a primitive past marked by superstition and religion) toward its ultimate goal of rational, evidence-based, clinical biomedicine—in short, *us*. It is an appealing narrative because biomedicine has made immense advances in eradicating diseases and in curing illness. There is a significant error, however, in a positivist history of medicine that skews the past in order to celebrate a steady, almost predestined triumph of science and of reason, as if the mortal doctor from the island of Kos simply won in a knockout over his slow-footed rival and ancestor, the drowsy healing god Asklepios.

It wasn't so simple. For many centuries, the two classic icons shared power.

Asklepios held a place in the ancient divine hierarchy just below the twelve chief gods residing on Mount Olympus. Some sources regarded him not as a god but a demigod, like Hercules, a human figure whose achievements merited godlike status. Most, however, recognize him as a god, and even as a demigod he could claim direct descent from Apollo. The awe that Asklepios inspired had material as well as mythic backing. Magnificent temple sanctuaries attested to his prestige, such as the famous Asklepieion at Epidauros that boasted an immense ivory and gold statue of Asklepios seated on a throne in Zeus-like majesty. Priests there, as at the other principal Asklepieion sites in Kos and in Pergamon, administered expansive bureaucracies that included amphitheaters and offered long-term accommodations. Treatments often began with ritual purification and sacrifices, for both priests and patients, but the most important therapeutic process was called *incubation* (Latin *cubo*, I recline). During incubation, patients slept in the temple precinct, or *abaton*, awaiting a dream contact from the god. The divine visitation might also come through contact with the sacred temple snakes, an impressive nonvenomous species four to five feet long.[5] This dream-based, snake-mediated therapy left some patients fully healed, as they attested in votive offerings (such as life-sized terracotta casts of a leg or hand) hung on the temple wall in thanks. The huge temple complexes constituted a significant material infrastructure that extended the power of Asklepios well into the Christian era. Tertullian (ca. 155–240 CE), an early Church father, praised Asklepios as proof that the medical arts were given by God.[6]

The magnificent statues, panoramic settings, crowds of rich pilgrims, and shrines that were strictly off-limits to the uninitiated gave Asklepios a presence in the ancient world that run-of-the-mill mythological figures could not match. He was, simply, a great god, and his godlike temple complexes stood as visible proof. The tenacious hold that Asklepios exercised over ancient medicine extended, at least in popular belief, to a power over death, as his biography gave rise to a powerful thematics of death and rebirth. Asklepios, it was said, could awaken the dead. He was also believed to have returned from the dead himself, after Zeus supposedly

killed him with a thunderbolt. Socrates, who served one term as priest at
the Asklepieion in Athens, said in his enigmatic last words that he *owed
a cock to Asklepios*—a statement that Christian exegetes read as affirming
a Socratic belief in eternal life.[7]

The high standing that Asklepios attained among the educated upper
classes is confirmed in the odd diary kept by a health-obsessed popular
Greek orator in the age of Nero, P. Aelius Aristides. Aristides had traveled widely throughout Egypt, Greece, and Italy, often in search of health,
and in his autobiographical *Sacred Tales* he consistently addresses
Asklepios as *Master*, *Savior*, and *Lord*. "Great and many are the powers
of Asklepios," he writes, "or rather he possesses all powers, beyond the
scope of human life. . . . It is he who guides and directs the Universe,
savior of the Whole and guardian of what is immortal."[8] Such claims suggest why the new Christian apologists emphasized the role of Jesus as savior
and healer and why it was as late as the sixth century that the Asklepieion
at Kos finally fell into disuse—no doubt partly due to the campaign of the
Christian emperor Justinian to root out signs of pagan worship.

There are distinguished historians today who propose a nonpositivist
account of ancient medicine in which Hippocrates and Asklepios coexist
as equals. In this revisionist history, ancient medicine for many centuries
embraced an intrinsic doubleness—a medical pluralism—with Hippocrates and Asklepios *sharing* power. Power sharing, however, is
rarely stable or equitable, and ultimately Asklepios (and medical pluralism) dropped from memory with the triumph of biomedicine. There
is nonetheless ample reason to reject the standard positivist narrative of
a Hippocratic knockout blow because the model of ancient pluralism,
maintained over many centuries, remains a durable legacy applicable even
today. The legacy of an unofficial medical pluralism survives alive and
well, for example, in modern rural folk medicine or within immigrant
communities, where people who remain largely outside the biomedical
orbit may also make irregular visits to primary care providers, purchase
over-the-counter medications, and consult osteopathic surgeons. Among
Native Americans, medical care often includes both tribal healers and
Western doctors. In affluent suburbs, where family doctors are a household
staple, shopping malls are also well supplied with acupuncturists, herb-
alists, and homeopaths.

Hippocrates rightly deserves his title as the founder of rational medicine, or medical logos, but, in a more comprehensive medical genealogy, Asklepios has every right to assert his former eminence as a power-sharing partner in healing. I would argue that Asklepios also merits renewed consideration as the unacknowledged founder of medical eros. Their shared power as a model of medical pluralism, however, truly becomes available for contemporary thought only after we unmask and reverse the historical campaign to all but erase the memory of Asklepios.

Illness as Intoxication

Anatole Broyard, the longtime book reviewer, columnist, and editor at the *New York Times*, found to his surprise that his imminent terminal illness was bound up with the double-edged bittersweetness of eros. A diagnosis of inoperable prostate cancer sparked in him an improbable erotic elevation of spirit so intense as to resemble the euphoria of falling in love.[9] He calls this response, which he did not anticipate, an *intoxication*. His experience cannot be dismissed as wholly eccentric, however, because it finds parallels elsewhere, as we will see. Perhaps it is only his open confession and wholehearted embrace of erotic intoxication that proved extraordinary. His essays collected (posthumously) under the title *Intoxicated by My Illness* (1992) both describe his encounter with medical eros and suggest the value in revisiting its now-forgotten classical progenitor, Asklepios. Broyard's account of his prostate cancer affirms erotic values that biomedicine, in its allegiance to the scientific method and to ethical norms of professional conduct, does not simply deny, avoid, or forget but actively represses.

The profession-wide repression of eros constitutes a specialized form of forgetting that not only forgets how illness intersects with desire but also forgets that it has forgotten. The forgetting moreover is culture-wide because biomedicine now dominates how most people in the developed world think and feel about illness. Broyard disconcerted his visitors as they arrived to offer consolation and found him, unexpectedly, so cheerful that they attributed his strange upbeat state to uncommon courage. "But it has nothing to do with courage," Broyard countered, "at least not for me. As far as I can tell, it's a question of desire. I'm filled with desire—to live, to write, to do everything. . . . While I've always had trouble concentrating, I now feel as concentrated as a diamond or a microchip."[10]

Desire, for Broyard, does not refer to the concept that classical philosophers so often warned against as suggesting an insatiable lack or gap, like a leaky bowl, nor does he share their sometimes contradictory view that regards desire as therapeutic.[11] His was a personal eroticism, more in the manner of William Blake, and he viewed desire as an abundant, transformative energy inseparable from sexualized excess. Anne Carson adds the important point that Greek lyric poets describe the lover's desire less as passive, unfulfilled longing—the sign of a voracious lack—than as an active force capable of transforming the lover who desires: it can offer access to a previously unknown or undiscovered self.[12] Contemporary writer and filmmaker Chris Kraus, narrating her own erotic obsession, observes that desire is not about *lack* (as in the *absence* of the beloved) but about a newfound "surplus energy."[13] Desire, perhaps like surplus energy rushing into (or out of) the gap left vacant by material and psychic absences, cannot guarantee zones of safety. It exposes almost everyone whom it touches to an unfixed experience of free-floating intensities where selves and relationships are always at risk—in danger of total breakdown—but open as well to astonishing discoveries and to unexpected transformations.

Broyard too found that serious illness, like love, intensified desire in a way that potentially transforms the self. Illness thus aligned him almost automatically with the position of a medical outsider, a stance he enjoyed, especially as he explored the freedoms of his new powers of microchip intensity. Not only did his illness put him outside social conventions surrounding the so-called sick role but it also conferred a new, wide-awake immunity from sentimental condolences and heartfelt sympathies, which his visitors imported from the world of everyday health. He was now the psychic stranger who inhabited an alien realm—a realm given over to unknown and newly savored sensations and desires from which the so-called healthy world is shut out. "I remain outside of their solicitude, their love and best wishes," he wrote of his consoling friends. "I'm isolated from them by the grandiose conviction that I am the healthy person and they are the sick ones. Like an existential hero, I have been cured by the truth while they still suffer the nausea of the uninitiated" (*IMI* 6).

Serious illness not only recruits and intensifies desire but, as Broyard insists, it also revalues apparently renegade decisions that flow from desire and run counter to prevailing biomedical wisdom. Broyard—the ironized existential hero of desire, consistent with his early reputation as a postwar Greenwich Village sexual legend—stands outside both medical traditions and the norms of bourgeois life. "My urologist, who is quite famous," he writes in deadpan, "wanted to cut off my testicles, but I felt that this would be losing the battle right at the beginning. Speaking as a surgeon, he said that it was the surest, quickest, neatest solution. Too neat, I said, picturing myself with no balls" (*IMI* 26). This breezy exchange merits a slow-motion replay. Broyard, that is, rejected the best biomedical judgment not because it was wrong but because medical logos failed to recognize the importance that he attributed to eros in his personal, psychic, and social identity. Medical eros, as Broyard offers his idiosyncratic spin, does not reject logic or reason but rather enlists them in the service of desire. "I knew that such a solution would depress me," Broyard continues, referring to his potentially testicle-absent state, "and I was sure that depression is bad medicine" (*IMI* 26). It was not freedom from medicine that he sought, but rather good medicine, which he redefined as medicine in league with the powers of eros.

Prostate cancer for Broyard, attacking a home territory of eros, was always more than a threat to the body. As he writes in a meaningful double-entendre, "When the cancer threatened my sexuality, my mind became immediately erect" (*IMI* 27). Illness as it intensified his desire also reorganized how he thought and felt. He recalled how the pursuit of a sexual liaison once focused his energies almost like (to cite his own image) a visionary experience. "Yet when I read about sex now," he reflected from the demystified stance of serious illness, "it seems to me that we've surrendered too much of that vision to the pursuit of orgasm" (*IMI* 28). Prostate cancer, in his illness-centered view, is not just a matter of cells and tissue damage, any more than sex is a matter of orgasm; bodies are inseparable from minds, and minds are inseparable from eros and the inner life. Eros here is not an addition to illness—an odd supplement, as when tuberculosis patients experienced heightened sexual feelings and a typical "hectic flush"—but rather an intrinsic part of his illness. Prostate cancer for Broyard was not about stirring up sexual hormones but about firing up his psyche, which turned out to be inseparably linked to sexual energies. "My libido," he explained, as if to correct a biomedical mistake, "is lodged not only in my prostate but in my imagination, my memory, my conception of myself, my appreciation of women and of life itself. It belongs as much to my identity and my aesthetics as it does to physiology" (*IMI* 27). A 1974 collection of his *Times* reviews received the provocative and punning title, no surprise to medical eros, *Aroused by Books*.[14]

Anatole Broyard will always remain something of a mystery: a black man who lived in the headiest circles of East Coast intellectual life and who chose to pass for white. He kept his racial identity secret even from his grown children—only his wife knew. Henry Louis Gates Jr. exposes with a fine sympathy the paradoxes in Broyard's artful self-fashioning during an era when racism in America meant that black skin, by default, allowed the white world to define (and to confine) you. Illness, too, tends to define by default. Broyard would not allow illness any more than race to define him, as if he knew that racism and racial disparities in health care have a dishonorable place in the history of biomedicine.[15] Just as he constructed an ambiguous racial identity that plays upon and subverts the opposition between white and black, he constructed a personal experience of illness that does not reject medical logos (as personified in his famous urologist) but also allows free play to medical eros and to the imperatives of desire. Prostate cancer became for Broyard the scene of an extravagant high-wire performance over the abyss—maybe an ultimate work of performance art—in which imminent death adds its incalculable erotic intensities. His embrace of eros in the grip of illness is far from unique, and it offers one model for constructing a personal conjunction of medical logos and medical eros. It also calls attention to a more than accidental absence amid celebrations of Hippocrates and rational medicine: the near-complete disappearance of Asklepios.

The Erasure of Asklepios

Asklepios, mythic son of Apollo and the putative founder of medical eros, held a revered and preeminent status in the ancient world as "the healing god *par excellence*."[16] The cult of Asklepios at its height, as classicist Bronwen L. Wickkiser puts it, reached "across the length and breadth of

the Greco-Roman world."[17] A savior-deity who, unlike the remote, aristocratic, unpredictable Olympians, cared for everyone irrespective of class
or social status, Asklepios achieved such a reputation that even into late
antiquity he was the chief pagan competitor of Christ.[18] His near total dis-
appearance constitutes a mystery with significant consequences for how
we experience illness today. It is an unusual mystery: it begins not with
discovering a body but—in a twist that might confuse Sherlock Holmes—
with the discovery that a body is missing. The missing body, in this
case, refers not to a person but to an entire medical legacy. The question,
then, is not *who done it?* Rather, *what in the world is going on?* How could
the chief pagan competitor of Christ—commemorated on coins, celebrated
in oaths, and worshipped in immense and impressive temple complexes
across the ancient world—simply disappear?

"One of the most impressive contributions of the ancient Greeks to
Western culture," according to historian James Longrigg, in a version of the
positivist narrative, "was their invention of rational medicine."[19] It is certain
that rational medicine ultimately won out over its indigenous competitors,
and it is certain that the invention of rational medicine in the Western world
can be credited to the Greeks. So far, Longrigg is correct. The triumph of
rational medicine, however, cannot be accurately represented as a clean victory for science, knowledge, and progress over religion and superstition.
Religion was inseparable from ancient medicine, as it was also inseparable
from civic life, governmental duties, and military excursions, which all invoked religious sanction. Medical practice among the Hippocratic doctors
thus required a delicate balancing act: rational medicine could oppose both
superstitious quackery and the medical high jinks of street magicians, but it
needed to make an accommodation with religion. Nonetheless, even with
such crucial revisions to the positivist narrative, no one is more important
in the redirection of ancient medicine than the mortal, empiricist physician
from the Greek island of Kos, Hippocrates.

Hippocrates (ca. 460–370 BCE) attained such eminence as a medical
practitioner in the age of Pericles that he justly receives credit for introducing an understanding of illness as based in a systematic, empirical
knowledge of the body. Although scholars no longer regard him as sole
author of the so-called Hippocratic Writings, a collection of medical tracts
by various hands, it is Hippocrates through his example and through his

eminence who stands as the official precursor of medical logos and as the distant father of contemporary biomedicine. To later ages, he comes to embody human reason and scientific medicine in their demystifying resistance to prerational magic, myth, superstition, quackery, and unreason. His victory and veneration are so complete that busts of Hippocrates today regularly adorn multiplex medical centers, celebrating not only modern rational medicine but also the positivist narrative that it sponsors, which explains illness and affliction, as medical historian Roy Porter puts it, "principally in terms of the body."[20]

Hippocrates justly receives credit, then, for establishing medicine as a body-centered, empirical practice and as a rational field of knowledge, leading to the scientific study of interior human workings through the now-famous nineteenth-century "clinical gaze." In providing the basis for contemporary biomedicine, Hippocrates thus provides a classical pedigree for the rational, materialist, biological, evidence-based understanding of illness that I am calling medical logos. Medical students today are trained, tested, and evaluated as scientists and technicians of the human body. Communication skills, empathy, patient care, and bedside manner—as distinct from differential diagnosis and treatment—take second place. The legacy of Hippocrates thus finds continuous reinforcement in a primary commitment to rational analysis, biological sciences, evidence-based practice, and a body-centered clinical gaze, as if there were no other training possible for an accomplished physician. Non-Western traditions, indigenous practices, and homeopathic approaches that fall outside the dominant biomedical paradigm simply do not merit full institutional respect, and Hippocrates assumes his eminence by virtue of an historical process that not only affirms the supremacy of rational medicine but also buries Asklepios in an oblivion where all that survives, if anything, is just a name.

The triumph of rational medicine, as I am arguing, occurred only after centuries when Hippocrates and Asklepios coexisted in a forgotten or misremembered *medical pluralism*.[21] Hippocrates very likely trained at the impressive healing complex at Kos called, as all such complexes were called, the Asklepieion; originally no more than a grove or glade regarded as sacred, soon it developed into a sprawling hilltop installation with views stretching seaward toward Asia. The Asklepieion was generally located outside city walls in settings where springs, vistas, and foliage made nature a participant in the rituals of healing. *Hippocrates the Asklepiad* was the formula that Plato and other contemporaries use to describe the famous doctor from Kos, and the Hippocratic Oath begins by invoking Apollo *and his son Asklepios*. Most early physicians referred to themselves as *Asklepiads*, and numerous patients made extended pilgrimages to the Asklepian temple complexes, often spending weeks or months in residence and leaving behind material signs of their gratitude to the god. What made Asklepios such a formidable presence in the ancient world? A full answer, I suspect, suggests how his legacy might make a significant contribution today toward a renewed understanding of the powers of medical eros.

Asklepios matters less because of his eminence in the classical world than because his near total disappearance prevents us from recognizing what the powers associated with his name contributed to the pluralism of ancient medicine. In the ancient world, even long after the advent of Hippocratic or rational medicine, in practice a two-tier system prevailed. Patients would consult *both* Hippocratic doctors and Asklepian priests, much as today many people consult both primary care physicians and therapists who practice alternative modes of healing. The Asklepieion moreover accepted patients with chronic and incurable illnesses that Hippocratic doctors avoided—the advice to avoid such patients was specified in writing—and in practice both the Asklepieion and the Hippocratic doctors often recommended identical or quite similar therapies that emphasized exercise, purgation, and dietary restrictions. Reason, then, had little more to offer than did dream therapies, and Asklepios meanwhile welcomed patients whom the Hippocratic doctors shunned.

Asklepian dream-based therapies, especially as they were quite similar to reason-based Hippocratic recommendations, did not strike the ancient world as irrational. Dreams held a sanctioned status (ever since the time of Homer) as a portal to revealed truth. Some dreams, of course, could be deceptive, so caution was required, much as reason too could go astray. Some dreams were regarded as truthful, however, and truthful dreams (like official omens and auguries) belonged to an authorized system of communication with the divine that was as intelligible to skilled interpreters as, say, semaphore is today.[22] In effect, ancient medicine was concurrently (without self-contradiction) both rational *and* religious. It had ample room for *both* the rationalist Hippocrates and the dream god Asklepios.

The cult of Asklepios is arguably as significant to the history of medicine as are the theories in the Hippocratic corpus, and for centuries the two healing traditions coexisted comfortably. As historian Vivian Nutton puts it, "For a doctor to reject Asklepios and his healings might also be for him to reject the very things for which medicine was thought to stand. In this way religious and secular healing reinforced rather than opposed each other."[23] The Hippocratic writers, pagans as well as budding clinicians, felt comfortable embracing a polytheistic cosmos, and Asklepian medicine had already won institutional status, unlike the magicians in the marketplace who sold nostrums to the gullible public. Thus, the ongoing struggle between rational medicine and magical quackery did not taint Asklepios, who held the stature of a god, and the Hippocratic writers by declaring themselves Asklepiads cagily invoked his authority and power. Asklepios thus remained a revered figure, remote in the divine power embodied in the marble, gold, and ivory Zeus-like statue at Epidaurus, but also he was an everyday presence depicted on the ancient coins that circulated his image for over 700 years.[24]

Asklepios and Hippocrates: The Traces of Eros

The contrast between Asklepios and Hippocrates, despite the medical pluralism that brought them together in the ancient world, in one respect could not be clearer. Hippocrates understood illness through a reason-based knowledge of the body and through the empirical study of disease; Asklepios cured through dreams, in temples, and through firsthand contact with divine power. The contrast between these two very different ways of understanding illness is captured in visual representations that help to illuminate the alternate values at stake. The comparison (which unjustly pairs images from widely different periods) cannot be more than illustrative—apples versus mock oranges—but the contrast helps to emphasize how Asklepios and Hippocrates embody a radical difference that extends to their implicit relations to eros.

The archaic Greek statuette of Asklepios (Figure 2.1) depicts a young, faunlike, sexualized figure still close to the natural world, accompanied by his totem snake and woodland rod. In stark contrast stands the older, intellectual, urbanized Hippocrates (Figure 2.2).

The difference is striking in other respects as well. Thick curly locks and a muscular torso give *Asclepius adolescens* (to use the Latinate, art-historical term) a youthful, sexual presence. Even when represented in manly middle age, Asklepios exudes a bearded, majestic, erotic power. Images of Hippocrates, by contrast, usually depict him as old and bald. Baldness became almost a visual signature for Hippocrates, prominent enough to require comment: one ancient text offers seven separate explanations

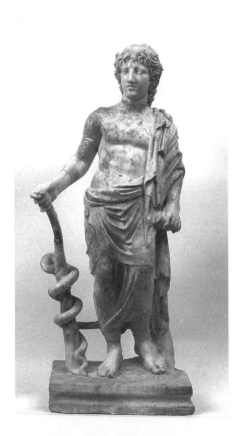 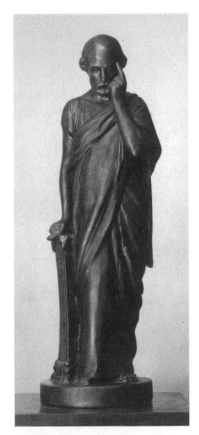

FIGURE 2.1. *Statuette of Asklepios.* 100–200 CE. Marble. National Archaeological Museum, Athens. Copyright © Hellenic Ministry of Culture and Sports / Archaeological Receipts Fund.
FIGURE 2.2. *Hippocrates.* Undated statue (Enlightenment Era?). Image courtesy of The National Library of Medicine, Washington, DC.

for the trademark felt cap (or *pilos*) that covered his bare crown.[25] The undated statue here is likely from the later European Enlightenment, but its representation is entirely traditional and telling. The old, bald, studious Hippocrates stands finger-to-cranium, like an icon of deep thought, suggesting how easily the eighteenth-century Enlightenment and its heirs assimilated Hippocrates and rational medicine within the heady reformist agendas associated with such intellectual enemies of superstition and friends of reason as Voltaire, Kant, Pinel, and Jefferson.

The contrasts keep proliferating. Because Hippocrates came to stand for a medicine based in reason, medieval illustrations regularly associate him with scholastic philosophy, often showing him with a manuscript or scroll in his hands. The scroll also links him with literacy, writing, and the entire Hippocratic corpus. Asklepios belongs instead to the preliterate oral tradition, where the main texts are dreams, where snakes and dogs embody divine healing powers, and where priests interpret the words of the god as patients recount their dreams. Only in retrospect does the triumph of Hippocrates appear inevitable. The Roman senate in 291 BCE, to stop a deadly plague, voted to summon Asklepios from Epidaurus, and ten senators brought the god, by ship, in the body of a large snake. The poet Ovid recounts the solemn event, and Romans chose the holiest date in their calendar, January 1, to dedicate the foundation of their new temple to Asklepios.

Asklepios, no matter if embodied in a large reptile or depicted as a sensual demigod, holds a place of honor and answers to basic human desires for healing. He gestures toward a sacred space: sanctuaries of a divine healing power. It was a gesture that heirs of the new guild-centered Hippocratic tradition—with apprentices bound by oath in order to prevent defections—needed to forget.

The forgetting of Asklepios did not require a showdown or a conspiracy but simply the advancement of science and the relentless triumph of a medical ideology that today finds expression in the molecular gaze. Rational medicine in its historical push for legitimacy needed to shed Asklepios, the barefoot nature god, who entered Rome in the body of a snake and cured through dreams. The ideological erasure is comically obvious in an Enlightenment engraving (Figure 2.3) designed to celebrate the new reformist ideals of medical progress.

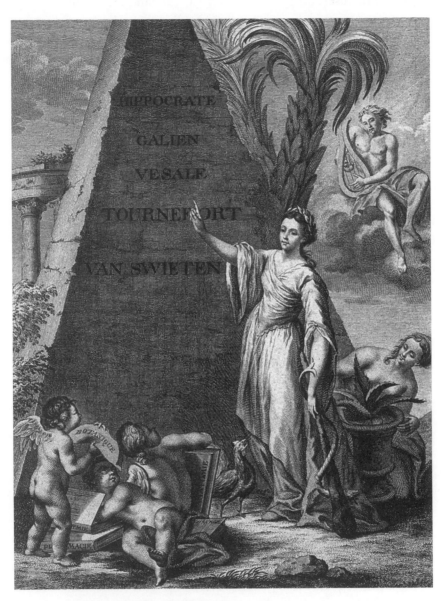

FIGURE 2.3. Hygieia stands before a pyramid engraved with the
names of famous figures in the history of medicine.
Etching by B. Hübner, 1777. Wellcome Library, London. (CC BY 4.0)

Hygieia, the mythic daughter of Asklepios, stands beside a pyramid engraved in descending order with the great names in medicine: Hippocrates, at the apex; then Galen and Vesalius; right down to celebrated contemporary doctors toward the base. Patricide is rarely performed by daughters, yet imagine the ideological gall or willed forgetting required to recruit the daughter of Asklepios for the purpose of endorsing a new medical genealogy that begins with Hippocrates—the man of reason and science—and completely erases her father's memory.

What matters most here is that Asklepios maintained an unofficial connection with eros, while Hippocrates kept a professional distance. The Hippocratic oath expressly forbids its followers to engage with their patients in "sexual contacts" (*aphrodisionergon*).[26] The erasure of Asklepios thus corresponds to a wider forgetting. Evidence confirming the close link between Asklepios and eros, if not obvious in the faunlike archaic statuette, requires gathering scattered sources. A woman named Nikesibule attests that Asklepios came to her in a dream, in which she copulated with his totem snake, giving birth within a year to twin boys, so Asklepios certainly shares some ground with eros as a fertility god.[27] Among the votive offerings preserved from the Asklepieion in ancient Corinth are images representing male genitalia as well as female breasts, ovaries, and uterus.[28] Physician Rachel Naomi Remen reminds medical students that Cicero describes a statue of Venus in the central courtyard of Asklepian temples, and the second-century Greek doctor Pausanias reports that the magnificent Asklepieion at Epidaurus included in its rotunda a picture of Eros.[29] Perhaps most significant: it is a physician, Eryximachus, who in Plato's *Symposium* proposes eros as the evening's sole topic. "It's from medicine, my own area of expertise," he says, "that I've realized how great and wonderful a god Love [*Eros*] is, and how his power extends to all aspects of human and divine life." The essence of medicine, Eryximachus instructs his fellow symposiasts, "is knowledge of the forms of bodily love [*somatos erotikon*]." It is Asklepios, "our ancestor," to whom he attributes the crucial discovery that "eros regulates the principles and processes of medicine." Medicine, Eryximachus declares, evoking its erotic lineage in a spasm of implicit self-regard, "is wholly governed by this god."[30]

The Resurgence of Medical Eros

"His erection startled me." This sentence opens a memoir-like essay by physician-poet Rafael Campo.[31] When he was a young intern in a San Francisco HIV/AIDS ward, one of his patients was a preoperative male-to-female transsexual, whom he calls Aurora. Aurora had advanced-stage disease, but their regular encounters concerned more than medical matters. Campo, then living as a closeted gay doctor, disapproved of Aurora's over-the-top colorful costumes, dazzling cosmetics, and kitschy seductions expressing an uninhibited, self-confident freedom. She liked to tease the straitlaced, somewhat puritanical, and monogamous gay intern with comments that hovered between pop psychotherapy and erotic play. "I know you're in there," Aurora teased Campo, safe behind his screen of medical duties, as he "mechanically" performed the examination, concealing his unease both with Aurora's promiscuous lifestyle and with his own erotic self-denials (*DH* 30). Aurora's erection that startled him called attention not only to the antisepsis of the hospital setting, where eros has no place, but also to his own sexual confusion.

Campo's visits with Aurora expose what he comes to regard as a mistaken view of medicine (the view he held as a young student) in which desire is the outlaw. "I began imagining myself as the model physician," he writes of this early self, "for whom desire was forbidden and in fact repellent" (*DH* 21). This medicalized rejection of desire, he decides, served as a convenient defense against his own growing sexual interest in men. The Hippocratic ideal of a physician who swears off "amorous acts" with patients—which seems a wise, rational, professional decision—fails to capture the mixed sense of loathing and of fascination implicit in Campo's earlier view of medical desire as both *forbidden* and *repellent*. His continuing medical education, thanks to Aurora, brought him face-to-face with the dilemma of his own sexual identity and with larger, related questions about the place of desire in medicine. His ultimate open self-affirmation as a gay Latino doctor (and poet) depended crucially on a recovery of desire. Desire, Campo acknowledges, is precisely what he had blocked both in his self-formation as a physician and in his own erotic life. Medical logos, in its sometimes wise rejection of desire, may also at times fail doctors as seriously as it fails patients. The turning point in Campo's transformation both as a doctor and as an openly gay man came through his daily, developing encounters with the flamboyant Aurora.

Desire, as the key to Campo's self-transformation, does not emerge without struggle. Aurora's comfort with eros initially frightened him, but even fear did not prevent Campo from valuing her vitality, excess, and sheer nerve. Nonetheless, he continued to ward off emotional awareness with the respectable talisman of medical professionalism: overwork and self-denial. "I was too busy," he explains, "to give much thought to what I had felt; my job was not to feel but to palpate" (*DH* 30). A doctor palpates by pressing on the patient's body in aid of diagnosis, but "feeling" implies an emotional engagement. Aurora, of course, was riding on an unstoppable trajectory toward death. Neither her campy, playful seductions nor the welcome visits of the young closeted intern could delay the relentless progress of HIV / AIDS. On one routine visit, which changed him forever, Campo arrived to find his patient almost immobile: "her face stripped of all her glittery makeup, expressing not recognition but a deeply subterranean pain." Frantically, in his role as physician, he listened to her heart and lungs. Whatever medical data he gathered through the stethoscope about possible blockages in respiration or blood flow did not register as primary. His own blockages were what he finally began to recognize: "I heard my own stifled desire surface for air in my long sobs" (*DH* 32).

Stifled desire is not a professional requirement in medicine. Medicine, however, if it does not *entirely* block or deny desire, redirects it toward sanctioned professional goals such as work, altruism, money, and power. These commonplace objects of desire seem so widely approved as to constitute almost desire-free self-evident goods, like air or water. It is as if our culture *already* desires such goods for us, automatically, so that (alienated from our own desire) we focus on rational, instrumental means to obtain whatever our culture desires us to desire. Campo's experience with Aurora, in its unwilled transgression of professional norms, unexpectedly affirmed his own direct, unalienated desire. It did not lead him to reject the Hippocratic abjuration of sexual contacts or amorous acts (*aphrodisionergon*). "Many doctors must fall in love with their patients," he speculates, "though far, far fewer would likely dare to admit it" (*DH* 25).

Admitting desire, however, differs from acting upon desire; admitting desire differs from stifling desire. The medical inadmission of eros, as Campo now sees, entails harmful self-denials and even self-betrayals—which extend, in his case, to the crippling disavowal of his own professional and personal identity as a gay doctor. It is this medical flight from desire that, as Aurora brought him to realize, limits or subverts his effectiveness as a physician.

Modern medicine, in its contact with the body, mostly serves an almost ascetic denial of desire. Doctors, as Campo put it, palpate rather than feel. My physician father liked to recall that the stethoscope originated in France in 1816 because its inventor, physician René Laennec, felt uncomfortable placing his ear (to listen to the lungs and heart) directly on a woman's breast.[32] Moreover, doctors are notoriously poor at self-care, which depends on feeling as well as on medical skill; my father burned out his body in the care of patients. It is medicine's intimate contact with the body during trauma and serious illness, paradoxically, that also allows Campo to make contact with his own feelings and desire—helping him give better care both to himself and to his patients. As his experience suggests, a medicine that deliberately ignores, denies, or stifles desire also implicitly disregards the fullest range of human function, including the emotional inner life of the body. Medical eros, if it believed in credos, would assert that desire matters. Desire matters—as a truth of the body and as a fact of the inner life—as much for doctors as for patients. The dangers always inseparable from desire are often less worrisome than the consequences that follow from a denial of desire.

Aurora died later the same day. It is worth paying attention to the bodily relation among sobs, breath, and desire as Campo listens to her chest. Eros calls inner life into play, as Bataille insists, but it is an inner life evoked in and through the body. The medical body, always more than a cultural construction, is understood as an intricate, interlaced, biological system of organs, fluids, heartbeats, and respiration. A neurobiology of electro-chemical flows and synapses underlies even such cerebral and culturally inflected desires as a longing for swimsuit models, fast cars, or luxury vacations. Campo describes Aurora's impact in a long, lyrical, penultimate paragraph where the memory of her qualities—qualities inseparable from her bodily life—now somehow enters into his own bodily life, almost as

easily and as invisibly as desire engages our thoughts and moves our feelings: "I find her voice in mine, like a lover's fingers running through my
hair; my voice sounds warmer, more comfortable to me now. I discover
her hands on my own body when I examine a person with cancer, or
AIDS, searching for the same familiar human landmarks that bespeak
physical longing and intimacy. Her glorious eyes return to me when I finally see someone for the first time" (*DH* 32). Seeing someone for the first
time, as physicians do on a regular basis, differs from, for the first time,
"finally" *seeing* someone. Desire for Campo is what allows him to recognize patients and to see himself in a way that far exceeds the norms of
professional knowledge. Desire is both what drew him to medicine and
what helped rescue him once he became a physician, as Aurora finds daily
presence in his altered voice and hands and eyes.

Virginia Woolf and Audre Lorde, writers separated by age, race, and
nationality, offer additional support for believing that the triumph of medical logos entails significant loss and that eros has a crucial place in the
medical encounter. Neither Woolf nor Lorde makes a claim for medical
eros, of course, at least not by name, but both recognize that biomedicine
has established its dominance largely through the work of physicians for
whom reason and science are regarded as the only appropriate tools. It is
hardly surprising, in retrospect, that two independent, creative women
in the role of patients feel at odds with the dominant medical system and
adopt strategies of resistance: resistance that Woolf expressed indirectly
in her writing through irony, metaphor, and misdirection, and that Lorde
expressed far more directly in a language of excess, transgression, and
defiance. They both stage a feminist or proto-feminist poetics of desire
in order to assert, finally, a healing role for eros in illness.

Audre Lorde in *The Cancer Journals* (1980) enters the arena of serious
illness equipped with a certainty about her sexual identity and an aggressive antagonism toward social and medical norms that differ markedly
from Campo's experience.[33] She describes herself in *The Cancer Journals*
as a black lesbian feminist poet, an identity that embraces multiple es-
trangements from mainstream American life. In contrast to Broyard's
ambiguous racial self-fashioning, Lorde celebrates her African heritage,
invoking as a personal mother-figure the South African creatrix Sebou-
lisa (*CJ* 11). Her experience of breast cancer, then, is inseparable from a

racial and sexual dissidence that extends to a political outlook familiar in the 1970s, much as Susan Sontag's opposition to military metaphors (as applied to illness) coincides with her opposition to the Vietnam War. Cancer, in threatening Lorde's health, that is, also threatens her identity as a black feminist writer. She actively opposes the silences, personal and social, surrounding breast cancer, much as the brash, hardline direct-action advocacy group ACT UP (an acronym for AIDS Coalition to Unleash Power) used aggressive guerilla-theater performances to give teeth to their slogan that "silence equals death." Lorde's impulse, when threatened, is to fight back. It is an unusual struggle nonetheless in which, especially through her open sexual embrace of other women, she discovers the creative power of eros to oppose the inherent destructiveness of illness.

Illness in its power for damage sets Lorde on a difficult journey in which eros proves crucial in the re-creation of personal identity. Breast cancer invisibly damages her sense of self as it visibly damages her body. While recovering from a mastectomy, she openly longs for a return to "*the old me*" (*CJ* 12). Like fellow writer Reynolds Price, however, she finds in cancer a turning point. Her only alternative to a loss so complete that it threatens to overwhelm both body and soul is a reinvention of the self. This self-transformation entails, if unevenly, erotic affirmations that lead to a hard-won sense of exhilaration, as if she has left an older, preliminary, unfinished self behind. There is soon no more talk of return to the *old me*. Rather, "*I feel like another woman*," she writes, "*de-chrysalised*" (*CJ* 14). Such glimpses of emergence and renewal later, however, prove problematic. Cancer can be a disease of wild swings, with its progressive natural history matched by a personal history of emotional change. At least for Audre Lorde, a new de-chrysalized self did not necessarily remain stable, much as eros does not guarantee a smooth, steady, or permanent self-transcendence.

Lorde's ultimate source of strength—far different from Reynolds Price's biblical inspiration to *choose life*—comes from her identification with a lineage of women warriors, the one-breasted Amazons. The Amazon warrior offers her a potent alter ego, damaged but undaunted, courageous in the face of enemies. Enemies, for Lorde, include medicalized social norms. A prosthesis, in covering up the result of a mastectomy, strikes her as no better than a lie. Many women will disagree, making different personal choices that do not reduce to a preference for lies. While Lorde's identification with one-breasted Amazon warriors adequately conveys her own militant stance, it cannot completely describe her strategies of resistance to cancer, which had to survive even intermittent episodes of soul-crushing despair.

The Cancer Journals, in its stop-and-go, diary-like, uneven journey through an ultimately fatal illness, nonetheless rounds at last toward a position in which the emergent figure with whom she identifies—never assigned a name or abstract specific character—might as well be eros. "Perhaps I can say this all more simply," Lorde sums up, as if done with the notorious changes and complications of illness: "I say the love of women healed me" (*CJ* 39). Lorde credits her recovery—the recovery of a whole new selfhood as much as her material healing—to an erotic force not only outside medical logos but also outside *any* system of containment. In describing her hospital stays, she frankly explains her need to masturbate, and she is equally candid about her sexual pleasures. She has no interest in a Christianized *caritas* or *agape* that might substitute compassion for pagan *eros*. She writes in an extended fugue about the emotional and erotic relations with the women who helped in her healing:

> Support will always have a special and vividly erotic set of image /
> meanings for me now, one of which is floating upon a sea within a ring
> of women like warm bubbles keeping me afloat upon the surface of
> that sea. I can feel the texture of inviting water just beneath their
> eyes, and do not fear it. It is the sweet smell of their breath and
> laughter and voices calling my name that gives me volition, helps me
> remember I want to turn away from looking down. These images
> flow quickly, the tangible floods of energy rolling off these women
> toward me that I converted into power to heal myself. (*CJ* 39)

Healing, of course, differs from cure, and healing is crucial especially when medical logos—as ultimately happened for Lorde—has run through and exhausted its repertoire of curative therapies.

Lorde died of cancer in 1992, a decade after *The Cancer Journals* first appeared, but her personal ring of support has since multiplied in women's centers, breast cancer clinics, and lesbian health initiatives, built upon an initial ideology of women caring for women, although women's health enlists professionals across the lines of gender. Eros still arouses distrust, of course, especially because, as Lorde says, "many of our best and most erotic words have been so cheapened" (*CJ* 39). Eros, uncheapened and rescued from silence, remains in her view a vital force for opposing illness. She stands with Anatole Broyard, Reynolds Price, and Rafael Campo as contemporary writers who see eros not as a panacea or substitute for biomedicine but as a crucial ally in the struggle against illness and against an implicit, willful, prevailing medical obliviousness to the powers of human desire.

Virginia Woolf in *On Being Ill*—published in 1926 as an essay and revised for book publication in 1930—wrote in the generation before Lorde, Broyard, Price, and Campo. Her endorsement of eros is less direct, but she is no less transgressive as she systematically reverses the established values associated with health and illness. Illness, for Woolf, alters how we experience the world and introduces us to an extravagant realm where ordinary rules no longer apply. Woolf, in fact, invents the ruling metaphor that Susan Sontag made famous—illness as *another country*—but unlike Sontag, who viewed illness as a biological condition fully reducible to the scientific knowledge of disease, Woolf describes illness as a radically alien psychic state, irreducible to biology and opening upon a strange landscape of excess, subversion, and unreason. Illness for Woolf resists all efforts to demystify it or to reduce it to medical knowledge; its otherness remains intrinsic and impenetrable. "The merest schoolgirl, when she falls in love, has Shakespeare or Keats to speak her mind for her," she observes in a celebrated passage, "but let a sufferer try to describe a pain in his head to a doctor, and language at once runs dry."[34]

Woolf set out to invest illness, in its resistance to language and in its absence from literary texts, with a new presence and a new language appropriate to its excess and uncanny otherness. Far from language running dry, the opening sentence in *On Being Ill* runs on for an extravagant, tour-de-force of *280 words*. *The Oxford Guide to Plain English* cites research indicating that the average English sentence contains nineteen words,[35] but plain English belongs to the world of health and reason and normal life. Illness, according to Woolf, transports us, far beyond reason, into an inherently excessive realm where ordinary language not only does not run dry but also, on occasion, overflows its banks in verbal transgressions that hold the power to expose all the illusions that underlie our everyday lives in conditions of so-called good health.

Woolf's multiple transgressions follow from her fundamental reversal that identifies illness as ultimate closeness to truth. Health, in her reversal of traditional values, emerges as a state of self-delusion, lies, and banalities. The truth of illness, in this transvaluation, lies in its absolute fidelity to the body and to its desires. For Woolf, the linguistic and conceptual systems that normally guide us through life in health are absent from illness. In their absence, illness confronts us with a familiar but newly estranged and even scandalous figure: the body ("this monster"). The body, grown monstrously present in illness, attains a material, immediate, sensual state utterly withdrawn from the meanings, including the medical meanings, that we usually superimpose on it. It is sheer presence alone, material and physical, always in withdrawal from ordinary life and its healthy pretenses. It relocates us in a flesh-centered state where mind and intellect cannot maintain a bogus dominance, where social abstractions such as duty and honor no longer rule, where the consoling illusions and self-deceptions that sustain us in health are exposed in their true and alarming insufficiency. Illness reintroduces us to the topsy-turvy tangible world of the body, where the ruling power (no matter how outrageous, excessive, nonsensical, and shamelessly pleasure-seeking) is now . . . desire.

Illness, in Woolf's subversive outlook, is firmly on the side of eros. Her new erotics of illness divides humankind into two opposing groups, whom she calls *the upright* and *the recumbent. The upright* (healthy but deceived) go to work, build cities, establish empires, wield power, and define orthodox values: a patriarchal, imperial enterprise that Woolf depicts as steeped in self-deception and illusion. Meanwhile *the recumbent* (enlightened by illness) abstain from patriarchy and power. Not surprisingly, given the gender inequalities built into the social system of Woolf's generation, the recumbent class is overrepresented by women, while the upright, healthy, self-deceived movers and shakers are, of course, mainly men.

The bedridden invalid (Woolf's female figure for illness) gains a decisive advantage in her alienation from masculine reason and power: direct contact with unalienated desire and unmediated access to truth. Illness, in effect, introduces the invalid to life naked, raw, blunt, true, and undefended by sentimental pieties. It confers a shocking irreverence: "There is, let us confess it (and illness is the great confessional), a childish outspokenness in illness; things are said, truths blurted out, which the cautious respectability of health conceals." One instance? "About sympathy for example—we can do without it" (*OBI* 11). Albert Camus would make bleak truth-telling a mark of the existential hero, but for Woolf truth-telling is not heroic, and heroism is one more masculine illusion, which she deflates by calling it as hollow as "the heroism of the ant or the bee" (*OBI* 16). From the disillusioned perspective of illness, even sympathy is a form of spurious feeling that the upright, healthy, male world overvalues precisely so it can be relegated to women: soft, weak, emotional, but, like piano lessons, an acceptable female accompaniment for masculine power and reason. Woolf's invalid sees through the gender-driven ruse of sympathy and of daily life, which she wholly rejects in favor of the body-centered truths of desire. Desire is what the invalid prefers to reason, and desire is what drives her into the outlaw realms of poetry and of love.

Illness thrusts the recumbent invalid ("outlaws that we are" [*OBI* 22]) into a territory where desire validates various forms of erotic transgression. The ill, in place of everyday prose statements, seek a new discourse—"more primitive, more sensual, more obscene" (*OBI* 7)—open to unstable ironies and to violations of syntactic rules. Much like Woolf's transgressive opening sentence. The outlaw reign of desire, for example, prefers poetry and stories, which skirt the hoary, male dictum that writers hold a mirror up to nature. The imitation of nature, from the perspective of illness, is simply another regulation, sent down from the office of health, while illness is life lived in full feeling with "the police off duty" (*OBI* 21). Stories and poems, for the recumbent, not only break the rules but also do no work. They transport us, like illness itself, to another country, an erotic refuge of the inner life, where the recumbent citizens are free from obsessions with reason, order, and linear, prosaic statements of what the upright patriarchs call fact. Even worse: in their link with eros and desire, stories and poems claim as their entire justification, if any justification mattered, a wholehearted pursuit of pleasure.

Eros appears in Woolf's essay mainly by indirection, which may be the only way it *could* appear, given her radical views of illness and her reluctance to engage in personal confession. *On Being Ill*, for example, omits any mention of her erotic feelings for Vita Sackville-West. Love and eros, however, obliquely govern her conclusion, which mirrors in its run-on final sentence the extravagant length of her opening sentence. The outlaw-ill in their choice of books, she asserts, reject Shakespeare for Augustus Hare. Augustus *Who?* Woolf's strange choice—Hare over Shakespeare—is doubtless meant to scandalize serious readers, such as the ultra-serious editor (T. S. Eliot) who solicited her essay. Augustus John Cuthbert Hare (1834–1903) wrote numerous biographies and historical accounts of British upper-class life, not omitting castle ghosts, and Woolf's conclusion proceeds, Hare-like, with the extended synopsis of an outdated novel about the upper-crust world of a fictive Lady Waterford. Hare, unlike Shakespeare, is pure escapist reading. Illness, however, has no tolerance for the high seriousness of Matthew Arnold, and a taste for escapist fiction simply reinforces the fundamental importance of pleasure.

Pleasure, as Woolf implies, holds an indirect but powerful relation to eros. Her long synopsis of the Hare-like foolish novel thus closes as Lady Waterford suddenly learns that her (numbskull) husband has died while, of course, out fox hunting. All at once, everything changes. The aristocratic world of Lady Waterford has schooled her in manners and in the public denial of unladylike feelings. Eros, however, finds a way to infiltrate and subvert even well-schooled, foolish norms. Woolf's excessive final sentence thus concludes with a telltale sign that eros (marking the body and its uncontainable feelings) survives even our most well-mannered efforts to regulate it. Publicly unbroken and with the dignity required of an upper-class woman who must stifle desire, Lady Waterford receives the news of her husband's sudden death as she stands beside a velvet curtain, which she holds with one hand and—in an almost imperceptible sign of raw emotion—silently *crushes*.

Illness and trauma for Woolf have everything to do with eros and desire. As she writes somewhat cryptically, illness "often takes on the disguise of love" (*OBI* 6). She means, I think, that lovers (like invalids) must often dissemble in order to maintain the truths of desire. Desire in its excess cannot always, in the social world constructed by health, take the form of outward public display. It must assume a disguise in order to live out the body's forbidden truths. It is the inexpressible presence of the body both as a sign of desire and as a conduit to the mysteries of the inner life of consciousness, beyond all rational knowledge or social codes, that for Woolf bonds illness inseparably with eros. Lady Waterford, even in upholding the expectations of a perverse and confining social code, offers an indirect tribute to how eros nonetheless holds a power to draw us beyond disguises, beyond what is seen and done, beyond what is said, and even beyond what is left unsaid—into alien, inaccessible regions of the unknown and the unsayable.

A New Philosophy of Medical Knowledge?

"We need nothing less than a new philosophy of medical knowledge," writes Richard Horton, editor of the distinguished British medical journal *The Lancet*. He specifically laments "a schism" in the understanding of illness that divides patient from doctor.[36] This doctor/patient schism in understanding, if he is correct, doubtless involves multiple causes and has no quick fix. One resolution, however, might lie in a twenty-first century medicine that addresses and corrects the historical, epistemological erasure of Asklepios. It might lie in openly acknowledging the legitimate claims of eros and its link to the inner life. Is a new philosophy of medicine possible that recognizes the legitimate claims of *both* Hippocrates and Asklepios? Perhaps it will take patients to supply the momentum for change, in insisting that medical logos and medical eros are not binary opposites, doomed to eternal conflict, but rather productive (or at least potentially productive and forward-looking) contraries.

The signs of a schism are evident. Doctors, on the side of medical logos, simply do not have a vocabulary or structure in which to value medical eros, while patients too often simply internalize the values and beliefs that they associate with biomedicine. A new and nonschismatic philosophy of medical knowledge needs to place biomedicine with its invaluable Hippocratic legacy into dialogue with Asklepian medicine and its erotic heritage. It is not necessary to imagine a merger, amalgamation, or sham equality. Rather, each tradition with its built-in incompleteness requires the other as a supplement and ally. Each tradition has distinctive virtues, virtues called for perhaps at different moments and in different degrees during the extended, changing course of illness. Partnership as contraries, however, implies principles that do not reproduce the mutual exclusion of logical opposites. Medical eros and medical logos, understood in partnership as mutually supportive contraries, offer together a pragmatic, if not strictly philosophical, platform from which to address the schisms separating doctor and patient. Together, they let us understand illness as both a biological and a cultural phenomenon, a condition that involves desire as well as genes, that involves the inner life as well as the life of the body—twin crucial elements of our well-being, like rain and sunshine.[37]

A new philosophy of medical knowledge, if it can imagine a partnership or dialogue of contraries, must also expand its concept of knowledge. Scientific, empirical, statistical knowledge does not exhaust the relevant range of knowing. Physician Rita Charon, as we will see, makes a strong case for a necessary complement to logico-scientific understanding. She calls this complement "narrative knowledge," and such narrative knowledge could well include an awareness of the dynamics of desire, especially as desire plays out not only on the patient side of the bed but also among physicians, where (as for Rafael Campo) it might take the inverse form of a well-schooled stifled desire, or desire deflected and misdirected. D. H. Lawrence, for example, writes a poetic goodbye to his "scientific doctor" upon realizing "what a lust there was" in the doctor "to wreak his so-called science on me."[38] Surgeon Richard Selzer, a generation later, offers a similar reading of desire misdirected. The great writing about doctors, he asserts, will be done only by a doctor "who is through with the love affair with his technique, who recognizes that he has played Narcissus, raining kisses on a mirror."[39] Narcissus, of course, never recognizes that he is the victim of his own erotic self-absorption.

There are grounds for hope that a new philosophy of medicine, or a pragmatic alternative to medical logos, is beginning to take hold. One sign is a new interest by the medical establishment in Asklepios. Various organizations within medicine, including the American Medical Association (AMA), had for years adopted as their defining symbol the classical *caduceus* or winged staff of Hermes. Hermes, however, had no mythological connection with medicine: his staff (with its two coiled serpents) was

likely confused with the rod of Asklepios, who also held a close association with snakes, although usually only one snake appears coiled on his
trademark rod. The editors of *The Oxford Illustrated Companion to Medicine* (2001), after weighing the claims of Hermes and of Asklepios,
decided that the staff and serpent of Asklepios have "the more ancient
and authentic claim to be the emblem of medicine."[40] In 2005, the
AMA introduced a stylized new logo, and the official announcement
describes its new emblem as "more than just a visually pleasing take on
the Staff of Asklepios." What, specifically, is this vague *more*? The new
AMA symbol, as the announcement continues, represents "many things
that are good about the profession and its organization, not the least of
which is continuity." Then comes the truly groundbreaking clarification.
In an assertion of continuity with its Asklepian founder, the new logo
makes "a statement about the transformation of the AMA" and about
changes required in a *"medicine for the 21st century."*[41]

A new medicine for the twenty-first century—which the AMA announcement invokes but does not describe—needs to take a solid stand
for medical pluralism. It must also be willing to take practical steps in the
direction that such a pluralistic partnership implies in pairing Hippocratic
and Asklepian contraries. It has to address the desires and the not-
knowing that so often accompany serious illness. Jennifer Glaser was
just twenty-four years old when her boyfriend was diagnosed with leukemia. "Cancer works very hard to make life unsexy," she recalls in a brief
memoir published in the *New York Times*.[42] Desire plays an increasingly
crucial role in proportion as medical knowledge has less to offer. "We
flirted, canoodled, talked about sex, and had sex when he was sick
because, well, sex wasn't death," she writes. "It was the antithesis of
death." A new twenty-first-century plural medicine must also find explicit
space for the uncertainties—the not-knowing—that desire and illness entail. Whatever such a twenty-first-century medicine comes to be, it needs
to reject both the obsolete positivist narrative in which rationalist Hippocrates supplants the dream-god Asklepios and also the supporting biomedical ideology (really a form of narrative) in which logico-scientific
knowledge is the sole, unquestioned, highest good in the pantheon of
values that biomedicine has the power to establish and to revise. It needs

to consider, above all, how the experience of illness and the practice of medicine almost inescapably coincide with eros, and how eros in conjunction with illness transports us into an uncanny nightside realm, where the inner life is preoccupied by desire and where the single almost guaranteed experience is the experience of not-knowing.

CHAPTER THREE

Not-Knowing: Medicine
in the Dark

I am obliged to perform in complete darkness
operations of great delicacy
on my self.
—*Mr Bones, you terrifies me.*

JOHN BERRYMAN, *77 DREAM SONGS* (1964)

*E*ROS, IN ADDITION to his shape-shifting powers, no doubt speaks perfect French. Writer, Jungian analyst, and activist Florida Scott-Maxwell recalls a telling episode as she traveled in France before the First World War. As she explains: "when the train stopped a middle-aged woman entered the compartment accompanied by a distraught-looking girl of perhaps seventeen who held a handkerchief to her eyes. The woman announced quietly but gravely and dramatically, '*C'est l'amour.*' At once the five or six other passengers rearranged themselves, leaving one side of the compartment vacant. The young girl laid herself down at full length, her head in her mother's lap, a cloak over her, and softly sobbed herself to sleep. The other passengers sat crowded in silent respect. A god had struck, and it was best to be wary."[1] It is not just the young who are vulnerable to eros. Scott-Maxwell wrote her memoir in old age during what she described as her surprisingly "passionate" eighties. Eros can lead almost anyone into passions that border on illness and even risk death. Americans over age fifty-five accounted for 5 percent of new HIV/AIDS infections in 2010 and constituted almost 20 percent of the people then living with HIV infection in the U.S.[2] Scott-Maxwell is right: best to be wary.

Eros is dangerous especially because the inner life of desire is intertwined with biology, including the biology of illness. Even prairie voles, whose inner life remains unknown, are at risk. A female prairie vole (the monogamous prairie vole *Microtus ochrogaster*, in particular) shows rapid attachment to the nearest male when scientists infuse her brain with the hormone oxytocin, which interacts with the same circuitry that in humans produces both euphoria and addiction.[3] Affective connections are equally powerful in humans. The risk of a heart attack on the anniversary of a bereavement is twenty-one times higher than normal. The risk of illness and altered biochemistry seem closely entangled with eros, although we manage to fall in and out of love (for the most part) minus trips to the emergency room. Nonetheless, brain scans show that love or romantic feelings activate cortical and subcortical circuits associated with motivation, reward, and addiction, much as romantic rejection triggers circuits associated with a craving for cocaine. In one study, the mere picture of a loved one reduced moderate pain in viewers by 40 percent.[4] Perhaps such processes with their underlying neural networks contribute indirectly to the appeal of pop music, with its insatiable appetite for lyrics that never manage to get to the bottom of love. The complex, interconnected biological and cultural systems involved in love mean that eros, like an apparently bottomless ocean or rift, confronts us with far more than we can understand.

Eros, even simplified as romantic love, plunges us into a condition of not-knowing that is not necessarily debilitating: we don't need to know exactly what love is to experience its power. Isn't love, asks the cultural theorist and psychoanalyst Slavoj Žižek, the supreme instance of "an enigmatic term"? *An unknowable X?*[5] Serious illness too involves an unknowable X. The enigmatic inner life of illness cannot easily be disentangled from its biological correlates, but neither can it be fully contained or explained as a phenomenon of bodies. Eros and illness at times share a common language. "At mere sight of you," writes Sappho in her famous ode 31, "my voice falters, my tongue / is broken. / Straightaway a delicate fire runs in / my limbs; my eyes / are blinded / and my ears / thunder."[6] The lover, inflamed, goes almost instantly deaf, dumb, and blind. Trusted senses betray us. Metaphors brush dangerously close to actualities. It is a state that the ill, like the lover, may experience as truly death-like. "I grow / paler than grass," as Sappho's final line confesses, "and lack little / of dying."[7] Eros and illness, not only in their brush with death, hold a power to induct us into the ultimate, enigmatic presence of not-knowing.

Not-Knowing and the Myth of Medical Knowledge

Suppose you are seriously ill. What do you most urgently need or desire? What can't you do without? I would want the best contemporary clinical knowledge—in short, medical logos. In valuing the best clinical knowledge, however, I would make a serious mistake to undervalue medical eros and the complexities (including possibilities for healing) associated with not-knowing. "I won't know for a while what treatment, if any, I'll need next," as I recall my friend Gail Lauzzana e-mailed after her breast cancer diagnosis. "Another period of waiting to find out. Well, it's a good lesson, to live with the unknown." Serious illness, her words suggest, almost requires patients to live in a protracted state of not-knowing.

Knowledge in medicine is the sovereign power. King Data rules. Knowledge rolls into one massive ruling principle the medical equivalent of state, monarch, constitution, imperium, and social contract. It is what confers legitimacy upon doctors and upon the diverse group of health professionals (from nurses to clinical psychologists) for whom doctors here stand as surrogate. The implicit authority of modern biomedical knowledge in effect backs up the physician like a reserve battalion. A practice or claim in biomedicine *without* knowledge behind it simply has no standing. The sovereignty of knowledge in medicine, however, may also serve as a reassuring myth erected by patients as much as by doctors. If we shadowed a physician through a normal workday, we'd likely observe hunches, jokes, missteps, empathic smiles, bursts of anger, fatigue, frustration, and multiple gestures—winks, hugs, handshakes, scrub-downs—where knowledge is secondary.

Like the distinctive type of knowledge that the ancient Greeks called *phronesis*, or "practical reason," clinical knowledge often bears less resemblance to laboratory science than to old-fashioned, trial-and-error, check-the-landmarks navigation.[8] Still, the mythic sovereignty of knowledge in medicine shapes not only the institutional delivery of medical care (which drives fully one-eighth of the U.S. economy) but also the implicit self-understanding of doctors and of doctor-educated patients. Surgeon and writer Atul Gawande distills the myth into a statement of everyday life in modern medicine when he explains, from his insider position, that doctors tend to have "a fierce commitment to the rational." If there is a credo in practical medicine, he writes, apparently believing that there is, it attributes prime importance to what is "sensible."[9]

Straw-man or mythic images of biomedicine as "all knowledge, all the time" do not acknowledge the pragmatic suppleness of individual physicians moving through a normal day, varying treatment options, for example, to suit what they sense or know about individual patients. In their books identically titled *How Doctors Think*, scholar Kathryn Montgomery and physician Jerome Groopman describe everyday medical practice as punctuated throughout by tentative judgments, by practical choices, and by the encounter with inescapable uncertainties.[10] Trial and error, in controlled settings, are basic to empirical knowledge. Nonetheless, biomedicine includes a built-in drive to reduce risk, to generate sensible options, and to circumscribe uncertainties in the pursuit of knowledge. Computers now provide automated estimates of risk factors adjusted by age, gender, race, and family history. Knowledge as a goal and achievement is already inscribed in the most basic terms of medical language: *diagnosis* and *prognosis* both derive from the Greek root *gnosis*— meaning knowledge.

Most patients wouldn't have it any other way. *You're the doctor.* This clichéd expression of deference does more than state the obvious; it reflects a patient's implicit belief in the superiority of medical knowledge. Even the cautious desire for a second opinion, as patients begin to understand their new role as medical consumers, does not destroy a trust in medicine as a body of knowledge. Patients still seek whatever opinion they consider the most knowledgeable. Doctors, meanwhile, have strong incentives to embrace the ever-expanding biomedical database, including a knowledge of the newest technologies, because professional respect, board certification, and hospital privileges are among the valuable byproducts of knowledge. Anatole Broyard evidently liked knowing that his urologist ranked as a "superstar." (His urologist was so famous and superior, Broyard claimed, that he barely spoke to his patients.) Biomedicine, as embodied in particular patients and doctors, values knowledge so highly that it seems almost quixotic to make a case for not-knowing. Medical eros, however, requires that we question not only the sovereignty of biomedical knowledge but also the neglected and devalued state of not-knowing. "It's only human to want to know more, and then more, and then more," says the narrator in Don DeLillo's novel *Zero K* (2016), which describes a secret compound where human bodies are preserved until futuristic biomedical technologies can return them to health. "But it's also true that what we don't know is what makes us human. And there's no end to not-knowing."[11]

Not-knowing, as we enter into the nightside of life, is both so inescapable and so native to the experience of illness that we tend to take it for granted, since physicians and patients usually share the common goal of removing medical uncertainties and replacing them with knowledge. Illness shares with eros the unsettling power to draw doctors, nurses, patients, caregivers, friends, and family into a state of less than perfect clarity. The not-knowing native to illness, however, no matter how temporary, not only remains distinct from ignorance but also holds a respected status in the psychology of cognition and of creative discovery. Montaigne gave the skeptical question *what do I know?* a philosophical turn in which reason doubts both received authorities and its own operations. *Negative capability* is a term that medical student and poet John Keats invented to describe the fundamental artistic need to entertain uncertainties, mysteries, and doubts without an "irritable reaching after fact & reason."[12] Donald Barthelme, a master of modern short fiction, defines the writer as "one who, embarking upon a task, does not know what to do."[13] A hospital emergency department, of course, cannot afford the luxury of philosophical skepticism or of endless poetic deliberation; not-knowing in a medical crisis (where inaction risks death) must give way to action. Yet, even *surplus* medical knowledge, as in the pharmacopeia of competing drugs, can thrust doctors and patients, full force, into the dim, uncertain twilight of not-knowing.

Medicine in its commitment to the production of knowledge (knowledge that it continually revises and updates) often gives little thought and less respect to not-knowing, even when not-knowing is part of the journey that leads toward new knowledge. (Willful, know-nothing ignorance is simply malpractice in any endeavor.) Not-knowing as a state quite familiar to patients as well as to doctors, even if less talked about, frequently bears little relation to the production of knowledge. Illness, like the 41 percent of the moon's surface not visible from planet Earth, has its own intrinsic *dark side*: mysteries of inner life that no Luna-3 mindcraft is likely to map with certainty. This mode of not-knowing—as basic to the experience of serious illness as it is to the erotic—may not produce distress; it can simply imply a respectful openness to incomplete understanding. Unlike systems of knowledge or reasoned analysis, it acknowledges a human desire to encounter what lies just beyond the limits of human knowledge. Eros, after all, regularly plunges off the deep end. It sees little more than comic futility in reason-based lists of a lover's good qualities and bad qualities.

Paul Kalanithi, a talented neurosurgeon, was diagnosed at age thirty-six with stage IV lung cancer. His remarkable memoir *When Breath Becomes Air* (2016), written during what he knew was an illness that he would not survive, describes both his chosen medical journey to become a doctor and his subsequent unchosen medical journey as a patient. He writes with deep respect for the science-based biomedical knowledge basic to his profession, but he understands too the limits of such knowledge and the importance of human affiliations that extend beyond the natural histories of disease. It is his wife, Lucy Kalanithi, who writes the epilogue to his unfinished book, explaining that he died surrounded by family in a hospital bed close to the labor and delivery ward where their daughter, Cady, had been born eight months earlier. "Science may provide the most useful way to organize empirical, reproducible data," Paul Kalanithi writes in a measured tone that fully appreciates both the accomplishments and the paradoxes of medical logos, "but its power to do so is predicated on its inability to grasp the most central aspects of human life: hope, fear, love, hate, beauty, envy, honor, weakness, striving, suffering, virtue."[14]

Illness, for doctors as well as patients, may always include an immersion in doubt, uncertainties, ambiguities, and imperfect knowledge. Not-knowing also often encompasses the patient's and the caregiver's crisis-born state—sometimes protracted until it feels like a native land—of *being at a loss*: without bearings, disoriented, barely standing, all systems crashed. Paul Kalanithi repeats in his mind Samuel Beckett's weary self-contradiction (a tacit clip of inner life that I, too, silently recited like a caregiver's mantra) "I can't go on. I'll go on." Illogic and self-contradiction are among the disconcerting veracities that belong to the lived experience of illness, where scientific reason and empirical data—despite their formidable powers—reach the outer limits of what they can tell us and of what we can know. It is nonetheless these exact same powers that are now redefining a new age of biomedicine.

Medical Logos and the Molecular Gaze

"A threshold has been crossed," writes Nikolas Rose, director of the BIOS Centre for the Study of Bioscience, Biomedicine, Biotechnology and Society at the London School of Economics. The particular threshold he refers to is what he calls "a molecular vision of life."[15] Medical logos—marked by its double-blind studies, peer-reviewed journals, grant agencies, statistical probabilities, scientific methods, laboratory analysis, and rational argument—certainly bases its power on the production of new knowledge, as opposed to the unruly, indefinite, emotion-rich erotic desires basic to not-knowing. Medical logos places us within an era when biomedicine (as the institutional practice of a molecular vision of life) holds power over human affairs comparable only to the role of theology in the Middle Ages. Unprecedented advances now mesh humans with machines and with altered forms of life (from the genetically modified livestock we consume to body parts manufactured from stem cells), propelling us rapidly into a cyborg era that some call *post-human*.[16] Eros too has shifted shape to keep up with the molecular vision. In 1954, the first human experiments using oral progesterone gave birth to a breakthrough female contraceptive; the Pill in effect helped launch the sexual, cultural, and political revolutions of the 1960s, with which it is inseparable. New pills have continued to alter erotic relations, as Viagra and its ilk initiate molecular-level changes rippling across sociosexual boundaries from Idaho to Iraq.

All is not well, however, in the brave new world of the molecular vision. Eros too seems to be staggering in the porn-on-demand era of virtual sex. Medical logos, despite its unparalleled institutional power and its new threshold-crossing alliances with biotechnology, nuclear medicine, and genetic therapies, faces serious and mounting discontent. "Wherever I lectured," writes surgeon and medical educator Lori Arviso Alvord, "people would come up to me afterward and tell me stories of their impersonal treatment by doctors, of problems getting appropriate treatment through managed care programs, and of doctors or hospital staff who had treated them insensitively. They felt powerless, often miserable inside hospitals, stripped of their dignity."[17] Alvord, who belongs to the Navajo nation, knows firsthand the costs incurred when people are stripped of their dignity. Western medicine, as historians have shown, served imperial powers in the nineteenth century as an instrument useful in delegitimizing native systems and in consolidating their hold over colonized populations. The molecular vision of life, in addition to its economic costs, may have human costs in colonizing patients that we do not yet anticipate.

Contemporary doctors such as Alvord now lend their voices to a growing rumble of discontent. "A crop of books by disillusioned physicians reveals a corrosive doctor-patient relationship at the heart of our health-care crisis." So claims a sobering 2014 review article in *The Atlantic* magazine.[18] Physicians in the daily practice of medicine encounter demands from senior associates, government bureaucracies, insurance carriers, hospital administrators, and attorneys, to name a few, while individual doctors also often work under pressure to generate specific levels of income for departments or for group practices. Medical salaries higher than the national average apparently do not ensure satisfaction, professional or personal. Physicians as a group experience high rates of burnout, alcoholism, and suicide, with the highest suicide risk awaiting women physicians.[19] "Physicians would tell me that they wanted doctoring to go back to the old ways, when they were known and trusted by their communities and families," Alvord writes. "They complained of health care systems that require them to see a new patient every fifteen minutes."[20] Of course, the old ways cannot survive unaltered in the age of the molecular gaze. All professions adapt to change. Rapid advances in biotechnology, however, while they have increased the speed and efficiency of medical procedures and have vastly improved the management of illness, seem to entail significant losses. Clearly, something has gone wrong in the high-speed, digital arena of medical knowledge.

The molecular vision of life is no doubt partly to blame. New medical technologies, while they increase access to information and speed up care, perhaps encourage unrealistic or false expectations that doctors will be as efficient and systematic as their machines, but—with the possible exception of Andy Warhol, who wished that he could *be* a machine—most patients and doctors resist assumptions that appear to reduce them to the status of biological clockwork. Medical eros would make the additional point that molecular biology, even when fully integrated into the flexible daily practice of medicine, does not preclude a more inclusive vision open to the inner life and to the mysteries of not-knowing. Much about illness and desire, in truth, remains unknown. The molecular gaze, uncoupled from reductive or narrowly scientific concepts of knowledge, holds at least one solid advantage for medical eros in demonstrating that the ancient division between reason and emotion—a split unfortunately reproduced in the biomedical flight from eros—is a longstanding neurological mistake.

The time-honored binary opposition between reason and emotion simply cannot survive research in cognitive neuroscience, which has shown how the processes involved in feeling come to interpenetrate the processes of reasoning—and vice versa—via complex feedback loops and neural networks.[21] Emotion and reason, while sometimes at odds, are also often mutually supportive, rarely proceeding in absolute separation. Rational thought, as we will encounter later in discussing pain, is far more fluid as a biological endowment than we see represented in analytic calculations or in logical systems; it is open to modifying input from the senses and the emotions. Feeling and emotion, in turn, are far from frenzied passions untethered from other modes of cognition.

Biomedicine certainly has every right to uphold its chosen standards of validity, and evidence-based medicine is a practice that most patients applaud. A molecular vision of life, however, crosses only a single threshold. Medical eros identifies an adjacent and connected threshold—not yet crossed—that leads forward into a twenty-first-century medicine that validates erotic dimensions for which the biomedical evidence is already strong. Medical logos and the molecular gaze may well remain fixed in a commitment to evidence-based knowledge, but medical eros reminds us that illness has its inherent dark side that resists microscopic mapping and rational knowledge. Illness, even in the era of the molecular gaze, places us in a world still shadowed by desire, where hope, fear, love, hate, beauty, envy, honor, weakness, striving, suffering, and virtue still interrupt the orderly progress of biomedical knowledge with their unpredictable erotics of not-knowing.

Medical Eros and the Fruitful Darkness

The worst error in a narrative that describes medical eros and medical logos as potentially productive contraries would be an endorsement of the Hollywood tradition in which the heart, after numerous tribulations, finally triumphs over the head. Medical eros refers to complex powers of desire originating deep in the brain, some hardwired in autonomic responses swifter than reason, but also recruiting complex experiences of *la vie intérieure* inseparable from the modifying forces of culture. These experiences invoke not only conscious modes of reflection but also experience-based, nonconscious emotional responses that are sometimes eye-blink fast or as involuntary as a bad habit.[22] Medical logos refers to a similarly complex set of cerebral processes that we cannot shrink down to a one-word noun, reason, the remnant of old-fashioned faculty psychology. Reasoning is a highly evolved, complex function receiving input from multiple brain systems and processing varied sensory data, as it seeks to understand experiences that range from the philosophy of Heidegger to night baseball. Even the vaunted credo of practical medicine ("a fierce commitment to the rational") contains a mild paradox in that *fierceness* must reflect an emotional engagement. *"Why so fierce, doctor?"* The road through medical school is long, hard, and paved with examinations. The desire to heal, however, as Rafael Campo insists, does not describe a state arrived at through a process of analytical reason.

Medical eros embraces *not-knowing* as an acknowledgment that illness evokes a matrix of nightside experiences that bear no relation to analytical calculation, logical deduction, or the processes of rational thought. This matrix takes darkness as its representative state. Darkness, of course, belongs to a venerable philosophical and religious tradition in which it signifies an absence of reason and a withdrawal from God. Historian A. Roger Ekirch in *At Day's Close: Night in Times Past* (2006) describes how numerous ancient civilizations represent darkness as a demon-filled source of evil: a trope for everything malevolent and fearsome. Light, in biblical and Christian traditions, represents Reason and God, which therefore means that Desire and the Devil must reside in Darkness. In Milton's *Paradise Lost*, Lucifer, the rebel angel (whose name means bearer of light) is cast out of Heaven and finally comes to rest (renamed Satan) on the garish, burning lake of Hell, a surreal inferno lit only by "darkness visible."[23] The punishments of Hell include darkness so fiendish that the Heaven-deprived souls have just enough illumination to recognize the pitch-black medium of their torment. The demonology and iniquity associated with darkness, however, tell only half the story. Gloom, graveyards, and gothic terror can also lay claim to their own historical and psychic attractions.

Traditional underworlds do not monopolize the meanings associated with darkness. Darkness as a matrix of productive forces and as a seedbed of creative not-knowing maintains associations with wisdom, awakening, and spiritual growth not only among traditional mystics (who make divine contact within the cloud of unknowing) but also among many indigenous peoples. Anthropologists report that such darkness constitutes a necessary access to primal forces: forces within the earth, within the community, within the self. This primal, creative darkness, so easily lost in the neon dazzle of modern life, continues to provide a rich resource for certain contemporary artists and counterculture traditions. Darkness, like the mysteries often attributed to religious faith, holds a power to draw its adherents toward nourishing, productive states in which not-knowing— at least in a temporary, restorative interval—proves as important as knowledge.

"We need the terrain of the half-solved, the half-solvable riddle, the distance between knowing and not knowing, and being aware of our own limits of understanding," writes South African artist William Kentridge.[24] Joan Halifax—Zen Buddhist, anthropologist, ecologist, social activist, and thanatologist—embodies a similar spirit of openness to experiences defined by their distance from what is solved or recognized or illuminated by reason. She is perhaps best known in certain medical circles as the founding director of the Upaya Zen Center in Santa Fe, which offers a groundbreaking program entitled "Being with the Dying." Light is not always what is most needed; a lifelong searcher after the wisdom that Western traditions of reason tend to miss or ignore, Halifax titles her book of autobiographical reflections *The Fruitful Darkness* (1993).

Medical eros would recognize in not-knowing a fertile or fruitful darkness that differs profoundly from the deprivation of reason and the absence of light. No one—at least no one I've met—wants a medicine of irrational quirks and whimsy. Medical eros, however, as a supplement and contrary to medical logos, can helpfully explore approaches that open access to the patient's full experience, especially to experience of the inner life and to the forces of desire that reason cannot fully monitor or control. The nightside of life plunges patients and doctors both into an experience that cannot eliminate darkness, ambiguities, uncertainties, contradictions, paradoxes, and impasse. Some patients will express a desire *not* to know the results of genetic testing that might indicate a predisposition to or even firm likelihood of (at some undetermined time) terminal illness. Not-knowing, in such cases, includes ethical—not merely cognitive—dimensions.

Medical eros, in its partnership role, can even draw support from the findings of medical logos that offer evidence for believing that darkness embodies positive, creative powers. Literal darkness appears to stimulate or foster inventive cognitive responsiveness, a result analogous to the creative possibilities that Joan Halifax and William Kentridge find in not-knowing. The *Journal of Environmental Psychology* in 2013 published a study demonstrating that a measurable diminution of light, at least under the controlled conditions of a scientific experiment, contributes to creative thought.[25] The authors recruited participants who were instructed to sit alone in a small room designed to simulate an office. A single bulb provided adjustable levels of light, from dim to bright. Participants in the dimly lit room solved significantly more assigned cognitive tasks than participants in brightly lit or normally lit rooms. Dim light, the researchers concluded, with perhaps a small creative leap of their own, "improves creative performance." Oddly, the correlation between darkness and creativity extends even to *thinking* about darkness: thoughts about the dark also measurably improve performance. Medical eros, in its attachment to not-knowing, doubtless suspected as much: What experienced lover would fail to dim the lights?

Not-knowing obviously cannot stand as a complete or valid description of what we expect of doctors. Medieval mystics found spiritual nourishment when enveloped in a cloud of unknowing, but surgeons cannot perform their work properly without a bank of intense lights. Nobody wants a doctor for whom the creative possibilities of not-knowing mean blowing off appointments, ignoring laboratory reports, and simply winging it. Patients, family members, and anyone who enters into the life-changing experience of serious illness will nonetheless likely recognize not-knowing as their new native territory, and they won't necessarily like it.

Patienthood can place formerly self-reliant adults in a position of relative dependence or even childlike helplessness. (Whoever designed butt-baring hospital gowns surely meant them as instruments of humiliation.) The darkness of not-knowing has both fruitful and frustrating dimensions, but it nonetheless helps define the situation from which the patient speaks. This situation is a space of partial understanding, gaps and fragments, even outright incomprehension, especially in the case of immigrant patients when translators are either unavailable or untrustworthy. Medical eros, at this intersection of the familiar and the not-known, is poised to make a valuable contribution. While medical logos is absorbed in the molecular gaze, medical eros can turn its attention elsewhere and enlist the sensory mode that biomedicine is regularly criticized for neglecting: the sense of hearing. There is much of value to learn from paying special attention to the *voices* of medicine: the patient's voice, the doctor's voice, and the interpenetrating cultural and personal discourses that shape our speech in implicit dialogue with the surrounding voices.

The Patient's Voice(s)

"He doesn't speak our language."[26] Perri Klass as an American medical student in India offers what she thinks is helpful information to the English-speaking Hindi attending physician. They are discussing an Indian father who has been tending his dying tubercular son, and their discussion concerns when to stop all drug therapies in what is, medically speaking, a lost cause. The father, as it turns out, perfectly understands the speech of the Hindi doctor—but not the doctor's medical point of view. The language of medicine, Klass brings us to understand, includes the values and attitudes of a professional subculture that often stand in asymmetrical relation to the values and attitudes of the patients it serves. Back in the United States, Klass as a young doctor and young mother discovers that medicine doesn't always speak her language either. She arrives with her team at the bedside to perform a neurological examination on a newborn. "This baby is poopy," she announces with a mother's hands-on experience. "He needs to be changed." The male doctors maintain an icy silence.

Klass assumes, incorrectly, that she has simply used the wrong vocabulary. The entry into medical care, for young doctors as well as for patients, is the entry into an unfamiliar linguistic domain governed by rules that are rarely brought to light. All languages work by means of such unarticulated structures. Klass tries again. "This baby has apparently had a bowel movement." She adds, "Let me just put a clean diaper on him."[27] Worse and worse. The doctors vigorously shake their heads. The medicalized language of "bowel movement" did not somehow work the desired magic. Diaper-changing, Klass finally learns, is a job that the male doctors regard as falling to nurses. The entire misadventure, of course, can initiate rich reflections on the sexual politics of medicine—a sexual politics increasingly in flux as women students now constitute a majority in American medical schools and as women doctors reassess their roles.

The most important insight, for Klass, comes with understanding that the language of medicine encodes assumptions, knowledge, and values that outsiders—including novice doctors—do not fully comprehend. The patient, as an outsider, speaks not only a nonmedical language but also a language of not-knowing that expresses a personal, subjective experience of illness that medical logos almost automatically discounts as less than authoritative and translates into its own official dialect: the test results—numerical, statistical, laboratory-validated, solid knowledge— will have the final say.

Medical eros will further perplex anyone with a staunch scientific mind-set because it is open to learning from fictive voices. Practical distinctions between fiction and nonfiction, of course, are easy to make in obvious cases. Only someone from Mars would mistake Little Red Riding Hood for a statistical study in *JAMA* on mu-receptors and opioid analgesics. The two specimens belong to radically different genres. However, even scientific genres dealing with data and fact are not somehow free from the artifices of narrative. The novelist E. L. Doctorow observed the inescapability of fictive techniques: "News magazines present the events of the world as an ongoing weekly serial. Weather reports are constructed on television with exact attention to conflict (high pressure areas clashing with lows), suspense (the climax of tomorrow's weather prediction coming after the commercial), and other basic elements of narrative." Reflecting on the relentless appropriation of fictional techniques by people who create, advertise, package, and market so-called factual products, among which we should include pharmaceutical medications, Doctorow concludes, "I am thus led to the proposition that there is no fiction or nonfiction as we commonly understand the distinction: there is only narrative."[28]

Medical eros understands that the voices of patients, whether actual or fictive, cannot emerge into language outside the structures of narrative. Even tax forms involve an encounter with the shaping artifices of language. In this sense, every utterance shaped by narrative structures and by narrative techniques is in part fictive—that is, constructed. It could be said otherwise. As medical ethicist Tod Chambers explains, "Every telling of a story—real or imagined—encompasses a series of choices about what will be revealed, what will be privileged, and what will be concealed; *there are no artless narrations*."[29] Some may wish to assign a relative greater authority to the voices of actual patients, as opposed to the voices of patients in works of fiction, but the grounds for such a decision are highly questionable. Medical eros contends that what matters most is the commitment to listening. Careful listening as a medical tool is as important, in its way, as scalpels, stethoscopes, and sutures.

The patient's voice, from the perspective of medical eros, always and inescapably takes the shape of narrative. Even the official medical "history" edits and transfers the patient's oral narrative into the brief form most useful to doctors. Flesh-and-blood patients are always singular, changing, historical persons, never fully knowable. Their voices and their narratives may differ significantly depending on context. For example, an unemployed single mother on welfare may use a different vocabulary and tell a slightly different story when she talks with a middle-aged nurse or with a young intern. Medical software programs and rules concerning confidentiality generate data that deliberately disguise or conceal individual identities so that even statistical studies, in effect, create or depend upon invisible miniature fictions. The fictional patients created by physician-writers from Chekhov to Perri Klass are no less compelling or instructive, in the view of medical eros, than the self-portraits in memoirs by patient-writers from Audre Lorde to William Styron, which also employ fictive or semifictive narrative techniques. In short, the patient's voice, even in a raw transcript or video reproduction, is always a narrative creation, and so, too, is much of the medical encounter. It is no wonder an entire new subfield has recently opened up called "narrative medicine."

Medical eros sees no need to carry out a rigorous winnowing that, once and for all, divides fact from fiction; they regularly mix and follow a narrative structure. Even the tubercle bacillus, as Susan Sontag showed, was once absorbed within framing cultural narratives that had a significant impact on people with tuberculosis. What's needed, instead, is to listen to selected voices in medical contexts to discover what they say that might prove of value to doctors and to patients. Their collective evidence, I am convinced, gives strong support to the values and attitudes associated with medical eros. Not-knowing has its own neglected value in a surrounding culture and in a medical profession that venerates scientific data and that understands patients and illness as necessarily falling under the supervision of the molecular gaze. In such a setting, the voices of not-knowing are especially worth listening to.

"I don't feel that it is necessary to know exactly what I am," said Michel Foucault. Foucault surely ranks among the most incisive modern thinkers, so it is significant that he also leaves space for not-knowing. His definition of humankind as "thinking" creatures, does not mean that Foucault imagined thought as a means for filling up the universe with knowledge. Knowledge always raised his level of suspicion because so often knowledge becomes a means for exercising control that easily edges over into oppressive forms of order. Most importantly, his life as a gay man and as a "militant intellectual" expressed a resistance to orthodox structures—resistance he explored in his writing. Significantly, unreason and sexuality are among his primary subjects, and both closely link with eros; they interest him particularly as they tend to disrupt settled systems of knowledge.[30] "There are more ideas on earth than intellectuals imagine," Foucault writes. "And these ideas are more active, stronger, more resistant, more passionate than 'politicians' think. We have to be there at the birth of ideas, the bursting outward of their force: not in books expressing them, but in events manifesting this force."[31] Impassioned ideas drew him, not knowledge; and not-knowing is the matrix for ideas that burst forth with the passion of events. Such not-knowing provides a crucial service in holding open a space for what is yet to come: the unseen, the unknown, the unforeseen. Foucault concluded his reflection on humans as "thinking" creatures with an endorsement of the need for not-knowing: "The main interest in life and work is to become someone else that you were not in the beginning. If you knew when you began a book what you would say at the end, do you think that you would have the courage to write it? What is true for writing and for a love relationship is true also for life. The game is worthwhile insofar as we don't know what will be the end."[32] Knowledge, which for Foucault is always organized like a game, proves worthwhile only insofar as it embraces within its structure a fundamental and ineradicable not-knowing. Anything else amounts to little more than dogma.

Not-knowing may strike some physicians and patients as mostly a nuisance, a state to be erased as soon as possible and replaced with knowledge, but such views simply repeat the ruling doctrines of medical logos. It is not a waste of time, however, to listen and to oppose business as usual if medicine reduces patients to a case, a room number, a disease, or an organ ("the gall bladder in room 305"), or worse, reduces the patient to an insulting acronym. GOMER is crude medical code for "Get Out of My Emergency Room." Listening to the voices of medicine can even direct attention to the commonplace collective nouns such as

"doctor" and "patient" that, under scrutiny, resemble semifictive con-
structions that erase meaningful differences: white or black, urban or
rural, male or female, young or old, Christian, Muslim, Jew. When "the
patient" is a frightened ten-year-old Syrian boy in an American medical
center, perhaps a war orphan who speaks no English, a Spider-Man
comic may prove as crucial as drugs to the process of recovery. Medical
eros is less concerned with whether various narrative voices are factual
or fictive, because narrative always blurs the line, than with how we
might profit from attending seriously to what such voices—even in their
blurred confusion and not-knowing—can tell us.

An Erotics of Not-Knowing: Narrative and Pleasure

John Cage, the avant-garde composer who challenged and changed
twentieth-century music, did not restrict his innovations to musical composition. In 1938 he invented the "prepared piano," inserting screws, nuts,
and bits of rubber between the piano wires, and in 1952 he debuted the
infamous work 4′33″ (three short movements lasting, altogether, four minutes and thirty-three seconds, in which, for each movement, the pianist
raises the lid from the keyboard, sits silent, then lowers the lid). At age 65
Cage exhibited a portfolio of prints, entitled *Seven Day Diary*, completed
during an invited one-week crash course on etching: "an activity," he told
interviewer John Ashbery, "that would be characterized by the fact of my
not knowing what I was doing." Ashbery, a poet and art critic who understood Cage's musical preference for including random sonic events from
street noise to radio broadcasts, then asked what the advantage is of *not
knowing what you are doing.* Cage replied, "It cheers up the knowing."[33]
    Not-knowing in medicine and in illness is, of course, never a steady
state. It exists, as if in counterpoint, only in relation to the knowledge that
it interrupts, as knowing and not-knowing alternate, collaborate, interpenetrate, or overlap in what is always an improvisation. The knowledge
that medicine at times must impart—the "bad news" that doctors hate
to tell patients—is sometimes so dire that it may well put us in need of
cheering up. Not-knowing, in turn, can offer the spiritual nourishment
that Zen teachers describe as a return to "the beginner's mind." Cage no
doubt owed much of his celebrated optimism to his study and practice of

Zen ways, and optimism—reconfigured as the biology of hope—makes a well-documented contribution to wellness. Medical eros, however, understands not-knowing as far more than a possibly therapeutic source of wellness and cheering up. Not-knowing (as crucial to eros and to illness) reminds us that medical knowledge and the molecular vision of life do not constitute an impervious, all-powerful, giant monolith, an Australian Uluru. They exist only in relation to forms of life and modes of knowing that go on, as it were, in another dimension, much as Uluru looms up against the sky, set off against the surrounding plain or bush, where aboriginal inhabitants know how to find water and food, inscribing their sacred stories and legends in pictographs where outcrops, overhangs, and occasional secluded pools offer shelter and instruction hidden within the 5.8-mile circumference of the ancient red-sandstone monument.

Philosopher and novelist Richard Kearney delivers the bad news to anyone who believes that narratives, even if they pass straight from a real patient to an actual physician, express the unvarnished truth. As he puts it, "stories are never innocent." What he means is that all narrative is open to "a continuing conflict of interpretations."[34] Who has the right to say, for certain, what a particular story means? The doctor? A computer program? Two literary critics? Suppose they disagree? Moreover, stories and narrative structures often knowingly or unknowingly support a particular point of view. Medical eros at least deals openly with such dilemmas, which medical logos prefers to ignore despite their scandalous presence in medical practice. "Uncertainty," writes Dr. David M. Eddy, a specialist in health policy and management, "creeps into medical practice through every pore." He adds, as if breaking a professional code of silence: "Whether a physician is defining a disease, making a diagnosis, selecting a procedure, observing outcomes, assessing probabilities, assigning preferences, or putting it all together, he is walking on very slippery terrain."

The cognitive slipperiness native even to biomedicine gives purchase to the uneasy thought that reason and science are not fully in control. Eddy summarizes the dilemmas that accompany diagnosis, treatment, and outcomes-assessment: "It is difficult for non-physicians, and for many physicians, to appreciate how complex these tasks are, how poorly we understand them, and how easy it is for honest people to come to different conclusions."[35]

Medical eros operates on the assumption that, no matter how much we know, knowledge in medicine always contains gaps, uncertainties, dark spots, and slipperiness. Mysteries remain that defy sense, elude reason, and baffle textbook logic: sudden deaths, flesh-eating bacteria, chronic pain with no identifiable lesion, spontaneous remissions, miraculous recoveries, and new diseases without cure. A tested therapy, successful in extensive trials, will suddenly fail a particular patient. Why? Drugs and devices prescribed by a generation of doctors suddenly vanish from the marketplace amid class-action lawsuits. Experienced physicians develop a sense for how to proceed amid uncertainties and the unknown, although generally they proceed on a path meant to produce answers and successful treatments. Even so, there is much that medicine, ultimately, *cannot* know. It cannot know, for example, the life story of every patient; it cannot peer deeply into the financial and personal struggles that every doctor faces. Illness brings the unknowns that surround individual doctors face to face with the unknowns that surround individual patients, and uncertain knowledge is the flimsy rope bridge swinging between these two dark immensities, with illness the abyss below. Medical eros, even when invisible and unacknowledged, has a place in negotiations that involve the not-knowns inherent in the triangular relation among doctor, patient, and illness.

Eros and not-knowing, it must be said, almost always carry a whiff of scandal in a profession that celebrates knowledge, reason, and scientific discovery. Medical students and nursing students, in my experience, find the rough, eroticized throat examination by the doctor in William Carlos Williams's "The Use of Force" totally unacceptable, as if to confirm Rafael Campo's early belief that, for a model physician, desire is repellent and forbidden. Can pleasure exist where there is no desire? Does a profession that outlaws desire also, even if unwittingly, outlaw pleasure? Medicine in its close confederation with science and knowledge can easily appear complicit in what scholar Wendy Steiner describes as the contemporary *scandal of pleasure*.[36] The sadomasochistic eroticism in the photographs of Robert Mapplethorpe, deliberately scandalous, of course draw attention to the extravagances of desire and suggest that pleasure can cross or erase boundaries as surely as eroticism (for Bataille) destroys the normal, self-contained character of the participators. *Should* medicine perhaps seek to outlaw pleasure?

Illness, like eros and like pleasure, crosses boundaries and erases constraints. It, too, destroys a sense of normalcy, which is why, to the ill, harmless pleasures can seem like a gift delivered from a forgotten homeland. Medical eros cannot avoid risking scandal in its relaxation of borders. It gives implicit permission to pleasurable human activities—sex, laughter, dreams, music, play, story—which may well constitute or contribute to Broyardian good medicine, even if, like most drugs, their power falls somewhere short of cure. Jennifer Glaser and her boyfriend bedridden with leukemia did not spend their afternoons in search of biomedical knowledge.

The pleasures that medical eros endorses, if just implicitly, can claim support from authorities that carry the endorsement of medical logos. Take dreams, for example. Dreams, despite a lurking possibility of nightmare, are a traditional source of pleasure, as reflected in the multiple ways in which we apply the adjective *dreamy*. Once a crucial therapy in the ancient Asklepieion, dreams still find a therapeutic use among certain specialists in mental health, and brain-imaging studies show that neurons in the cerebral cortex are far more active during the stage called rapid eye movement (REM) sleep, which is the period when we experience vivid dreams. Whatever such dreams may mean or do, we go through the REM sleep cycle five or six times during eight hours of sleep. Research has suggested that prolonged deprivation of REM sleep is associated with depression and other illnesses. Dreaming—as it accompanies REM sleep—would seem important to human health, and so too are the pleasures of sex. Sexual activity is a source of illness when seriously disordered or pathological, of course, but otherwise it is a function of the healthy adult organism. Its erotic pleasures, for many people, involve a plunge into darkness and not-knowing. Knowledge mostly just gets in the way.

Medical eros would propose laughter and music as two other sources of pleasure, and both have demonstrable value in reducing pain and in opposing illness. Research into the neurobiology and psychology of laughter has long shown its power to reduce pain, in part through the role of laughter in distraction, but researchers have offered other, less well-documented claims of health benefits of comic laughter, from improving blood flow to strengthening the immune response. Music, of course, can intoxicate an entire audience. Oliver Sacks, from his perspective as a neurologist, has described how music is effective in helping patients with certain neurological disorders such as Parkinson's disease and advanced dementia.[37] The close association between music and emotion is enshrined even in the history of military bands, and this immediate link with emotion is surely part of what Sacks's patients respond to. Medical logos has every right to remain skeptical about specific claims until they are proved. Medical eros, however, stands as the icon for an intuitive recognition that pleasure—as an object, by-product, and component of desire—has a positive role to play in health and illness.

The pleasures of not-knowing might even claim to tap into a higher-level spiritual or sacred dimension. Joy, invoked as a very specific concept distinct from simple pleasures, certainly holds a power (almost like music or group prayer in a Baptist church) to unite people in a communal spirit that has its own demonstrated health benefits. Joy, we might say, resembles the ecstatic states associated with Hassidic or Sufi worship. The ecstatic visions of Saint Teresa of Ávila, memorably represented in Bernini's marble statue in the Cornaro Chapel in Rome, bring the intense pleasures of a mystical communion with the divine scandalously close to an image—or fantasy representation—of female sexual orgasm. It is not necessary, however, or perhaps even possible to remain for long periods in a state of unrelieved ecstasy, whether spiritual or profane. Simple free play, meaning a pleasurable expression of ludic desire outside regimented or professional playgrounds—from Little League sandlots to multimillion dollar sport complexes—has ramifications so basic to healthy human function that it's surprising all hospitals don't encourage it.

The evolutionary value of play, as musician and author Stephen Nachmanovitch contends, is that it makes us flexible: "Play enables us to rearrange our capacities and our very identity so that they can be used in unforeseen ways."[38] Play is now highly valued for its role in childhood development and might be said to reaffirm its presence in adult, social existence through the institution of the theater. *Plays*, as we call the performances staged from ancient Greek amphitheaters to Broadway, not only enlist the pleasures of fiction but also hold, as evidence now suggests, important therapeutic powers. Aristotle saw pleasure as basic even to tragic drama and invokes a broadly therapeutic value for dramatic productions, no matter whether we translate *catharsis* as purgation, purification, or clarification. With an even more directly therapeutic aim, driven to respond to the alarming rate of suicides among veterans of recent U.S. military conflicts, the contemporary company called Theater of War performs scenes from classical drama for audiences of wounded veterans.[39] Suicide may mark the ultimate failure of eros, and whatever power opposes suicide can be regarded as life-affirming. Sophocles, as the Theater of War reminds audiences, was an Athenian general, and Aeschylus produced his *Oresteia* with Athens at war on six fronts. Classical tragedy enfolds experience that is not foreign to modern combat veterans, and its account of human suffering can spark post-performance discussions among audience members that prove extremely valuable. Theater of War Productions has by now presented many hundreds of performances of Sophocles's *Ajax* and *Philoctetes* for military audiences worldwide, from Guantanamo Bay to the Walter Reed Army Medical Center.[40] How many other companies have performed at both the Guggenheim Museum and the Pentagon?

Pleasure is not always a direct goal of drama, and playwrights may prefer to challenge audiences with an experience of outrage, alienation, or confusion. The mixed impulses that bring us to the theater or to the playground, however, cannot be entirely detached from a desire for pleasure. It is a pleasure, too, that often depends upon a willing, if temporary, encounter with not-knowing. The dark woods in *A Midsummer Night's Dream*, for example, are an easy journey from Athens, which Shakespeare represents as the citadel of reason, patriarchy, and law. (Athens, through association with its famous resident Hippocrates, might count as the home of medical logos.) As the Athenian duke, Theseus, and his captive bride-to-be quarrel, the amorous discord extends even to the tutelary rulers of the woods, the king and queen of the fairies. Meanwhile, four young lovers leave Athens and spend the night lost in the woods, where the eros-surrogate Puck embroils them in misunderstandings. When Puck eventually intervenes once more to set things right, the lovers awake, pair off in the proper combinations, and the royals (both in Athens and in fairyland) mirror the new concord. Everyone then returns to Athens for the Duke's wedding, including Bottom the Weaver (whom actor Kevin Klein plays as endowed with a touch of the artist). Bottom wakes alone, semiconfused, from a magical night spent enfolded in the arms of the beautiful queen of the fairies, which of course he can't wholly recall, so he imagines that he must have dreamed it: "I have had a most rare vision. I have had a dream, past the wit of man to say what dream it was."[41] Dreams, as medical eros would contend, are a resonant image for the therapeutic pleasures of not-knowing. As if they had spent the night in an Asklepian abaton, Shakespeare's quarrelsome lovers achieve a happy ending only *through* their immersion in darkness and in dreamlike confusion, and the pleasures that await them take the time-honored comic image of marriage. Eros, for all the discontents it can provoke, also leads to harmonious resolutions and to pleasurable renewal. It offers a force for healing even the rifts and wounds it might cause. Tragedy offers a sterner perspective, but we proceed at our peril if we ignore the healing power of eros, of not-knowing, and of comic pleasure: in short (a caution to all who struggle with serious illness), if we fail to dream.

Few events in clinical medicine are more basic and less often discussed than *not*-knowing, and patients, too, are often in the dark. *A Midsummer Night's Dream*, in its encounters with disorder, invites us to consider how the dark struggles and confusions that typify illness—including the altered states of inner life—require an acknowledgment of mutually fruitful contraries: nightside not-knowing along with daylight rationality. Eros and illness immerse almost everyone, sooner or later, in the unknown and in the unknowable, but the experience need not be permanently disabling. Parallels with medical eros and medical logos seem relevant. Medical practice cannot somehow exclude encounters with not-knowing and disorder, despite the preference of biomedicine to emphasize its astonishing technical innovations and its scientific knowledge of diseases. Doctors cannot stop work at the bright lines that mark off perfect and certain knowledge, and patients live within the shadow of uncertainties and not-knowing that biomedical floodlamps will never completely dispel. A serious question in medicine is not how to stamp out every known disease but rather how to proceed in the inescapable presence of the not-known. The unknown and the unknowable are as common in illness as the presence of its mostly invisible companion eros. Shouldn't *somebody*—doctors, patients, caregivers, families, administrators, grant agencies, politicians— eventually take note?

The note or annotation is a genre so negligible (if it even rises to the level of a literary event) that it might provide a fitting emblem for the invisibility of eros in illness. As a brief written record often for future reference, the note also has an established role in medicine. Progress notes, according to one standard guide, are the core or heart of most clinical records: a repository in which health-care professionals enter details concerning a patient's status during hospitalization or outpatient care.[42] The note is also, however, a legal, actionable document, and one authority recommends that trainees, in self-protection, imagine a hostile prosecuting attorney reading the note in court. The margins of most of my books, safe from litigation, include handwritten annotations that might rate the technical term *marginalia*. The lowly annotation even generates its distinctive contemporary forms, such as the indispensable sticky note, and it is thus instructive to observe what a recipient of the Nobel Prize in Literature makes of this modest, everyday, fragmentary record or reminder.

Wislawa Szymborska, the poet, essayist, translator, and 1996 Nobel Prize winner, begins her brief poem "A Note" by focusing on almost the opposite of epic or the sublime: "Life is the only way / to get covered in leaves, / catch your breath on the sand, / rise on wings; / to be a dog." Her list of casual, ordinary, unexpectedly strange experiences, animal and human, ends with another apparently miscellaneous sequence that just might catch us up short. Life, she concludes on a quiet note, allows you to "mislay your keys in the grass; / and to follow a spark on the wind with your eyes; / and to keep on not knowing / something important."[43]

Does the value that we automatically place on knowledge in effect keep us from understanding the value of not-knowing? A note, of course, captures only a fragment; it is a form disrespected precisely because it specializes in the partial, the fleeting, the tentative, and the incomplete. It is also, in its distance from the certainties of authorized knowledge, where for Szymborska the truly important experiences of life seem to reside. The note coincides with a realm in which we wouldn't need a note to remind us if human knowledge weren't so often piecemeal and so often given to a slide back toward not-knowing. Not-knowing, in effect, is what we do every day, without knowing we do it; without knowing how important the everyday things truly are; without knowing—Szymborska's ultimate paradox—how important not-knowing is. Knowledge may be power, as thinkers from Jefferson to Foucault assert, but knowledge can also solidify into oppressive power, as Szymborska, who in Poland lived under a dictatorial regime for many years, pointed out in her Nobel Prize lecture. "This is why I value that little phrase 'I don't know' so highly," she said in her talk. "It's small, but it flies on mighty wings." "Poets," she added, "if they're genuine, must also keep repeating 'I don't know.' Each poem marks an effort to answer this statement. . . . Whatever inspiration is, it's born from a continuous 'I don't know.' "[44]

Medical eros in its role as contrary seeks to recover—to take note of, rather than to deny or forget—exactly those aspects of health and illness that medical logos and the molecular vision tend to overlook or dismiss as not worth knowing. Paradoxically, with its embrace of not-knowing, medical eros can offer at least one source of support that physicians and health-care professionals have increasingly come to value. Distinguished pain specialist Scott Fishman puts it this way: "When somebody comes in with 25 years of chronic pain, I might sit with them for 90 minutes to get the beginning of the story, to really understand what's happening. The insurers would rather pay me $1,000 to do a 20-minute injection than pay me a fraction of that to spend an hour or two talking with a patient."[45] Insurance providers adopt (as in their financial self-interest) the technical procedures favored by medical logos and by the molecular gaze, which entail an almost automatic aversion to getting the story. Stories or narrative, despite the varieties of not-knowing that they entail, belong also to the native terrain of illness. A distinguished line of modern doctors and modern patients, in opposition to the insurers, are beginning to reclaim, revalue, and redirect the ancient interest in narrative. The next frontier in biomedicine might well lie in rediscovering the everyday importance of narrative and in talking with patients to hear their individual stories of illness.

Part Two

The Stories

CHAPTER FOUR

Varieties of Erotic Experience: Five Illness Narratives

Compared with this world of living individualized feelings, the world of generalized objects which the intellect contemplates is without solidity or life. . . . We get a beautiful picture of an express train supposed to be moving, but where in the picture . . . is the energy or the fifty miles an hour?

WILLIAM JAMES, *THE VARIETIES OF RELIGIOUS EXPERIENCE* (1902)

*E*ROS IS THE ENERGY and the fifty miles an hour—desire as an express train that blows past whatever eros-concept or eros-picture the intellect prefers to contemplate. Medical logos, on the side of intellect, devises strategies of containment and speed limits, perhaps a patient's bill of rights or an ombudsman, but these sensible concessions to the bill-paying patient hardly conceal where the real power lies. Patients, to receive treatment, sign consent forms acknowledging almost every possible risk, absolving physicians and institutions of predictable harms that seem to stop short only at criminal negligence, while doctors sign nothing except large checks to cover malpractice insurance. This imbalance of power is not grounds for a people's revolt. Doctors, like patients, face serious dangers. It is also the unspoken duty of institutions and professions to protect and to perpetuate themselves, in which obligation hospitals and medical staff are no less self-regarding than universities or big-name golf tournaments. What makes this common situation worthy of note is that patients, despite their position of dependency, have recently begun to assert a modest power as they publish books, articles, blogs, and random tweets about their experiences of illness. While biomedicine still rules the institution and while the molecular gaze brings back ever more detailed pictures from the interior of the body, the medical eros express train—long neglected or invisible—is picking up speed.

The shifting social dynamic in twentieth-century medicine, proceeding alongside the explosion of new biotechnologies, has thrust into prominence a new figure whom sociologist Arthur W. Frank aptly calls "the wounded storyteller."[1] Book-length accounts of illness written by patients were uncommon before 1950, as scholar Anne Hunsaker Hawkins observes, and they were rare before 1900.[2] Starting in the second half of the twentieth century, however, the patient as wounded storyteller began to fill the bookstores and airwaves and Internet chat rooms with personal illness narratives. The reversal of position is important to recognize, even as biomedicine solidifies its power. Doctors in their role as medical scientists or as designated scientific-minded authorities on the body had long possessed a monopoly on writing about illness. Illness was their precinct, almost like a cop on the beat, and writing about illness was just what doctors did—mostly in arcane papers published in peer-reviewed journals read by other doctors. The medical profession controlled the discourse of illness.

Today each new best-seller list contains memoirs in which patients, family members, or lovers recount their stories and report their personal truths. In these new patient-centered narratives, doctors no longer hold a privileged position as science-minded authorities on the body. Biomedicine can still report amazing scientific breakthroughs and announce unimaginable cures, but such news reports must now compete with off-setting narratives describing misdiagnosis, medical bungling, bureaucratic delay, and fatal outbreaks of ever-new viral diseases. The new world of medical narrative is a site where patients no longer accept a passive, voiceless role. Doctors, too, and other medical insiders have begun to join the narrative jamboree, writing less from an elevated position as scientists of the body than from a level playing field as first-person participant-observers in the drama of modern health care. In 2015, for example, the *Annals of Internal Medicine* published an anonymous article entitled "Our Family Secrets"—in which an intern and doctor recount similar stories of inappropriate sexual language and sexual behavior among male physicians in obstetrics and gynecology.[3] Other prominent medical journals now publish brief first-person narratives by doctors and other health professionals, recognizing a value in narrative that extends well beyond its use in exposé. The work of contemporary physicians from Richard Selzer and Oliver Sacks to Atul Gawande, Danielle Ofri, Abraham Verghese, and Siddhartha Mukherjee demonstrates that doctors rank among the most talented writers of our times. Verghese's self-described "love of medicine," for example, plays out in complex novels where desire and erotic impulses prove crucial to the operations of empathy and of healing.[4]

The professional epicenter for this new interest in medical narrative is the Program in Narrative Medicine, founded in 2002 by physician Rita Charon at the Columbia University College of Physicians and Surgeons, a beacon and model for proliferating medical programs and journals interested in narrative. Psychiatrist and anthropologist Arthur Kleinman helped mark the path in his trailblazing book *The Illness Narratives* (1985), and Arthur W. Frank, in addition to *The Wounded Storyteller* (1995), has added a suite of influential studies on stories and illness. Narrative, almost overnight, has turned into a rich field of medical research. Psychologists have conducted some of the more remarkable recent studies: James W. Pennebaker, for example, shows that writing about trauma correlates with *measurable health benefits*; Richard G. Tedeschi and Lawrence G. Calhoun pursue narrative-based research into the "posttraumatic growth" that many times accompanies or grows out of crises such as serious illness.[5] (As many as 90 percent of survivors, they report, experience at least one aspect of posttraumatic growth, such as a renewed appreciation for life.) Well-tested psychometric instruments and software programs for analyzing speech now give narrative researchers the ability to transform stories and first-person discourse into the quantifiable, statistical data that most medical journals expect. Meanwhile, however, not-knowing remains a hard sell in medicine, as it makes for a feeble research agenda and a career that looks dead on arrival. The molecular gaze automatically privileges visual data, where seeing is believing, and what can't be seen (or converted into pie graphs) isn't really believable. My aim, minus the computer analytics, is to examine five illness narratives and to ask in an exploratory spirit (that privileges words over images and not-knowing over knowledge) what is it that patients *desire* and what is it they desire *to say*?

Depression: *Darkness Visible*

"I felt my heart pounding wildly, like that of a man facing a firing squad, and knew I had made an irreversible decision." So wrote famed American novelist William Styron as he describes the moment, one cold early December, when recurrent, ever-deepening depression pushed him to the edge of suicide.[6] He had just stuffed his writer's notebooks into the trash bin. Only a few technicalities remained to settle: a rewritten will, a suicide note, the method of self-execution. Other illnesses, Styron felt, allow a hope of improvement or the faith in an eventual return to health, but not serious depression. "In depression this faith in deliverance, in ultimate restoration," he writes, "is absent. The pain is unrelenting, and what makes the condition intolerable is the foreknowledge that no remedy will come—not in a day, an hour, a month, or a minute. . . . It is hopelessness even more than pain that crushes the soul" (*DV* 62). Eroticism, Bataille had written, is "assenting to life up to the point of death."[7] Assent (*l'approbation*) means approval: finding good. Depression—with its dark, unending, soul-crushing, life-renouncing despair—constitutes for Styron almost an official anti-eros.

Medical logos meets its limits for Styron in the soul-crushing moment when despair turns suicidal. The molecular gaze offers no solace when doctors, drugs, and therapies have exhausted their powers, leaving Styron alone to face the ultrarational, binary choice between hopeless, endless suffering or a quick end. The rationality of suicide is what Styron chose to emphasize in a controversial op-ed piece that he published in the *New York Times*. His circle of literary friends included several famous writers whose suicides Styron staunchly defended against detractors who attributed the deaths to momentary irrational acts. His heart pounded wildly, but Styron's decision to end his life was not a sudden response. Suicide is for Styron the opposite of an impulsive, mad, or delirious act. It is more like the conclusion to a logical syllogism, the ultimate coldly rational decision of a reasonable man with no other option.

Darkness Visible: A Memoir of Madness (1990) is Styron's account of his life-threatening illness. In its chilling inside look at depression, Styron provides facts and figures that make his narrative more than the memoir of a strictly personal dilemma. In its shape as well as its subject, it stands as a seminal document in the development of narrative medicine. Depression, even twenty-five years after Styron wrote, is according to the National Institutes of Health one of the most common mental disorders. The figures for 2014 show that about 6.7 percent of all U.S. adults experience a major depressive disorder.[8] Women are far more likely than men to experience depression. Such alarming numbers mark a significant crisis in public health, and Styron's achievement is to take us inside the numbers in order to understand the personal or lived experience of depression. Serious, clinical depression for Styron means that he arrives at a moment when, with medical knowledge and medical assistance now no more than a hollowed-out husk, he methodically completes the necessary preparations for suicide.

Medical eros might be described as the secret hero of *Darkness Visible*. This tendentious description, however, requires some acquaintance with the knowledge that Rita Charon calls *narrative competence*. Narrative competence, as Charon describes it, is "the competence that human beings use to absorb, interpret, and respond to stories." Her account, slightly expanded, leads us straight back to Styron. "The narratively competent reader or listener," Charon sums up, "realizes that the meaning of any narrative—a novel, a textbook, a joke—must be judged in the light of its narrative situation: Who tells it? Who hears it? Why and how is it told?"[9] The narrative situation in *Darkness Visible*, as we know, involves a famous writer (Styron), gripped by depression, who tells his story in retrospect. The retrospective stance allows him to compose a highly literate memoir of his experience, a legitimate contribution to his prize-winning career as a writer, complete with references to Milton and to Dante. Why? *Why* is implicit in *how*. Styron tells his story in a way that traces a well-crafted arc from descent to emergence. *How* he tells the story, then, involves describing an action in which the well-crafted arc reaches a crucial turning point. Styron's *turning point* (*peripiteia* is Aristotle's technical term) occurs when the downward arc reaches its nadir and the upward movement begins. This turning point has little to do with reason and everything to do with eros.

It is a compelling story told by a master storyteller. Late at night, bundled up against the bitter cold outside, knowing that he cannot make it through the next day's pain and with preparations complete for his self-destruction, Styron (solitary in his depressive state) sits alone watching a film. It is the equivalent of a prisoner's last meal. His wife, Rose, he tells us, is upstairs in bed. Suddenly, from the soundtrack, he hears a "soaring passage" from the Brahms *Alto Rhapsody*. The music, he writes, "pierced my heart like a dagger." This heart-piercing music does not belong to the world of reason. Rather, it opens up "a flood of swift recollection" (*DV* 66). The prize-winning writer—lionized in Paris with a prestigious award as the book artfully opens—now finds his thoughts returning to the daily pleasures of love, work, and family life. The turning point, then, evokes multiple events so closely linked as to constitute a complex knot. Soaring music. Heart pierced like a dagger. Memories of house, love, children, work, and family life. "I am convinced that this was the moment that saved him," Rose Styron later wrote about her husband's sudden decision to abandon his well-planned and nearly completed suicide, "and I'm certain his thoughts of our family did finally nullify his resolve to kill himself."[10]

Styron's turning point stands as a reversal of everything that reason had argued in favor of suicide. It overrides even all his detailed and sharply argued skepticism about doctors, hospitals, and the limits of medical logos. It also exposes the complex role of emotion in illness and in healing. The soaring passage from Brahms's *Alto Rhapsody*, as we learn, reminds him of his mother, who had died when he was thirteen. She was an opera singer who had sung the same soaring passage. The memory of family joys also proves inseparable from a somewhat sentimental passage that he recalls from a poem by Emily Dickinson. "I woke up my wife," he writes, "and soon telephone calls were made. The next day I was admitted to the hospital" (*DV* 67). Styron remains vague about the details and about exactly how hospitalization restored him. Depression, as he indicates, rarely yields simple explanations, biochemical or psychological, and he remains skeptical about the hospital therapies. What he gives us, in effect, is the account of a near-fatal illness arrested at the last moment by a rush of emotion—what I might compare to a heroic rescue at the hands of medical eros. The memoir concludes its well-shaped arc with a line from Dante as he at last emerges from his dark underworld journey (through the seven circles of Hell) and once again beholds the stars.

Stories, never artless or innocent, always embody the shape of a narrative situation. They are constructed by someone, for someone, with a specific point of view, and often with a particular purpose. Styron's youngest daughter, Alexandra, accurately terms *Darkness Visible* "a tale of descent and recovery."[11] Tales or fables, of course, often achieve their power through radical simplification. Rose Styron points out that *Darkness Visible* does not mention her husband's relapse in early 1988, when he again grew depressed and, in her words, "violently suicidal" (*S* 135). (Styron died of pneumonia in 2006.) Was Bill Styron really alone—Rose asleep upstairs—when he heard a soaring passage from the *Alto Rhapsody?* "In *my* mind," Rose Styron writes, "I never slept if Bill was not in bed beside me" (*S* 133). Rose Styron, a fellow writer, does not suggest literary deception; memory is imperfect, and all writing requires shaping artifice. It is telling, however, that she chooses a significantly different title for her essay-length account of their shared experience of his depression: "Strands." Strands, especially loose strands, are what *don't* get neatly tied up as a well-constructed plot concludes. They are the surplus—untethered filaments, tangled leftovers—that resist a full and final account. Rose Styron's experience (as spouse and caregiver) takes as its title and metaphor an untidiness or incompletion that does not trace a mythic trajectory from darkness to light.

Narrative competence, if it deems medical eros the unseen hero in *Darkness Visible*, requires that we also notice the cost that stories may or may not acknowledge. Eros is not unfailingly kind, and Styron omits a full account of the darkest hours when, as we learn from his daughter, he tried to tell his wife "the names of all the women he had slept with over the course of their marriage" (*RMF* 222). Medical eros, if we do not romanticize it, will contain fractal moments of strain, conflict, paradox—in effect, *strands*. Alexandra Styron, as she examined letters from grateful readers in her father's archives at Duke University, struggles to reconcile the book's generally sympathetic narrator with the difficult father she grew up with: "How could a guy whose thoughts elicit this much pathos have been, for so many years, such a monumental asshole to the people closest to him?" (*RMF* 11). Hard words, but they indicate how far illness and its effects ripple through the surrounding supra-dyadic spaces in which children and families struggle to make sense of experiences they imperfectly understand—which grow darker in retrospect—where knowledge must rub up against its limits in the darkness of non-knowing.

While no panacea, medical eros, even in its raggedness can offer solace amid the wreckage. "He'd spent more than twenty years pushing her away," as Alexandra Styron observes the change in her parents during her father's depression; "Now he wouldn't let her out of his sight" (*RMF* 221). Her father's recovery transformed his obsessive clinging into what she regarded as a new closeness. Rose Styron seems to agree in the poetic fragment—another loose filament—that she includes toward the conclusion of "Strands": "*Love that lay hidden under/yesterday's monstrous breakers/in the pounded dunes/walks with us*" (*S* 135–136). Her final paragraph offers a similarly muted testament to eros: "Looking back, I would say that sticking with the person you love through the stressful dramas of mood disorder can eventually be incredibly rewarding" (*S* 137). Medical eros would advise that we do not overlook the strandlike modifier *eventually*.

Breast Cancer: *Cancer in Two Voices*

"I shut my eyes and saw absolute black," writes Barbara Rosenblum of the day—November 20, 1985—when she learns that her breast-tissue biopsy has tested malignant: "no lines of red or purple, pure black." Barbara Rosenblum is, strictly speaking, not in her right mind. "My agitation lifted me off the table and I started walking around the examining room in small steps, working off the tension," she writes. "I thought I might put my fist through the wall." She pauses—for a paragraph break—as if to catch her breath. "And then, when I opened my eyes, I couldn't see too well. Or hear too well either" (*CTV* 10). Betrayal by one's own senses, which Sappho describes in the lover, is *mutatis mutandis* the state of the patient, too.

Sandra Butler, as surviving partner of cancer patient Barbara Rosenblum, begins their unusual coauthored narrative with a direct address to the reader: "We wanted to tell you our story."[12] The narrative situation here is inseparable from the act of storytelling, and the pronoun "our" signals that this particular illness narrative is unusual in its double narrators. Through the formal structure of alternating narrators, illness displays its power to enfold more than the patient alone. In addition, the opening address (we wanted to tell *you*) not only affirms what theorist Richard Kearney calls the "intersubjective model" of narrative discourse but also enfolds the reader too in the supra-dyadic force field of illness.[13] The reader is an especially important figure for Rosenblum and Butler, who write with the specific purpose that their story be "of use." The uses of narrative, however, ultimately include what writing (in the triangular bond linking teller, tale, and reader) does *to* and *for* authors. As Sandra Butler explains directly, "We wanted to tell our story, finally, because this writing made us visible to ourselves as we were living it" (*CTV* i).

Barbara Rosenblum died at age forty-four, February 14, 1988, on Valentine's Day, three years to the week after she learned of the diagnosis: stage-three breast cancer. Based on data covering 2010 to 2012, approximately 12.3 percent of women in the United States at some point in their lifetime will be diagnosed with breast cancer.[14] In 2013, over 3 million American women were living with the disease. The prospects in 1985 when Barbara Rosenblum received the awful news were even more dire. Although the death rate from breast cancer among all ethnic groups has been declining in recent years, some 39,620 American women died from breast cancer in 2013. Happy endings do occur, with unexpected remissions and difficult, protracted cures. The valiant friend who had e-mailed me with the news of her diagnosis with breast cancer is now—after a long arduous course of treatment and thanks in large part to the fine biomedical care she received—cancer free. Medical logos, nonetheless, cannot yet remove the looming threat of death from breast cancer. *Cancer in Two Voices* offers an indirect tribute to medical eros not in its power to extend individual life expectancy but in its power to improve, in crucial nonmedical ways, the *quality* of life.

The possible conflict between medical eros and medical logos (always implicit in their role as contraries) finds representative figures in Barbara Rosenblum and Sandra Butler. Rosenblum, who grew up in a Brooklyn lower-class, immigrant, Jewish family, describes herself as a secular, academic rationalist. A no-nonsense, problem-solving sociologist, she refuses to view her mastectomy as a crisis of womanhood or a blow to her self-esteem. "Losing my hair has been much harder than losing my breast," she observes in her face-the-facts, rationalist mode. "No one can see underneath my clothes. But everyone can see my hair" (*CTV* 130). Sandra Butler comes from a different Jewish background—middle-class, activist, assimilated—and she is far less given to rationalization. Emotions regularly drive her experience, and she is quick to voice her distress. "Cancer swallows up the air of my life and insinuates its presence everywhere," she writes. "Nothing remains untouched" (*CTV* 48). Medical logos, while it provides a road map for rationalist Rosenblum, has little to offer Butler. In dealing with the stress of her caregiver role, she rejects tranquillizers in favor of a therapist and a support group, where she can vent face-to-face about feeling "invisible and misunderstood" (*CTV* 108). It is understandable that the visibility conferred by narrative might prove crucial to the often-neglected caregiving partner, whose social identity illness relentlessly thins out, but it is not as evident what narrative visibility and medical eros have to offer the less expressive Rosenblum.

Rosenblum and Butler in *Cancer in Two Voices* (1991), creating a remarkable dialogic narrative that describes their three years living with breast cancer, offer a compelling vision of how serious illness continuously alters and recalibrates the experience of two loving partners. Butler, the healthy partner, never breaks free from the confining, dynamic circle of Rosenblum's illness. Their dual voices thus do not belong to separate worlds of the sick and the well but instead embody a new, conjoined reality. The narrative is most powerful in shaping its account not as a traditional story about "struggle and courage," as Butler puts it, but rather as unscripted, unfolding, journal-like entries that reveal how serious illness plays out within the shifting dynamics of a loving, two-person relationship. Their narrative thus explores ground with almost no interest for medical logos—the patient dies—but with complex and far-reaching significance for medical eros.

Cancer in Two Voices develops through irregularly alternating passages in which each partner records her experience, but their voices also record a simultaneous underground contest between medical logos and medical eros. This subterranean theme soon takes a dark turn as Rosenblum's cancer spreads. Both women swiftly adapt to their newly medicalized conversation about intravenous fluids, chest X-rays, and chemo-embolization. Rosenblum, who wrote a pioneering scholarly book on the sociology of aesthetics, laments the change as she trades theories of beauty for daily talk of Adriamycin, Cytoxan, and Prednisone. Her formidable reason also begins, slowly, to turn against the daily regimens of medical logos: "I hate how my life has turned into a series of doctor appointments, treatments, side effects, blood tests, CAT scans, liver scans, and bone scans" (*CTV* 125). Biomedicine keeps Rosenblum alive, as she knows, and she grudgingly accepts its enlarged presence— until the moment when her now-cancerous liver suddenly no longer responds to chemotherapy. A rationalist still, she makes a sober cost-benefit analysis of further treatment: terrible side effects, great risks, and very few rewards. Curiously, reason brings her to the same decision that Butler reaches with no more than a momentary burst of emotional intelligence. They both agree to exit the world of medical logos and to enter the new and uncharted territory of medical eros and not-knowing.

"Now medicine has no more knowledge to offer me," Barbara Rosenblum writes. The nadir of medical logos and the dead-end of knowledge nonetheless initiate, as for Styron, a crucial turning point. "So I have decided to face this period with the wisdom that love and friendship provide and use the time I have left to write and to have fun" (*CTV* 163). Medical eros might seem a desperate last resort—Rosenblum's white flag of surrender—but perhaps eros and logos for Rosenblum have simply changed places. Once her cancer spreads out of control, the love and friendship basic to this introspective relationship between women who met in middle age (after failed marriages) simply assert their sometimes unseen dominance. The illness narrative turns into a distinctive and hotly contested dialogue in which, as death nears for Barbara Rosenblum, it is medical eros that speaks with a dominant voice.

Medical eros takes a deep interest in topics such as pleasure and sex that hold little value for medical logos. Cardiac surgeon Larry Zaroff worked near miracles to repair the damaged heart of an underworld boss; his patient, Zaroff told me, was unimpressed and complained that the surgeries did nothing to fix his impotence. Medical logos, despite its skill in repairs, does not always recognize what the patient truly wants or fears. Rosenblum writes frankly about how the side effects of her cancer treatment involved changes in vaginal tissue, loss of vaginal moistness, and finally a complete absence of sexual desire. "I confess I was still nervous about not making love" (*CTV* 132), she admits, and Butler too confesses that she missed their former sexual intimacy, feeling vaguely cheated, as if she were back in her sexless marriage. Rosenblum knew what was going on. "I suspect Sandy would have liked it better," she writes, ever the rationalist, "if I experienced the life force as erotic energy, as libido. But I don't" (*CTV* 132). At this dangerous flash point in their strained relationship, who is the unexpected champion who saves the day with an erotic solution?

"We make love at the typewriter, not in the bedroom," writes Rosenblum about their new way to express intimacy through writing (*CTV* 132). "We typed, interrupted, criticized, added, paced, drank coffee, laughed, then grew thoughtful, intense, or joyous with relief when just the right word or image emerged. It was a making of love. An honoring of our bond. Lovemaking" (*CTV* 141). The passage captures the spirit that makes *Cancer in Two Voices* such a striking if indirect contribution to the literature of medical eros. "The work we did had the focus, the passion, the sense of completion our lovemaking once had," Butler also concludes, but this labor had nothing in common with industrial or commercial production, and it offered a knowledge that differed from the products of instrumental reason. As Butler reports on their erotics of literary coproduction, "I often felt similarly spent when a work session ended. But so loved. So known. So deeply connected to this woman" (*CTV* 141). Eros, in its embrace of not-knowing, provides access to a form of personal erotic knowledge: the lover "so known" by the beloved. It is an imperfect but crucial knowledge, whose truth lies not in repeatable experiments or in falsifiable hypotheses but rather in the power of the human connections that it permits and strengthens.

HIV: *Stories of AIDS in Africa*

Is there a politics of medical eros? Biomedicine certainly lobbies hard in its own professional and political self-interest, but not-knowing brought me to this open question because I thought I knew something about AIDS. I was wrong. I knew something about AIDS *in the developed world*. I knew nothing, however, about AIDS in Africa. Not-knowing, in this case, meant culpable ignorance—there was much I needed to learn—but I suspect that it was ignorance widely shared. How many people in Europe or North America understood the crisis in Africa? My not-knowing, as it turned out, was more than a state of ignorance. It was also a condition, basic to AIDS in Africa, that no amount of learning could stamp out. My abrupt wake up came when I encountered a book by Stephanie Nolen entitled *28: Stories of AIDS in Africa* (2007). Nolen, as the award-winning Africa bureau chief for Toronto's *Globe and Mail* newspaper, traveled extensively in Africa, and her book offers the story of one person to represent each million of the 28 million Africans infected by HIV at the time she wrote. The twenty-eight illness narratives were my belated introduction to the international, geopolitical complexities of medical eros.

Any sexually transmitted disease holds an opportunistic relation to eros. As Nolen writes, HIV targets the topics that people generally least like to discuss: "the drugs we inject, the sex we have, especially the sex with people we aren't supposed to have sex with—and the interactions least open to honest discussion or to change."[15] Traditional societies in Africa often regard the discussion of sex as taboo, which greatly inhibits prevention and treatment. Most important, Nolen emphasizes that HIV thrives on "imbalances of power" (*AA* 5). It got its foothold in Africa among sex workers, drug users, gay men, and migrants—the poorest and most marginalized members of African societies—but it also had easy access to politicized power imbalances crisscrossing the continent, much like the network of highways traveled by long-distance truckers that provided ideal transmission routes for the disease. In 1986, Rwanda did the first national survey of HIV prevalence. The nightmare result: among city-dwellers, 17.8 percent were infected. Twenty million Africans, within two decades, died from the disease. Twenty million deaths can depopulate the entire state of New York. New York City would resemble the empty postnuclear urban wastelands in disaster films. It was devastation on a scale almost impossible to understand.

Eros revealed another layer of political complication when I spent four months on a round-the-world educational cruise where my shipmates included the charismatic Emeritus Archbishop of Cape Town, Desmond Tutu. Tutu—a former lecturer and board member of the academic program Semester at Sea—is a veteran of many voyages, and he is beloved by students, whose affection he returns. I met him by virtue of signing on as faculty for the spring 2013 voyage, which included ports of call in Japan, Vietnam, China, India, and Africa. I knew about Tutu's Nobel Prize awarded for his crucial role in the transition from apartheid rule as the head of the South African Truth and Reconciliation Commission. He is less well known, however, for his role in the Desmond Tutu HIV Foundation—now housed within the Desmond Tutu HIV Centre at the University of Cape Town. The Tutu HIV Foundation provided the first and only effective treatment for HIV/AIDS in the early 1990s, when antiretroviral drugs were almost impossible to obtain elsewhere.[16] It was a time when the stigma of HIV/AIDS had turned many African patients into (socially speaking) nonpersons. Stigma in Africa operated with special cruelty because Africans do not share in the cultural legacy of rugged individualism. *Ubuntu*, a Bantu word, refers to the traditional African form of life that situates our basic humanness in social connections.[17] "*Ubuntu*," as Tutu once explained, "says that we cannot exist as a human being in isolation. We are interconnected. We are family. If you are not well, I am not well."[18]

Descartes taught Western philosophers to believe that being is identical with reason: I think, therefore I am. This ultrarationalist proposition was almost guaranteed to catch the attention of generations of professional thinkers and reasoners. Archbishop Tutu translated the founding principle of *Ubuntu* into a paradoxical, anti-Cartesian statement that subordinates human reason to human connection: "*I am because you are.*"

Eros, among its multiple influences, contributes to the affective bonds not only between individuals but also within communities. HIV / AIDS, however, held the anti-erotic power to unravel *Ubuntu*. Just as HIV / AIDS attacked the individual immune system, it also attacked the social cohesion at the heart of African identity. Nolen provides heartbreaking stories of gaunt villagers, demonized, left alone to die because fellow villagers suspected them of wasting away with Slim—the local name for AIDS. As the number of AIDS victims mounted, the number of AIDS orphans also mounted, alarmingly, as villages could no longer look after the multitudes of orphaned children. Grandmothers were unable to carry the burden of so many young castaways, and the AIDS orphans were increasingly left to fend for themselves. How does an impoverished ten-year-old girl care for her two younger siblings? Prostitution—a common solution—simply perpetuated the dilemma. HIV / AIDS, in short, held a distinctively African profile, and thus it also exposed the ways in which diseases always take the sociopolitical shapes implied by specific cultural and historical contexts. Eros was the primary vector for spreading HIV from reservoir to host, and eros in Africa seemed powerless to help mitigate the social chaos it caused. On a scale unlike the dramas that unfolded in American living rooms and with little or no organized gay resistance, in Africa it was eros against eros.

We can learn from stories. Although medical logos relegates anecdote to the lowest level of evidence-based knowledge, Kathryn Hunter has shown how medical education is, in practice, shot full of narrative, from attention-grabbing lecture material to cautionary tales swapped around the watercooler.[19] Public-health narratives can also spread the word and teach strategies of prevention. Narrative education failed badly in Africa, less from failures implicit in narrative than from African geopolitics. "Put simply," Nolen writes, "millions of Africans are living with a virus from which they might easily have been protected if they had had access to education about it, or to the means of defending themselves" (*AA* 11). Africa, she notes, consists of fifty-three countries with very different traditions, resources, languages, and political structures, and these continent-wide separations helped discourage or defeat effective responses, both narrative and medical.

True, major improvements have occurred since Nolen published her book in 2007, but such improvements (funded in part by the U.S. $15 billion Emergency Plan for AIDS Relief) possess not only a biomedical signature—medical logos as answer—but also a political and narrative subtext. While Nolen's eyewitness stories help us learn about HIV/AIDS in Africa, they also embody and describe the power of narrative, especially when the narrative is a brief speech by an eminent and beloved African hero.

"We have called you today," Nelson Mandela began in his slow, dignified style—the imprisoned political militant who became the first black president of free South Africa—"to announce that my son has died of AIDS" (*AA* 313). Mandela is justly revered worldwide, but his term as president, from 1994 to 1999, reflects the failures, blindness, and confusion marking the distinctively African story of AIDS. "While he was in office," Nolen writes of Mandela, "South Africa became the most infected nation in the world. Yet Mandela himself rarely spoke the word *AIDS*" (*AA* 316). The HIV infection rate in South Africa rose from less than 8 percent of adults when he took office to nearly 25 percent, and his personal silence as president translated into governmental paralysis. His silence—to be fair—reproduced the domestic silence that gripped villages and families, where men refused to use condoms and AIDS was a forbidden topic. "Even in 2005," Nolen explains, "when eight hundred people a day died of AIDS in South Africa, no one liked to say the word" (*AA* 315). Then on January 6, 2005, five years after he had stepped down as president, everything changed when Nelson Mandela walked slowly from his house, as if bearing the full weight of his twenty-seven years of political imprisonment—and so much more—to address the media assembled on his Johannesburg lawn and to announce the death of his son Makgatho from HIV/AIDS.

"Let us give publicity to HIV/AIDS and not hide it," Mandela continued, and his statement registered like an earthquake. This was more than a family matter. As videotape recorders rolled and cameras clicked, Mandela offered the full weight of his personal reputation in an effort to change the African culture of HIV/AIDS. Mandela spent the rest of his life—joined by his activist wife and former nurse, Graça Machel—deploying his worldwide fame in campaigning boldly, tirelessly, and effectively for social change to repair the damage that HIV / AIDS had caused and to eliminate its further threat. He kept well informed about biomedical advances, especially new drug therapies, but he was far more than a champion of medical logos. Wasn't there a trace of eros in the perpetual smile of the well-dressed, elderly, ex-president who always insisted, smiling, that he was no saint? Mandela's story of change—about the social power of one leader's late awakening—belongs to the full narrative of HIV / AIDS in Africa. It is a story that includes the revelation about how narrative possesses the power to address and to repair the damage that eros, illness, and narrative (like the narrative of stigma) can also cause.

Locked-In Syndrome: *The Diving Bell and the Butterfly*

Imagine that you wake up completely paralyzed. The only bodily motions that you control are your eyelids, and somebody just now—you don't know who—is sewing your right eyelid shut! Eventually you learn that you have spent the last several weeks in a muddled stupor, following twenty days in a coma. Well, your left eyelid works, so you have at least the blurred half-vision necessary to appreciate the absolute existential bleakness of your condition. "In one flash I saw the frightening truth," as Jean-Dominique Bauby reflects on the moment when—as his metaphors of ruin suggest—he sized up the full grimness of his situation. "It was as blinding as an atomic explosion and keener than a guillotine blade."[20]

Medical eros would seem wholly irrelevant to a patient who has recently suffered a massive cerebral stroke that knocked out his brain stem and paralyzed his motor system. The rare event, known to medical logos as "locked-in syndrome," has no standard treatment and no cure. All but 10 percent of patients with locked-in syndrome die within the first four months. The occupational therapist informs him, with a euphemistic phrase, that he is destined to live out his days in a wheelchair. His life as he has known it—as the bon vivant, forty-three-year-old editor-in-chief of the glossy Paris-based fashion magazine *Elle*—is effectively over. Biomedicine, although it can provide life-support, speech therapists, and minimal physical rehabilitation, has no answers and nothing to offer. At this impasse where reason and logic fail, his only effective recourse, solace, and hope would come from medical eros.

Locked-in syndrome, while paralyzing almost every motor function short of Bauby's left eyelid, spares his inner life—*la vie intérieure*—and thus leaves open an unanticipated passage to the erotic. "Individuality," wrote the psychologist and philosopher William James, "is founded in feeling; and the recesses of feeling, the darker, blinder strata of character, are the only places in the world in which we catch real fact in the making."[21] The *real facts* of Bauby's life, as distinct from a mere official diagnosis of locked-in syndrome and a prognosis of imminent death, have far more to do with feeling than with the natural history of disease. Helped by his speech therapist and by an incredibly patient young woman, Claude Mendibil, who served as transcriber, Bauby composed an amazing memoir by spelling out every word, letter by letter, with a blink of his one functional eyelid. That is, he would blink when Claude's finger landed on the right letter in the alphabetic frequency chart she supplied.

Narrative often takes the shape of a particular genre or subgenre, from detective fiction to horror films, but there may be no weirder illness narrative than a memoir (written by a man who cannot move) that invokes the form of travel literature. "I loved to travel," Bauby spelled out blink by blink (*DB* 103). Love of travel identifies another role for eros; this glimpse into Bauby's inner life is more than just a random bit of autobiography. He explicitly describes the book, at the outset, as "beridden travel notes" (*DB* 5), and the concept of bedridden travel captures both the ironic spirit of his crazed blink-by-blink writing project and the Gallic wit inseparable from his identity and inner life. Travel literature as a genre often involves a threat to life that ushers in the creation of a new or much-altered identity. The journeys of Bauby's inner life—from flamboyant excess to deep despair—create a one-of-a-kind document in which identity is always under threat, including the threat of death, while it is writing, ironically, in the improbable genre of travel literature that somehow sustains him.

The book's framing paradox—a travel narrative written by a man unable to move—extends even to the droll last line: "I'll be off now." Bauby, of course, has nowhere to go and no way to get there. He died two days after the French publication of his book. His inner life of airy "butterfly" excursions, as he calls his brief chapters, always returns to an immobile diving-bell body. Nonetheless, travel narratives include a long history of erotic adventure, and desire itself provides unexpected travel-related pleasures. Paralyzed, deformed, and reduced in his own unromantic account to the status of a jellyfish, he nonetheless sets off on nightly erotic adventures. "You can visit the woman you love," he says of his mental travels, "slide down beside her and stroke her still-sleeping face" (*DB* 5). Eros regularly deserts him, but also continually reappears and keeps him company. The entire chapter that he devotes to a journey he once took with his girlfriend to Lourdes—which Bauby calls the "world capital of miracles" (*DB* 61)—focuses on a romantic breakup. An unapologetic hedonist, he does not spare his own faults, and he also refuses consolation, religious, moral, and medical. He understands that his journalistic rivals in the world of Paris fashion now dismiss him as a human vegetable. He understands that medical logos has already written him off. Eros is what remains, and for Jean-Do (as his friends called him) eros proves as vital as any vital sign.

Desire is what keeps him going: "I need to feel strongly," Jean-Do confesses, "to love and to admire, just as desperately as I need to breathe" (*DB* 55). His need for strong feeling—desire raised to the level of an existential requirement—takes two main forms. First, abiding affections and friendships help constitute what he explicitly calls "the chain of love that surrounds and protects me" (*DB* 41). This chain of love includes his ninety-three-year-old shut-in father, his eight-year-old daughter, his current girlfriend, his ex-wife, his speech therapist, and the person to whom he dedicates the book, his transcriber Claude Mendibil. The imagery of love as a chain sometimes gives way to a lighter, airy, butterflylike imagery. "A letter from a friend, a Balthus painting on a postcard, a page of Saint-Simon," he writes, "give meaning to the passing hours" (*DB* 55). The "meaning" of such miscellaneous scraps and tatters of human friendship embrace an erotic dimension that he not only recognizes but also devises fantasy plans to celebrate: "One day I hope to fasten them end to end in a half-mile streamer, to float in the wind like a banner raised to the glory of friendship" (*DB* 84).

Medical eros takes a second basic but indispensable form implicit in the image of a kite-tail tribute: pleasure. Memory and imagination both transport Jean-Do on erotic mental journeys in which pleasure, as an affair of inner life independent of his locked-in state, still retains its power to excite. Such memories are, like eros, sometimes bittersweet, but they can also call up and almost reproduce the delight he took in books, warm baths, or a glass of scotch. Dreams and daydreams also carry an erotic charge. Wrapped up in blankets, he imagines that he is a director re-shooting scenes from famous films. Or he is both the film star and the character: "I am the hero of Goddard's *Pierrot le Fou*, my face smeared blue, a garland of dynamite sticks encircling my head" (*DB* 29–30). Writing held erotic, almost sexual pleasures for Barbara Rosenblum and Sandra Butler, but Bauby's nighttime travels in *la vie intérieure* (as he pre-pared for the next day's writing) temper erotic pleasure with an ironic self-awareness. As he knows, Goddard's film concludes with the hero (madman, bourgeois runaway, and philosophizing criminal) struggling to defuse the garland of lit dynamite sticks—but too late. Eros, despite the pleasures of imagination, cannot for Bauby completely ignore or erase its equally strong link with approaching death and the not-known.

The bittersweetness of eros is finally the best that Bauby can hope for, since pleasure so often comes mixed with melancholy, like the piquant scents he recalls (*DB* 103). In his mental travels, he imagines flying to Hong Kong, where a French designer had, in fact, added Bauby's image (in tribute) to a chair at the Peninsula Hotel. Would a miniskirted Chinese beauty, he wonders, choose to sit in his chair if she knew how he looked now? (*DB* 106). He creates fleeting substitute identities for himself as a race-car driver, a Roman soldier, a long-distance cyclist. Travel, real or imaginary, is not just about observing foreign cultures from an objective position of relative safety and detachment. Travel also contains a subver-sive dimension.[22] It allows us space to try on new identities. As we change place, the new places (in ways large or small) tend to change us. The unforeseen outcomes may threaten or topple identity. All travel, in this sense, is mental travel, unpredictable and dangerous.

"I am fading away," writes Bauby as his travel narrative proceeds. "Slowly but surely . . ." (*DB* 77). Neither medical eros nor medical logos can offer him a way out. The narrative shards that imagination, memory, and desire conjure up cannot erase the nightmare, regret, and futureless future that are also salient facts of Bauby's inner life. *The Diving Bell and the Butterfly* contains enough moments of surplus dread—"irrational terror swept over me" (*DB* 53)—to offset any sentimental wish to read the book solely as a feel-good testament to the human spirit. Travel in its structure usually implies a return home, if only as an object of desire, like Ulysses willing his return to Ithaca, but in Bauby's butterfly excursions the only return home is to the paralyzed diving-bell body. Pleasures are temporary; eros notoriously comes and goes. In place of optimism or edification, Bauby (antihero of the inner life) creates the narrative self-portrait of a man who struggles against horrible misfortune using as resources only desire, wit, and ironic self-awareness. His mental travels, he knows, are a kite-tail of scraps. There is no arc, no trajectory, no emergence, no homecoming. It is storytelling alone that must sustain him, like Scheherazade, until the stories give out. His jaunty, hard-won, traveler's farewell—"I'll be off now"—is a tribute to what medical eros can accomplish when medical logos gives out.

Palliative Care: *Still/Here*

"In its beginnings," wrote the famed dancer and choreographer Bill T. Jones, "dance was something that we, as a community, enjoyed. It was a way we told our stories."[23] Medical eros extends its status as contrary and supplement to medical logos far beyond written or even oral narrative: it embraces the nonverbal, bodily, communal expressiveness of dance. Jones's famous multimedia performance piece *Still/Here* (1994), created in collaboration with video artist Gretchen Bender, returns dance from purely formalist movement to what Jones considers its origins in narrative and in community, but the return takes a surprising contemporary turn. Jones based *Still/Here* on the so-called Survival Workshops that he conducted in eleven cities, enlisting as participants ordinary people who were living with serious, even terminal, illness. Medical eros has now crossed an edgy line from private bedside or personal memoir to dance—public bodies on stage engaging serious questions about illness, disability, death, and dying. Jones is undeterred. *Still/Here* also holds very personal significance because he had recently disclosed his own status as HIV-positive.

Still/Here engages bodies and dance in exploring the delicate, explosive, subsurface terrain always implicit in the links between eros and death. Eros, of course, has an ancient affinity for dance, as both rely on the allure of bodies and on a nonrational drive as primal as Dionysian rites. Narrative has long held a respected place in classical ballets, which often reenact familiar stories; but contemporary dance (like abstract art) frequently minimizes or eliminates narrative. Still, Jones might argue that even abstract contemporary dance retains some basic narrative elements, such as the couple and the romantic triangle, with their jealousies, conflicts, and gender variations. Explicit storylines are superfluous, but *Still/Here* in its bold multimedia encounters with eros and death creates a mixed form in which bodies, music, visual images, and recorded speech collide and sometimes coalesce within an interruptive, fragmented narrative frame set free from plot or story. "Bill T. Jones has always liked to talk to his audience," writes the British dance critic Judith Mackrell, "taking a moment mid-dance to entertain or lecture us about his special concerns. Even when he doesn't open his mouth, his shows still speak loudly of the politics and passions of their subject matter, whether they be sex, race, art or death."[24]

Politics and passions give *Still/Here* an erotic charge that underlies Jones's entire multimedia performance. Videotape projected onto moveable screens brought the images and voices of participants from the Survival Workshops into the live dance. That is, while his professional dancers performed stylized movements that Jones drew from observing participants at the workshop sessions, spectators simultaneously saw the faces and heard the speech of people struggling with serious illness or with the prospect of imminent death.

"My name is Tawnni Simpson," says a videotaped Survivor Workshop participant, a cystic fibrosis patient. "I'm twenty-five and I think about sex" (*LN* 264). Tawnni Simpson worries that she may never find a lover: "Sex is something that's hard for me because of my lung illness." Jones writes that it was important for him to focus on her desires, which matched the desires he recognized in his healthy young dancers. The collaborative result onstage is an extended visual *ménage à trois* in which two handsome young male dancers flirt with, flip, vie for, and fondle a petite but hardly passive female dancer "with the will and ambition of a professional quarterback," Jones adds (*LN* 264). It was the "spirit" that workshop survivors expressed in facing serious illness that Jones said he wanted to embody, as a visual metaphor, in the vitality and power of his dancers. Such spirit, too, belongs to eros and the inner life.

All this provocation was too much for Arlene Croce, the dance critic for *The New Yorker*, who ignited instant controversy starting with her first sentence: "I have not seen Bill T. Jones's *Still/Here*, and have no plans to review it."[25] In explanation, Croce asserted that Jones's work belongs to what she regarded as a misguided cultural trend toward "victim art." Richly deserved dissent poured in from celebrities in the arts, but in one small, significant area her comments are useful. *Still/Here* is remarkable because Jones based it on workshops conducted with people who might easily be placed in the class of victims, and *Still/Here* aggressively de-victimizes them. More positively, the bodies and voices both on screen and on stage celebrate an erotic passion and desire affirmed even in the face of serious illness or of imminent death. *Still/Here* both frees serious illness from the dominance of medical logos and—while never denying the struggle that illness entails—manages ultimately to celebrate a joyful, indomitable, and even erotic will to live. The videotape images, projected on three giant screens, return toward the conclusion to dwell on the faces of workshop participants—among them a young girl ("Lucy") seen at the start wearing a baseball cap. As Jones described the scene, "The electronic blue of the third screen suddenly blossoms into the moonlike visage of Lucy, a young cancer survivor wearing a cap; she smiles enigmatically, drops her eyes, and appears to float up and out" (*LN* 259). The enigmatic smile, like the embraces that Jones shared with workshop participants, offers an unspoken assent to life that leads beyond speech or reason, beyond logos, into a realm of erotic not-knowing.

An assent to life, in Bataille's account of eroticism, cannot deny or ignore death, which participates in the erotic as well as marking its limit. Death, of course, takes many forms: as the mother of beauty, aching melancholy, autumnal fullness, or even as Sadean night journeys into the abject and horrific. *Still/Here* does not deny or ignore death but rather celebrates the life force that endures even in the shadow of death and dying. The only voice that it denies is the personal or social narrative of victimization. *Still/Here* is not victim art, whatever that might be, but rather an art that gives body, voice, movement, some measure of grace, and full human status to people whom critics such as Croce might classify as victims. Jones had a personal motive to face the dehumanizing aspects of serious illness. In a televised interview Bill Moyers asked what

Jones most feared. Jones instantly replied, "Pain." He had watched his long-time lover and artistic partner, Arnie Zane, die of HIV/AIDS in un-bearable agonies that left Zane (as Jones says) "bleating like an animal."[26]

Palliative medicine is a relatively recent subfield that has grown in stature and in importance since *Still/Here* opened in 1994. The U.S. Academy of Hospice Physicians was formed in 1988, and it took its present name, the American Academy of Hospice and Palliative Medicine, in 2000. Hospice has its roots in the United Kingdom through the work of Dame Cicely Saunders. Palliative medicine defines its scope more broadly as the prevention and relief of suffering, especially in patients with serious and life-threatening illnesses. The World Health Organization both widens and narrows the focus in stating that palliative medicine attends to the assessment and treatment of pain and other problems, "physical, psychosocial and spiritual."[27]

Physicians trained in the biomedical model still complain that pallia-tion implies merely "covering up" symptoms, as opposed to the biomed-ical emphasis on prevention, treatment, and cure. The Latin root *palla* does refer to an outer cloak or covering, but cloaks in earlier eras—before sidewalks and paved roads—had a job to do: offering protection against the assault of dirt, mud, rain, and sleet. Palliative medicine might be de-scribed as protecting patients against the assault of symptoms.[28] Its rise coincides with a period when attitudes toward the treatment of dying or terminally ill patients are changing faster among doctors than among fam-ilies, who are more often now the source of demands for every available drug and procedure. Too many patients delay the choice of hospice until the last week of life and so miss out on the solid advantages that hospice care provides. Ruth, for example, has received a greatly improved wheel-chair with braces installed that prevent her head from slumping to one side. Some patients actually improve after declining further biomedical attention. The staff, almost like proud parents, say that the patient has "graduated" from hospice care. This is a topic, however, that for me stirs nightmarish emotional conflicts, as hospice now keeps oxygen and mor-phine ready at Ruth's bedside, and I simply wait.

Bill T. Jones in *Still/Here* offers more than a bold performance af-firming life in the face of serious illness and death. He also points up the larger personal and cultural need to invent compelling new narratives of death and dying.

What might new narratives of death and dying look like? Medical logos here lacks tools and resources for change, since it in effect authorizes (even if it does not actively promote) the prevailing end-of-life narrative that enfolds patients in the frontier myth of fighting to the bitter end. Dylan Thomas put this American myth in more poetic imperative: *Do not go gently*. In truth, patients at the end of life are often too weak to fight, lying semicomatose, hooked up to blinking, beeping biotechnologies. The biomedical narrative also implicitly endorses a spare-no-costs approach, until the medical ammunition runs out. The social and economic costs are massive: medical care at the end of life now consumes 10 percent to 12 percent of the total U.S. health-care budget. It consumes a whopping 27 percent of the Medicare budget. The biomedical or frontier narrative is not only ruinously expensive but also, as many frustrated physicians will tell you, inhumane. Why order more tests for patients in their nineties dying of end-stage cancer? Barbara Rosenblum had to create her own personal narrative frame when she decided to discontinue further medical treatment. "I will not fight loudly into the night," she asserts, perhaps with a nod to Dylan Thomas. "I will go softly and with love."[29]

We like to say *cost is no object* when it comes to medical care, especially at the end of life, but we are deceiving ourselves. Cost is a crushing burden, and cost-related medical decisions about limiting care are made every day, if not publicized. Suppose a new narrative of death and dying saved significant sums, in addition to its primary focus on compassionate end-of-life care? Hospice and advance directives (specifying end-of-life choices) can offer significant cost savings if used effectively. Between 25 percent and 40 percent of health-care costs at present are incurred during the last month of life.[30] What changes might persuade people to make end-of-life decisions that are not only in their own best interest but also in the interests of the nation? Medical eros, as the power that holds sway over narrative, might offer two narrative possibilities with real hope for transforming the way patients choose to die.

Narratives of healing can offer a valuable alternative to the biomedical emphasis on treatment and cure. Ira Byock, a palliative medicine specialist, makes a critical distinction between cure and healing, emphasizing that many forms of healing can take place even as patients enter their last weeks of life.[31] In terminal illness, *cure* is by definition not within reach, but dying patients can experience rich and vital *healing*—families reconciled, feuds ended, friendships honored, blessings spoken. Many patients and families, when offered access to such narratives of healing, will likely prefer them to hospital exits in which their loved ones die in extreme pain, unresponsive, worn down by futile, invasive, agonizing medical treatments with no real hope of recovery or cure. Such narratives would certainly include Barbara Rosenblum's softer turn from cure toward "love." Love is undoubtedly a primal agent of healing, and a new end-of-life narrative that emphasizes healing would allow more patients to make a timely, worthwhile, informed choice of hospice care.

Narratives of contract sound more like legal documents than stories, but they can both offer guarantees and create a new end-of-life story. Modern life is already regulated by legal contracts, and legal documents are commonplace in medical settings. Some providers now require signed contracts, for example, from patients who receive prescription opioid painkillers. Moreover, good deals run smoothly along the American grain, and a new end-of-life contractual narrative has the advantage of offering patients a deal some will be unable to refuse. For the American grain includes one specific end-of-life idiosyncrasy: it turns out, as one survey found, that Americans are not afraid of dying—they are afraid of *dying in pain*. Both hospice care and palliative medicine, with their focus on symptom relief, are very well supplied (thanks to medical logos) with established methods to reduce and to control pain. Suppose, then, as an alternative to the biomedical myth of cure, medical eros offered patients an ironclad contract for a pain-free death. No death panels, no coercion, simply a contract and a choice. Patients who choose to accept the contract can dismiss one massive fear, and a pain-free death is well within the power of palliative medicine to guarantee. (The contract would be unavailable, however, in a tiny fraction of medical cases where pain control is very difficult.) The narrative of a contract at least respects the rights of patients. It gives patients and families a choice, it can facilitate opportunities for healing, and it helps eliminate or address the unbearable fear of dying in pain. The authors of a book-length study of hospice patients did not expect what they found: "We were amazed," they report, "at the examples of the therapeutic power of human presence, honesty, compassion, humility, humor, and the affirmation of life."[32]

Eros holds a close—uncomfortably close—relation with death and dying, but it can also transform even our last moments into an affirmation. Keatsian longing for transcendence ("half in love with easeful Death") may not strike the right tone today, but it suggests that end-of-life desires often yield unique personal narratives: stories that we invent and live out, right up to The End. Doctors may be caught in the impasse between their professional desire to preserve life and a dying patient's desire to accept death. Medical eros, among the gifts of narrative competence, at least offers patients the option to write their own endings, which have increasingly less to do with biomedicine and with hospital settings.

Oliver Sacks wrote his last slim book, *Gratitude* (2016), in his eighties, when a fatal melanoma had metastasized to his liver.[33] In its quartet of brief essays, the book ignores the biomedical details of his illness. Instead, it revisits moments from his own individual life story: from the early rejection of his Jewish heritage to the much later embrace of his gay sexuality. As if in silent tribute to Asklepios, *Gratitude* opens with a dream—"huge, shining globules of quicksilver rising and falling"—while its final sentence ends on an equally internal and personal note, in his private truce with Old Testament laws. "I find my thoughts drifting to the Sabbath, the seventh day of the week, and perhaps the seventh day of one's life as well, when one can feel that one's work is done, and one may, in good conscience, rest." The movement from "I" to "one" erases any hint of egotism from Sacks's summation of a life spent in the tireless service of medicine, but a life spent, too, in writing his distinctive "clinical tales" that affirm remarkable human powers demonstrated even amid the experience of illness and disabilities. Eros nourished him as much as logos. He loved music; music and chemistry were his twin abiding passions. *Gratitude*, for me, ranks with Schubert's great D-minor string quartet *Death and the Maiden*, composed when Schubert, too, knew that that he was dying—personal, bittersweet, but not bitter.

Eros offers the possibility for narrating the individual, personal, even idiosyncratic conclusions we most desire, even amid fears and not-knowing. We know what Bill T. Jones feared most. *Pain*. What did Jones *love* most? Bill Moyers put this unexpected question to him in an interview. Jones moved in a graceful arc and replied simply, "This." His bodily response underlines the affirmations, despite pain and serious illness, that *Still/Here*, too, embodies in its fragmentary multimedia narrative of dancers in motion. Perhaps, as individuals if not yet as cultures, we are already constructing the new narratives we desire. The Cedars-Sinai Hospital complex in Los Angeles—covering almost two city blocks—displays along its corridors original paintings and limited-edition prints donated mostly by former patients and families, in gratitude. "How do you cope with grief?" an interviewer asked Jones after Arnie Zane's death. *"Locate your passion,"* Jones responded, *"find out what you love, and give yourself to it"* (*LN* 249).

CHAPTER FIVE

Eros Modigliani: Assenting to Life

Stripping naked is the decisive action.

GEORGES BATAILLE, *EROTISM* (1962)

NARRATIVES OF PASSION and eros are not hard to find in Modernist Paris. "I will never forget Modigliani's funeral," wrote the sculptor Jacques Lipchitz of the bitter-cold January day in Paris 1920. "So many friends, so many flowers, the sidewalks crowded with people bowing their heads in grief and respect. Everyone felt deeply that Montparnasse had lost something precious, something very essential."[1] Montparnasse, as spiritual home to the painters, writers, musicians, and dancers who transformed twentieth-century art, knew very well the disappearances, wasting illnesses, and abrupt suicides that, among the survivors, failed to extinguish a will to create. Notice how Jean Cocteau, writer, artist, filmmaker, and right-bank outsider who seemed to know everyone in Montparnasse, begins the honor roll of great contemporaries: "Modigliani, Kisling, Lipchitz, Brancusi, Apollinaire, Max Jacob, Blaise Cendrars, Pierre Reverdy, Salmon, all those men who barely understood what they were doing, but who were causing a real revolution in art, literature, painting and sculpture."[2] Poverty was not shameful for the often penniless Amedeo Modigliani and his comrades but almost an

135

ideological precondition of art: the mark of a shared freedom from middle-class values that allowed them to stand apart while they pursued a revolution into the not-known. Better to give away drawings for a glass of wine, like the Italian hothead Modigliani, than to take the safe, well-known, commercial route. *Was Modigliani a madman?* an interviewer asked Cocteau. He must have been mad, Cocteau replied, to give away his drawings.[3] Modi, as friends called him, often said he wanted a life "brief but intense."[4] He got what he wanted—dead at thirty-six, with unseen costs. Two days after he died, Jeanne Hébuterne, his pregnant, common-law wife, leapt to her death from a fifth-floor window in the home of her bourgeois parents. Her body lay unclaimed on the pavement below for hours.

Famous and soon-to-be famous contemporary artist-friends walked in the funeral cortège. Picasso, Kisling, Salmon, Ortiz, Brancusi, Vlaminck, Derain, Soutine. The coach carrying his body was smothered in flowers, courtesy of his absent brother, a socialist deputy back home in Italy, whose telegram read, "Bury him like a prince."[5] The same police who had so often run him in for public intoxication now stood at attention. "D'you see?" said Picasso, referring to the nemesis-police lining the street. "Now he is avenged."[6] The belated payback extended to Paris dealers who overnight jacked up prices on his previously unsaleable works. Today, spectators crowd his blockbuster museum shows, somewhat to the dismay of elitist art critic Robert Hughes. Modigliani's painting, he jabs, is "modern art for people who don't much like modernism." He describes "a queue of pilgrims"—another jab—lined up halfway around a New York City block and adds, from his knowing height, "The nudes are, of course, what the general public most likes, but they tend to be overvalued."[7]

Modigliani's nudes are precisely what I want to take as my subject, in a sideways or slant approach to eros and illness. Questions of value, artistic or financial, are not my main focus, although it is worth noting that in November 2015 Modigliani's *Reclining Nude* sold at Christie's for $170 million—then the second-highest price ever paid for a painting at auction.[8] Modigliani was Ruth's favorite painter, both Jewish, both born on July 12, and his understudied nudes allow us to pursue eros and illness from writing and dance—from Anatole Broyard through Bill T. Jones—into the visual arts. Modigliani is almost unique and truly distinctive among Modernist painters for his focus on the human figure, especially in his melancholy signature swan-necked portraits, but the nudes are where he emerges unmistakably as the painter of eros: eros as a life-affirming, life-enhancing, life-giving power. Bataille described eroticism as assenting to life up to the point of death. Eros in Modigliani's series of glowing apricot nudes is the power of assenting to life up to, or including, the point of death. His nudes give him a central place in the narrative of medical eros as it enters the era when medical logos is just beginning to secure its professional power and when death takes on shapes never before witnessed in the history of Western civilization.

Nudes and Nakedness: The Artist Stripped Bare

"There's only one man in Paris who knows how to dress," said Picasso, "and that is Modigliani."[9] Personal display and performance, which extended to what he wore no matter how threadbare, played a crucial role in Modigliani's style. He cut a memorable figure in his trademark dark brown corduroy suit and red silk scarf, which as he doubtless knew simply accentuated his handsome features and smoldering brown eyes. "Women," as one observer put it, "could not take their eyes off him."[10] Picasso early on favored the blue overalls worn by zinc miners or, for photographs, dressed up like a college professor, but he never underestimated Modigliani's talent. The single crime with which Picasso reproached himself (in a life remarkable for acts worthy of self-reproach) occurred when once, dirt poor, he painted over a Modigliani canvas. Dress and self-display mattered to the ragtag multinational artists reinventing modern art in Paris, and not just as statements of fashion. Acts of covering and uncovering—abrupt exposures of the hidden truth—carried new significance in an era seeking to create not only a new art but also a new society. Dress expressed a sense that the veneer of an old world—formal academic art and a staid bourgeois social order—was peeling away, in decadent layers, right before their eyes.

"Paris," according to Gertrude Stein, who knew about such things, "was where the twentieth century was."[11] Paris is certainly where Modigliani was, despite several trips back to Italy to recover his health. Paris and the twentieth century also included private rituals and not-safe-for-public-view displays. As the Montparnasse evenings passed deeper into alcohol and drugs, the impoverished young Italian painter with, as several friends observed, the bearing of an aristocrat or prince, would begin to remove his clothes. Maybe it was at Marie Vassilieff's canteen, where the Russian painter (who had studied with Matisse) converted her second-floor studio into a cheap refuge for the painters she loved. All the regulars knew the ritual. Modi would stand upright and start by un-wrapping the long red scarf—four or five feet long—coiled around his waist in the style of French workers. Sometimes, knowing what was about to happen, friends seized him and tied up the scarf. But they were not always so quick. The trousers slipped down to his ankles as he simul-taneously pulled up his shirt. Modesty was not his style: "Aren't I hand-some? Beautiful as a new-born babe or just out of the bath. Don't I look like a god?"[12] Then came verses recited by heart from Dante, his Italian poet-hero, or passages from *Les chants de Maldoror*, a prose hallucina-tion by the obscure nineteenth-century French poet Isidore Ducasse, who published under the name Lautréamont, died young, and vanished without a trace. Modi carried a copy of *Maldoror* everywhere, and it soon became the sacred book of surrealism.[13] A cynic-outlaw at war with bourgeois society, Maldoror spoke for the torment that many friends rec-ognized in Modi despite the charade of brash self-exposure. "A dark fire," as Cocteau wrote, "lit his whole being."[14]

The public display of Dionysian excess, for Modi, was both strategic and intimately connected with private concealment, if only as a smoke-screen, and the truths hidden by his erratic public displays quite often centered on eros, including its self-destructive range. The affectionate nickname Modi is indistinguishable in spoken French from *maudit*, or *cursed*: an epithet bestowed on writers and artists in the dark romantic tradition of Baudelaire (another Modi favorite). His charm and aristocratic bearing, when stripped away by anger, drugs, or alcohol, exposed the brooding temper and scornful laugh that made him such a mercurial com-panion. He famously greeted strangers to the city of Notre Dame with the aggressive announcement "I am Modigliani. Jew!"[15] Certain truths, for Modi, could not remain hidden and still remain true. Exposure was a necessity. Or—fissured by self-contradiction—he exposed surface emotion in order to keep deeper passions in protective concealment. The young Russian writer Ilya Ehrenburg observed Modi's plunges into "unrest, horror, and rage" but noted also how he spurned the usual café art talk in favor of discussing literature and philosophy. Philosophy and rage, literature and striptease. The multiple layers or strata kept something forever unseen. "I was always astonished by the scope of his reading," Ehrenburg expanded. "I don't think I have ever met another painter who loved poetry so deeply."[16]

The secret to Modigliani's art is its interest in what remains secret. "It was human beings that interested him most of all and the invisible forces that were at work in them," said Léopold Survage, a perceptive French painter who met him at the artist-café La Rotonde. "Behind the physical appearance he imagined . . . a mysterious world."[17] Modi never painted a still life, and he painted only one landscape, derivative and unsuccessful. Individual human beings are his subject and especially—if one credits Survage—the "invisible forces" at work within and behind them. Such an explanation helps account for his insistence on working with a living model: academic plaster casts preserved the form but not the human vitality. Vital models also meant *untrained* models, and several sources confirm that he "loathed" professional models.

His portraits leave no doubt that Modigliani was in pursuit of something beyond an accurate representation of physical appearances, as his usual method involved dismissing the model after a few sittings in order to "complete the work from his imagination."[18] What did this imaginative supplement reveal or suggest? A "mysterious world" behind appearances? The swan-necked portraits might yield many responses, but I am concerned with the nudes only. One fact is undeniable: he painted no male nudes; his nudes are all women. His work, moreover, is distinctive even within the long painterly tradition of the female nude. In an exploratory spirit, without presuming to offer definitive claims, I want to pursue the thought that eros—both in its life-affirming desires and in its almost requisite immersions into not-knowing—stands foremost among the invisible forces somehow exposed in Modi's series of astonishingly exposed female nudes. First, some background and an interlude.

Some Background

The nude in Western painting is an academic exercise as predictable as the still life, but Modi's nudes explicitly flout academic traditions, and he held such a lofty view of art and of the artist's role that it is impossible to regard the nudes as potboilers for a bourgeois marketplace. The nudes enter Modigliani's work only at a specific period—late in his life—when his friends were alarmed at his sudden visible deterioration after years of alcohol, hashish, hard living, poverty, and illness. Eyewitnesses described him in the midst of a meal doubled over coughing. Spitting blood as he painted, cigarettes and rum close by his palette, Modi doubtless understood his work on the luminous, glowing nudes within the context of his devil's bargain for a life short but intense.

The intensity is photographic. A late image shows the formerly handsome, clean-shaven artist, who had been so obsessively well-dressed, now looking like a gaunt, bearded, wild-eyed figure out of Dostoevsky's underground. "He would thump his chest," according to one report, "saying: 'Oh, I know I'm done!' "[19] In the harsh Paris winter, Modi's devoted dealer Léopold Zborowski, a cash-strapped Polish Jew with a poetic sensibility and a heart of gold, sold his only overcoat to buy painting materials for his client. He then installed Modi in a studio—a room in Zborowski's apartment—supplying rum, models, and a small daily stipend. It was Zborowski who commissioned the nudes that Modi thereafter painted (as Cocteau reports) *"ceaselessly."*[20]

Something is at stake here, in this ceaselessness, beyond a painterly interest in form or in ideologies and manifestoes. Classical nudes by definition uncover the female body, but in some sense they cover over or clothe the body's nakedness with the trappings of high art. Are Modi's uncoverings, nonclassical in the extreme, a mode of concealment? Might nakedness leave space for the unknown or unknowable? Or, a direct personal question, why am I so drawn to these nudes? Artists whose work Modi knew well (Botticelli, Titian, Ingres, Manet, Degas) painted masterly nudes that don't particularly move me, so female nudity or artistic skill cannot entirely account for my response. Some art critics find female nudes an oppressive expression of male power: the male artist clothed, the female model naked, and the infamous "gaze" of the spectator unequivocally gendered male. Modi recognized a time-honored gender politics of the studio, with its erotic imbalances of power. "When a woman poses for a painter," he explained, "she gives herself to him."[21] Picasso produced an entire near-pornographic suite in which Raphael paints while he simultaneously fornicates with his mistress-model. Ruth, not one to tolerate oppression or gender imbalance, loved these Modi nudes as much as I do. My questions, right or wrong, do not concern gender or gaze. I keep asking what is it that gives these mysterious, calm, milky-orange nudes such amazing power?

An Interlude

I have somehow arranged a private visit to a Modigliani nude owned by the Guggenheim Museum and currently stored in a New York City warehouse. Precautions for my visit are worthy of a spy novel. The curator telephones me the address only a few hours before my appointment. A taxi winds through semideserted industrial streets to a nondescript brick building with a single steel door in a windowless, fortress-like façade. I have been granted a one-hour audience alone with the painting.

Eros preoccupies me as I lie stretched on the cement floor of the warehouse—in the almost deserted, echoing, industrial space, no museum etiquette is required—gazing underneath a sunny third-floor side widow at a priceless Modigliani painting from 1917, entitled simply *Nude* (Figure 5.1). I recline inches away from the creamy hues and surprisingly rough textures of a woman painted with eyes closed, wearing a necklace that only emphasizes (in its minimalist semicircle of beaded concealment) her absolute and totally serene nakedness.

Nakedness differs from nudity, according to Sir Kenneth Clark in *The Nude: A Study in Ideal Form* (1956).[22] Nudity, for Clark, belongs to high art. It concerns the perfection of form as represented in classical statuary, mostly male nudes, and it calls for a calm, contemplative, aesthetic response. Nakedness, in Clark's influential contrast, belongs to the unideal messiness of actual human flesh: it concerns kinetic desire as opposed to static contemplation. The difference between nudity and nakedness, at least as Clark proposes it, resembles the geometrical repose of a perfect circle compared with the turmoil of a sexual affair. Clark views the

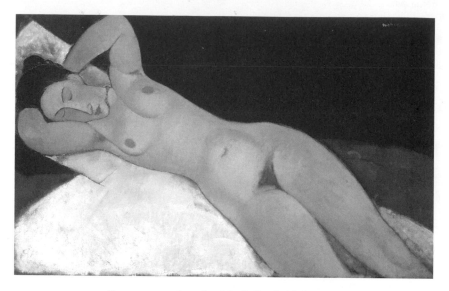

FIGURE 5.1. Amedeo Modigliani. *Nude.* 1917.
Photo Credit: The Solomon R. Guggenheim Foundation / Art Resource, NY.

idealized nude as representing the power of art to transform bare life. As I recline beside Modi's reclining nude, I am having none of these stale Clarkisms, and neither is art historian Lynda Nead in *The Female Nude* (1992). Nead offers a feminist critique of Clark's distinction, emphasizing that the naked body is never simply bare: "Even at the most basic levels," she writes, "the body is always produced through representation."[23] Nakedness represents one body, nudity another, if you even buy such a bogus Clarkian distinction.

A distinction between nakedness and the nude silently reproduces earlier theological distinctions that construe nudity (as, for example, in Eden) as representing Adam and Eve in a state of ideal innocence: "clothed," as the explicit theological paradox runs, with divine grace.[24] The Fall of Man, in this theological reading, is what introduced nakedness, fig leaves, and material clothing once the immaterial clothing of divine grace was lost. Modi's nude propped by the window is certainly not clothed in a Christianized divine grace, as far as I can tell. Its power is inseparable from its transgressions. It is, in a poetic paradox that Modi could appreciate with his knowledge of painterly tradition, a truly naked nude. The erotic creamy rich sensual flesh tones are sufficient to turn

Clark's outdated formula inside out, upside down, and backwards. These are nudes somehow set free from tradition.

I am gazing at the necklace. The necklace sends an erotic signal, much like a red scarf or stripper's veil, as the modest strand of jewelry here only serves to highlight an absence of clothes: it turns nakedness hypernaked. It also raises questions. Why does she wear a necklace? Self-expression? Self-adornment? Or a calculated erotic lure? I recall Édouard Manet's *Olympia* (1865) and its shocking revision of Titian's *Venus d'Urbino*, in which Venus reappears as a high-priced prostitute, utterly naked except for the black silk ribbon around her neck, perhaps a sign of her genteel enslavement as a kept woman or simply another prop in the bedroom where eros is on display and for sale. Modi's necklace, by comparison, seems innocent in its ambiguities, even as he depicts the woman as suspended in a private, indeterminate space, defined only by swatches of solid color free from the social details that mark Olympia's expensive boudoir. Formalists might admire how Modi's semicircular necklace enters into a geometry repeated in the pubic triangle. Form did not occupy the Montparnasse regular Francis Carco, penname for French writer François Carcopino-Tusoli, who owned several Modi nudes and whose response was far more kinetic than Lord Clark's aesthetic allows. "I had these nudes in my home like a lover," he writes, "they were women I loved and I felt alive beside them. And they were alive: their presence excited me."[25]

Aliveness—represented in the painting and communicated to the viewer—is a quality absolutely central to Modigliani's art. He saw the artist as a privileged benefactor of aliveness. *"Life is a gift,"* he wrote on the back of a painting, *"from those who have it and know it to those who don't have it and don't know it."*[26] This grandiose statement, which he borrowed from a favorite popular Italian novelist, defines the artist's gift not as a talent or genius for making art but rather as the possession of a power to awaken and to revitalize: to bestow an aliveness on sleepwalkers who don't have it and don't know they don't have it.

But there is more to ponder as I recline on the cool cement. What about the eyes? Closed eyes are a recurrent feature in Modigliani's work, but in the nudes they suggest a private and interior state: the woman is not asleep but rather given over to her own inwardness, as in daydream or meditation.

In contrast to Olympia's brazen stare as she gazes directly at the viewer or customer, the closed eyes of Modi's nudes suggest an inner life to which the spectator has no access. Modigliani creates a hypervisible nakedness and absolute exposure, down to the pubic hair, but nonetheless also manages to convey a sense of something still withdrawn and inaccessible. His mystical Catholic poet friend Max Jacob once said that Modi's portraits, which frequently depicted specific individuals from Cocteau to Diego Rivera, did not seek to capture appearances or personality but rather "the splendour of the soul."[27] As I continue to gaze, Modi's nude seems to embody a self-possession that eludes all categories of control or of understanding. The standard female images embodying male desire—earth mother, virgin, whore, showgirl, sex goddess—just don't apply as they run up against an enigmatic surplus they cannot account for. What is it, then, that keeps me coming back (what kept Modi coming back) to these erotic, sensuous, mysterious end-of-life nudes?

Eros *Ensemble*: The Nudes as a Series

I realize, once outside the warehouse, after passing through at least three layers of security to reach the exit, that my question contains its own response. Modi kept coming back because he understood the nudes as a series. Series are defined by the assumption that one is not enough: completion or at least fullness requires repetition. Art historians, in mostly ignoring Modi's nudes, naturally ignored the crucial fact that he conceived of the nudes as a series. Modigliani, as his work indicates, *thinks* in series. The series constitutes his basic unit of composition; it corresponds to periods or styles for Picasso. When asked once what school or style his work belongs to, Modi replied, "Modigliani!"[28] His portraits all bear a family resemblance as Modiglianis, whether the sitter is Cocteau (thin, prim, and well-dressed) or a stout nameless working-class girl, and in this sense they also comprise an undisclosed series. The nudes are not curious outliers, then, but belong to Modigliani's serial imagination. The importance of seeing the nudes as a series lies in the ensemble-effect that alters the impact and understanding of any single work, much like the limestone heads that he displayed in the Salon d'Automne exhibition of 1912. The catalogue describes them as "*Têtes, ensemble décoratif.*" Individual heads are impressive, but, set in a semicircle, together they create a new and distinctive artwork that one observer compared to archaic gods from an unknown religion. When sculptor Jacques Lipchitz encountered several of the heads set in the open courtyard of Modigliani's studio, Modi explained directly that he had conceived of them "as an ensemble."[29] So, too, were the *ensemble nudes*—or, as I prefer to think of them, slightly adapting a title now affixed to one of the major paintings in the series, the Grand Nudes.

The decision to paint a series of nudes placed Modigliani in a role he relished: direct opposition to authority. *"We demand, for ten years, the total suppression of the nude in painting."* So insisted Modi's fellow countrymen, the Italian Futurists, in the manifesto of 1909. The nude, they insisted, was "as nauseous and as tedious as adultery in literature."[30] Modigliani pointedly refused to sign their *Futurist Manifesto*, published in *Le Figaro*, which sought to demolish museums, declared an intent to "glorify war," and openly announced its "scorn for women." A racing car is more beautiful than the Winged Victory of Samothrace, they proclaimed. This is the artistic context within which the deliberate decision to paint not just one nude but a series of nudes marks a significant individual stance. Poet André Salmon, who spent his early years wandering Paris with Modigliani and Picasso, put it quite simply: "Modigliani is the only painter of the nude that we have."[31]

Modi's opposition to authorities extended to his relation to the painterly traditions old and new. His love of the Italian old masters meant that opposition did not take the form of direct rejections but rather of indirect revisions. Art historians sometimes detect allusions in Modi's nudes to previous works such as Giorgione's *Sleeping Venus*, but Modi's nudes are deliberately unlike the goddess of love, or any goddesses, whose ghostly remembrance serves only to emphasize the gulf separating classical deities from Modi's flesh-and-blood women. Their sensual radiance and repose are less evocative of divine grace or goddess worship than of postcoital glow. On the other hand, he equally keeps his distance from Picasso's angular, distorted, sometimes misogynistic images of women, often former lovers, much as he avoids both the celebrated Cubist dismemberments of the body and its depictions of crude sexuality. Picasso, asked to explain the difference between art and sexuality, replied bluntly: they are "the same."[32] Modigliani rejects Picasso's absolute equation between art and sexuality. Modi's nudes affirm a sensuality in which the women in their dreamlike suspended radiance explore, through an unconcealment oddly detached from sexual desires, rich variations in the free play of eros.

The series of nudes marks a very distinctive turn in Modigliani's lifelong devotion to eros. It all starts with his own sensual presence. On approaching Modi's hut-like studio at night, an observer reported seeing a woman in a kimono, breasts uncovered and hair down, dancing madly in the moonlight. Modi, "like a faun," was opposite her, leaping and yelling. Then, as the observer says, "the woman dropped her kimono and the two danced nude."[33] The same body-centered intensity carried over to the act of painting. The Japanese painter Tsuguharu Foujita, another Montparnasse veteran, said that Modigliani painted in a manner almost "orgiastic": "he went through all sorts of gesticulations . . . his shoulders heaved. He panted. He made grimaces and cried out. You couldn't come near."[34] His faithful dealer Zborowski was banished from the studio (in his own apartment) whenever Modi worked on a nude. Although many nudes explore more serene variations of eros, some are so open and uninhibited in their self-display, with an almost calendar-art sensuality, that painting seems momentarily given over to the limb-loosening, category-rending, classical power of desire, as in his *Reclining Nude* (Figure 5.2).

"All he did was growl; he used to make me shiver from head to foot," wrote the famed Montparnasse model and baker's daughter, Alice Prin, better known as Kiki, as she told of her encounters with Modi.[35] She did not omit to mention that she found him unusually "good-looking." Eros circulates through Modi's nudes in ways that are finally uncontainable, like the erotic impulses circulating through Montparnasse, where Kiki not only refused to wear panties but also turned public cartwheels calculated to distress the same bourgeois culture that strives to contain eros. No panties, she said, gave her the same freedom as men to piss outdoors. Eros affirms a private license that necessarily subverts settled hierarchies, regulations, and restraints. The nudes in their Kiki-like less-than-subtle ways affirm an escape from the authority of reason.

Eros, while central to Modigliani's assertion that the artist bestows on sleepwalkers the gift of life, nevertheless entails a distressing proviso. As Anne Carson explains, eros depends on a geometry of lack. We desire

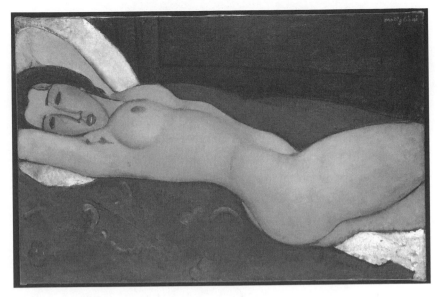

FIGURE 5.2. Amedeo Modigliani. *Reclining Nude*. 1917.
Oil on canvas. The Mr. and Mrs. Klaus G. Perls Collection. The Metropolitan
Museum of Art, New York, NY. Image copyright © The Metropolitan
Museum of Art. Image source: Art Resource, NY.

only what we don't possess—and what perhaps is permanently out of
reach. Between the lover and the beloved, then, a gap opens and an obstacle emerges.[36] Comedies overcome all obstacles and unite the lovers,
but comedy is only one mood of eros. Eros, in the intensified aliveness
that it imparts as its gift, cannot prevent a recognition that the ultimate
immoveable obstacle is of course death. Unlike the vacuous kitsch knock-
offs circulating on the Internet, Modi's nudes in their glowing vitality
cannot finally break away from this darkening embrace with death. Eros
and thanatos, love and death, meet in the luminous Modigliani nudes
in as-yet unexplored ways that confront us ultimately with serious questions about illness and about its possible relation to medical eros.

Eros as Action: Disturbances in the Field

Bataille in his account of eros describes stripping naked as "the decisive
action."[37] His statement deserves at least modest unfolding. First, the erotic
involves action, and thus it is far more than a mere attitude or feeling.

Second, the actions of eros entail an exposure far more uncivilized than simply disrobing for bed: stripping naked returns us to a primal or primary condition, both of bodies and of minds. Third, such primal exposures imply serious threats or disturbances. Eros does more than put inner life "in play," as Bataille's English translator puts it; as the French text says, eros puts the inner life "in question" (en question). According to Francis Carco, when his female concierge discovered a Modi nude on his bedroom wall, she "nearly dropped dead."[38] Parisian gendarmes were equally disturbed—perhaps for different reasons or feelings—and took counteraction to restore civil order and social equilibrium. The police commissioner, unluckily stationed across from the gallery where Modi's one-artist show was scheduled to open, had noticed crowds milling about the gallery. The source? A Modi nude in the gallery window. The commissioner sent an officer to demand its immediate removal. Berthe Weill, the gallery owner, crossed the street to ask why. "Those nudes," the commissioner stammered, "they have . . . hair!"[39]

The hypernakedness of Modi's nudes—nakedness doubly intensified by the exposed pubic triangle—constituted even in Modernist Paris of 1917 an affront to official values: the violation of an implicit taboo and an invocation of eros that threatened (as eros in its excess regularly threatens) a disturbance of the peace and an implicit danger to public order. Eros in its actions not only disturbs the peace. The whole business of eroticism, as Bataille says, is to destroy the self-contained character of the participators as they are in their normal lives. Such destruction, whatever the outward consequences, is an act of inner life, and actions of inner life often proceed in a private space, almost in secret or by stealth. The real danger posed by Modi's nude hung in Berthe Weill's gallery window had nothing to do with crowd control and everything to do with internal actions. It is thus worth exploring briefly, for their ultimate relevance to issues of illness and health, what specific internal sources of disturbance Modi's nudes threatened to uncover or uncheck.

The nakedness of Modi's nudes posed a particular threat in its suggestion of a stealth female agency no doubt disturbing well beyond the police force. The nudes, that is, depict individual women in the quiet, self-assured acceptance of their own sexuality. The women are no less subversive for their dreaming or meditative repose, especially because in their stillness they also appear enveloped in a private state of pleasure. They implicitly challenge the bourgeois norms that expected women to deny any personal erotic pleasures in favor of depersonalized duties to family, nation, and God. The ultimate threat enfolded in this erotic stripping naked—free from the invisible garments of middle-class ideology— is carried by the suggestion that Modi's nudes, in their stealth refusals, depict a female pleasure so self-contained and self-sufficient that men, too, as traditional agents of female pleasure, now appear unnecessary. Yes, by all means, call the police.

The stealth action of Modi's nudes also extends to the (subversive) rejection of a narrative frame. Female nakedness, in Modi's paintings, breaks free from the confining and domesticating limits of story. Much as the idiosyncratic bodies of his women resist the golden symmetries of classical art, Modi's nudes refuse to cover their nakedness with the fig-leaf contrivance of mythological and biblical narratives, especially narratives of shame, degradation, rape, or narcissistic, coquettish self-display. The absence of *any* narrative frame is arguably as impudent and antiauthoritarian as the presence of pubic hair. Modi reinforces this narrative framelessness by situating the nudes in a strangely ambiguous placelessness. Rooms, furniture, and visual backgrounds dissolve into swatches of rich color, liberating the women from locations that might explain—and explain away—their nakedness, even as studio models. A bed or sofa offers less an explanation than whatever colorful platform is necessary to prevent the erotic (as in Figure 5.3) from drifting off the face of the planet.

Modi's women, if based on models, are not *represented* as models, or as fallen women, or as shameless wives. Prostitutes in a hotel where Modi once stayed, knowing that he was too poor to afford models, sometimes posed for free, but his paintings never depict the nudes as whores, unlike Picasso's *Les Demoiselles d'Avignon*, which practices its breakthrough cubist style on women conveniently identified as prostitutes. Modigliani's nudes stand defiantly outside time, place, and story, as free from Edenic innocence as from canons of sin. He does not transform the women into objects or into angular blocks of color on a canvas. They simply *are*. Their erotic presence—*being*—is complete and sufficient.

The stealth action or inaction of *being*—simply existing in the fullness of what *is*—includes a subversive disturbance that links the nudes with

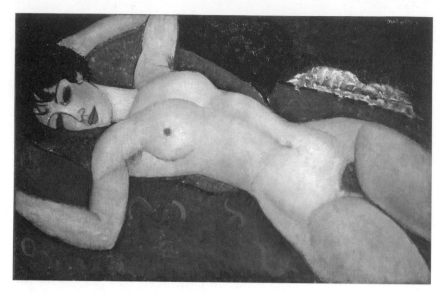

FIGURE 5.3. Amedeo Modigliani. *Reclining Nude (Nu couché)*. 1917–1918.
Oil on canvas. Formerly in the Mattioli Collection. Sold at Christie's on
November 9, 2015, for $170.4 million. Photo Credit: SCALA / Art Resource, NY.

ideologies of Modernist art and poetry. "A poem should be palpable and
mute / As a globed fruit," as the American poet Archibald MacLeish began
his "Ars Poetica" (1926), which ends with the famous line, "A poem should
not mean / But be."[40] *Being*, as a state of self-sufficient fullness unaccount-
able to meaning or reason, is the quintessential subversive state toward
which eros leads. The unseen action of Modi's great nudes, as the
ideology of "Ars Poetica" might contend, is not to *mean* something but
to be. They confront us with unmediated, unapologetic, erotic *being*.
Being, however, does not remain *entirely* undisturbed in Modi's luminous
nudes, even if the obstacle or lack or absence implicit in eros remains no
more than a hint or shadow. The intimate connection between eros and
death, however, also shadows the great nudes, even unseen, if we remember that these dazzling canvases were painted by an ill and emaciated artist, worn down to the bone, spitting blood and swilling rum as he
painted, cigarettes close by his palette. What happens in the studio, of
course, happens as if in secret, privately, by stealth—off the canvas—but
Modigliani's nudes (while set free from story, liberated from meaning,
allowed to repose in a subversive fullness of being) never entirely break

free from a shadowy link with death. Ironically, it took a storyteller, novelist Philip Roth, to bring this underground disturbance up into the light.

Roth's novel *The Dying Animal* (2001) unfolds the continuing erotic education of his regular protagonist, a middle-aged Jewish professor named David Kepesh. Born before the sexual revolution of the 1960s, Kepesh makes up for lost time by seducing his ex-student Consuela, who (born after the revolution) is quite willing to be seduced. They enter into an unusually intense eighteen-month sexual liaison until Consuela initiates a breakup. Then, after six years of silence, Kepesh receives a postcard from Consuela bearing on one side the image of Modigliani's *Reclining Nude*—also sometimes known as *Le Grand Nu* (Figure 5.4).

Does Consuela, Kepesh wonders in a dark mood, intend the image as a stealth invitation to resume their sexual enthrallment? He imagines that Consuela's invitation comes directly from the woman depicted in Modi's painting: "A golden-skinned nude inexplicably asleep over a velvety black abyss that, in my mood, I associated with the grave. One long, undulating line, she lies there awaiting you, still as death."[41] The always self-absorbed Kepesh does not know how uncannily prescient he is. Conseula is even then dying of cancer.

Modigliani's *Reclining Nude*—a treasure of the Museum of Modern Art in New York—finds its ideal critic in the eros-centered Philip Roth, although of course Roth fits his description of the painting to the mood and mind of the fictive David Kepesh. Still, who better situated than Roth to recognize the covert link in Modi's nudes between eros, loss, and death? Death also enters indirectly into Modigliani's portraits as a distinctive undercurrent of melancholy and a mute embodiment of loss that many observers sense. Ilya Ehrenburg, his young Russian contemporary in Paris, describes the sitters represented in his portraits as resembling "hurt children." "I believe that the world seemed to Modigliani," Ehrenburg concludes, "like an enormous kindergarten run by very unkind adults."[42] If so, the portraits help us recognize how the nudes (with their beautiful, vulnerable curves, their youth, their glowing vitality, their milky orange tones and dreamlike serene expressions) seem to emerge from some erotic alternative universe: an artificial paradise with no address, where the unkind adults seem magically absent. The nudes make

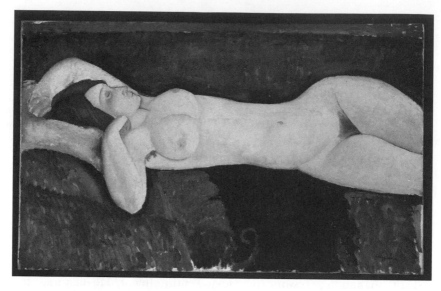

FIGURE 5.4. Amedeo Modigliani. *Reclining Nude* (*Le Grand Nu*). Ca. 1919.
Digital Image © The Museum of Modern Art / Licensed by
SCALA / Art Resource, NY.

contact with an authentic aliveness, as Francis Carco testified, with life as
a gift, but—the crucial point—this contact occurs within a surrounding
politico-social context where *being* or the inner life of eros is always under
threat. Modi's portraits often depict individuals sitting rigid, almost stone-
faced, expressionless, as if a vital spark has gone missing. The threat of
death and loss does not always announce its presence in art with a medieval hooded skeleton. It can lie concealed in a velvety abyss of blackness,
or linger just beyond the canvas, like Consuela's cancer or like the hag-
gard, ravaged artist.

A Politics of Eros: War, Dream, and Death

Death was not only hovering nearby in the studio as Modi spat blood,
doubled over coughing, heaved his shoulders, and painted his extraordinary series of nudes. World War I changed Paris forever as the new
German sixty-nine-foot-long "Paris Gun" fired its payload twenty-six miles
high before hitting its random targets and rattling windows almost nightly
in Montparnasse from March to August 1918. An evening curfew turned

the artist quarter into a ghost town. Art dealers fled and galleries closed.[43] Modi's alarming ill-health spurred Zborowski in 1918 to take him (with a war-weary entourage) to southern France, but even when Modi temporarily escaped wartime Paris his escape was predicated on illness and war. The Parisian crowds that in 1914 had shouted deliriously "To Berlin, To Berlin" soon gave way to amputees limping back from the Western front. Modi's friend Apollinaire now wore a huge turban of bandages over his head wound. Braque, too, suffered a head wound; Salmon and Carco were mobilized; Cocteau joined an ambulance unit; Foujita left for London; Kisling was stabbed with a bayonet; and Blaise Cendrars lost his right arm. (Where was Picasso? In Rome, a set designer for Sergei Diaghilev and the Ballets Russes.) Opposed trenches, so close that enemies shouted insults back and forth, crisscrossed the waterlogged terrain for 25,000 miles. *Shell shock* enters the medical lexicon in response to mechanized killing on an unprecedented scale. Over six days, British forces at the Somme took 300,000 casualties. It is politics that ultimately establishes the bounds of personal possibility and entangles individual inner lives in the filaments of historical desire, as AIDS in Africa has made painfully evident. The politics of historical desire constitutes the lost backdrop of Modigliani's nudes: the so-called Great War lies just outside the canvas.

The wartime nudes in their serene embrace of eros in effect constitute a rejection of the mechanized state violence: an erotic affirmation made in the teeth of the war machine. Modi had no use for this war, which historians argue was the utterly improbable result of statesmen, institutions, and nations bungling into horror like sleepwalkers.[44] Italy, although by treaty allied with Germany, entered the war on the side of Britain and the Allies in 1915. One report says that Modi tried to enlist but was rejected for poor health. Another report, more in character, says that after an hour waiting in line to enlist, he walked off in a rage. His politics, when not openly anarchist, found no real difference between the two vast armies of the bourgeoisie. Alert to Modi's self-contradictions, one observer called him a "violent pacifist." "Down with the Allies! Down with the war!" he was heard shouting.[45] This stumblebum catastrophe was not an occasion for demonstrating love of country—"Cara Italia" were supposedly Modi's last words—or for mounting an all-out defense of civilized values. The war, for Modi, was a pitiful deathtrap opposed to everything that the vocation of art (as a gift of life) stood for. His nudes stand as a silent protest: art as the opposite of war.

Nakedness has a modern history of protest that Modi's nudes might be thought to anticipate. In certain political contexts, it creates a powerful emblem of unconcealment that, paradoxically, exposes the concealments and fig-leaf fictions that nation-states employ in order to organize and justify mass killing. As protest, however, nakedness serves not only as a resistance to concealment, lies, and restrictions but also as a revelation. It reveals, as if bringing to light a long-lost truth, something fragile, vulnerable, and infinitely valuable: the undefended, poor, bare human body. The rock-musical *Hair*, for example, which debuted in 1967 during the height of the Vietnam War, concluded with a theatrical metaphor of its anti-war, peace-and-love protest in a then-shocking scene of brave, vulnerable, on-stage mass nakedness. Is it significant that Modi's nudes, like Virginia Woolf's invalids, are women who inhabit a political world run as anti-erotic or anerotic expressions of male power and reason? Modi's series of great nudes deploys nakedness, we might say, not only as a gift of life offered to the sleepwalkers and to the hurt children but also as a personal affirmation of eros. They affirm the value of life amid a conflict so horrific and life-denying that nakedness—in reducing human beings to an image of their primal (almost infantile) unprotected helplessness— in effect reverses its traditional erotic coding and stages a deliberately shocking protest against every form of wartime dehumanization.

"For over two years," writes the World War I historian Modris Eksteins, "the belligerents on the Western Front hammered at each other in battles, if that old word is appropriate for this new warfare, that cost millions of men their lives but moved the front line at most a mile or so in either direction."[46] Modigliani had thirteen months to live—and a few more nudes to paint—when the November 1918 armistice exposed the gruesome totals: over 8 million dead, 21 million gassed, maimed, and shell-shocked. Apollonaire died of his wounds on Armistice Day. The peace that followed such pointless carnage did not fill Montparnasse with joy even though, in the booming postwar art market as the 1920s roared in flush with cash, many bohemian artists soon enjoyed international reputations and immense financial success. His formerly destitute Russian-Jewish friend Soutine, whom Modi passed on to Zborowski, now drove a fancy car. Montparnasse artists complained that the old spirit was gone, and Modi's funeral—an event unparalleled since 2 million people had walked in the procession for Victor Hugo in 1885—had registered like the end of an era. His death in 1920 at age thirty-six seems the foregone conclusion to a life in which his fierce commitment to art and to the bohemian existence that his art-making required ultimately burned out the body. It did not, however, extinguish the era's passionate interest in dreams that Modi's nudes also, indirectly, affirm.

"What I am searching for," Modigliani wrote in an entry in his sketchbook, "is neither the real nor the unreal, / But the Subconscious, the mystery of what is Instinctive in the Race."[47] The nudes, in their opposition to the surrounding political landscape, take up a position somewhere between the real and the unreal: a dreamlike space where eros seems to transcend sexual turmoil, as if sedating turbulent emotions in the quieter pursuit of mysteries, desire, and the not-known. Dreams, of course, were serious stuff in Modernist Paris, both as an alternative to politics and as a privileged route to the inner life. Baudelaire stitched theological cliché to scandalous revisionism in the opening sentence of *Les Paradis artificiels* (1860): "Good sense tells us," he wrote, "that earthly things are rare and fleeting, and that true reality exists only in dreams."[48] Good sense said no such thing: it called dreamers *fools*. Devoted to Baudelaire and fluent in French, Modigliani shared the view that dreams and drugs opened up the route to an artificial paradise. Dreams and opium, since at least the time of the British Romantic poets, had acquired a contemporary reputation as a conduit of creative power. Modi used hashish and opium in pursuit of artistic ends, once claiming that they opened him up to a new sense of color, and some see a drugged vision behind the swan-necked portraits. But it is Cocteau, a reformed opium addict, who holds particular interest here because he argued *against* the myth that opium is a source of creative visions. "Opium," as he corrected the record, "nourishes a state of half-dream. It puts the emotions to sleep, exalts the heart and lightens the spirit."[49] Modi's nudes, as if in a state of *half-dream*, might well be in semicontact with the oneiric realm that Baudelaire would call "true reality."

Modigliani produced only a single self-portrait. Significantly, it does not depict a post-Byronic, torment-driven outcast or cursed dark-Romantic *poète maudit*—Maldoror-Modigliani—but rather it represents the artist at work, holding a palette, a gentle, pensive figure with (like many of the nudes) closed eyes and a half-dreamlike expression.

Consider the irrepressible Kiki. Alfred Maury had argued in his influential book on sleep and dreams, *Le sommeil et les rêves* (1861), that dreamlike fantasies are marked not by an extravagant departure from external realities—as the surrealists later believed—but rather by an uncanny closeness to what is external and real. Kiki, for example, had a distinctive feature that for modeling assignments she sometimes disguised with dark crayon. This trait, a visibly absent slice of pubic hair, was sufficiently well-known among artists that Foujita once joked about it, and Man Ray (her lover) later made Kiki's signature trait inescapably obvious in a photograph. There is no record that Kiki posed for Modigliani, but Zborowski often climbed the stairs to see her posing nude in Moïse Kisling's studio.[50] More than a few Modi nudes represent the woman's pubic triangle as strangely offset or askew. This erotic irregularity constructs certain Modi nudes as doubly unideal, declassicized, asymmetrical, and gently disfigured, in a half-dreamlike conjunction of the actual and the unreal: paradisal but earthbound, too. Modi's nudes do not edit out real-life traits, from teeth to rolls of fat or Kiki's offset pubic triangle, but instead occupy the mysterious erotic border where what is neither entirely *real* nor entirely *unreal* somehow meet in the creation of a female image that offers an artistic, critical alternative to the illness, injury, war, and death that nonetheless indirectly shadow it.

Tuberculosis: Art and the Limits of Medical Logos

Tubercular meningitis was the cause of death listed on Modigliani's death certificate at the Hôpital de la Charité. This fact, long known, seems to his most careful and resourceful recent biographer, Meryle Secrest, the key to Modigliani's well-publicized erratic, wild, and drunken self-display: "the explanation for the puzzle."[51] Self-display, of course, even offensive self-display, belonged to Modi's deliberate fashioning of a public persona. Picasso asked, not so innocently, why when Modi was drunk he always just happened to be drunk in front of Le Dôme and La Rotonde, cafés where tourists came to gawk at the bohemian artists. "More or less deliberately, he created his own 'legend,' " says a contemporary source.[52] The display of somewhat obnoxious excess as part of his public character might well seem puzzling as a deliberate choice, expressing a deep psychic contradiction. For Secrest, however, the hospital certificate identifying tuberculosis as the cause of death "changed everything." She astutely observes that Modi's dark alter ego, the antihero Maldoror, was also tubercular. She also documents the twentieth-century culture of illness that featured tuberculosis as a feared, contagious killer; patients were isolated and often stigmatized. She argues that Modigliani deliberately concealed his diagnosis beneath a veneer of public drunkenness. "The received wisdom," she writes, "was that he drank himself to death." Her tuberculosis-inspired revisionist view is that, instead, he used alcohol and drugs as an anesthetic, the means by which he kept functioning as an artist, and, most importantly, as a smokescreen to conceal "the great secret"—tuberculosis—that he must hide at all costs.[53]

Is Secrest correct? I don't know. It is a plausible argument. Modigliani's life was certainly shadowed by serious illness. Devastating childhood bouts with typhoid and with pleurisy almost killed him, weakening his lungs so seriously that he abandoned his early work in Paris as a sculptor, unable to withstand the constant stone dust. His health crashed so dangerously following his first extended stay in Paris that in 1912 he returned to Italy, where his mother nursed him back to health. On returning to Paris, he turned from sculpture to painting, living in unheated garrets and shack-like studios, during one period taking turns with Soutine to sleep in their only bed while the other painter slept on the floor. A shared bed constituted almost a luxury. Often, as one observer put it, he led a "vagabond existence," spending the nights "here, there, and anywhere."[54]

Medicine, too, was a luxury that destitute artists could rarely afford, and everyone, especially in winter, fell ill with something. Ilya Ehrenburg, when he learned of Modi's death a year later, offers only a brief and vague description with no sense of shock. "Modi was always coughing," he recalls, "always felt cold. He contracted a lung disease. His organism was exhausted."[55] Less than a decade after Modi's death, tuberculosis merited no more than a parenthesis in Jean Cocteau's account, which also embeds cultural myths surrounding tuberculosis: "Refined by illness (he was tubercular), he had the air of a true aristocrat."[56] If tuberculosis could isolate, it could also—so the myth held—lend an elevating, ennobling air of refinement, as the disease wasted away the flesh to expose pure spirit. One fact seems beyond argument. Even if Modi did not possess certain knowledge that he had contracted tubercular meningitis, he believed that the shadow of serious illness hung over him like a death sentence with the date of execution left open.

Modi's desire for a life brief but intense expressed the sense that his fierce devotion to art played out against a rapidly expiring timeline. Self-destructiveness, even beyond his deliberate public contributions to myths of the *poète maudit*, expressed almost a parallel sense that death was always hovering nearby. Just weeks before his death he stood outside for two hours, unprotected, in a freezing Paris winter drizzle. His actual death, officially caused by tubercular meningitis, stands as the final, lurid episode in a series of life-threatening illnesses and of body-killing deprivations compounded by alcohol, drugs, and poverty as he and Jeanne somehow endured the glacial winter of early 1920 in a heatless garret. His imminent death—looming as he "ceaselessly" painted his radiant apricot nudes—remains significant here as it testifies less to tuberculosis as a smokescreen than to his lasting affirmation of eros. Medical logos at the end of World War I had no cure to offer Modi; it had myriads of badly wounded veterans to care for. Eros, in the face of death, left open to Modi an alternative that exactly suited the darker range of his personal artistic temperament: a life brief but intense devoted to paintings that assent to life.

Medical eros might be described as Modigliani's life-sustaining alternative to a personal history of illness then beyond the reach of medical logos. In France, it was not until 1921 that the Calmette-Guérin vaccine was first used on humans, when one in six deaths was still caused by tuberculosis. If tuberculosis was Modi's great secret, it was a secret widely shared among the urban poor, who had nowhere to go except into voluntary *sanatoria* that resembled prisons. Modi instead kept painting, coughing up blood in a squalid, stone-cold, two-room garret he shared with Jeanne, and his nudes thus stand in opposition not only to the bourgeois war machine—grinding up artists and civilians and soldiers in its maw—but also to his own illness and death. The nudes in their erotic health and dreamlike serenity contradict or hold at bay the hacking cough and blood-red sputum. Their robust, fleshly well-being has nothing to do with the hectic flush typical of tuberculosis—sometimes falsely regarded, in myths surrounding tuberculosis, as a sign of hypervitality—but arises rather as a sheer erotic pronouncement: eros less as a god to be wary of than as, despite the inescapable costs, a life-affirming human gift.

Medical eros might nominate *Nude on a Blue Cushion* (Figure 5.5) as the antithesis of Modigliani's illness-exhausted organism in wartime Paris: the image of a woman reclining in a timeless, voluptuous ease, nowhere in particular except beside a strangely discordant blue cushion that shares top billing.

What to make of the ample curves, audacious sexuality, masklike and vaguely cubist nose, and open-eyed, come-hither look? Maybe the blue cushion holds a suggestion. Blue has a long history of association with the Virgin Mary, and Vassily Kandinsky, writing about the spiritual element in art, described blue as "the typical heavenly color."[57] The blue pillow, set against the adjacent dark, red-brown hues, might also recall the theory of complementary colors (he called them "laws") developed by French chemist Michel Eugène Chevreul in 1828, whose work became "an essential manual for painters."[58] Chevreul showed how primary colors look brightest in contrast with dissimilar or complementary hues. The bright color of the woman and her blue cushion carries its own mute subtext. Modi's quest for the mystery of "what is Instinctive in the Race" might also start and conclude with an ambiguous spiritual/erotic image featuring breasts so prominent as to be simultaneously erotic and maternal: the eternal feminine. No one could mistake *Nude on a Blue Cushion* for a classical portrait of Venus or for an image of virginal innocence. Isn't that the point? Modi's female nude, in all her ambiguity, is an homage to the power of art and to the power of women to make a crucial and redeeming affirmation of life and of eros.

Modigliani's erotic "dreamgirls" (as David Kepesh calls them) observe a single rule that does not shift: always, full frontal nudity. The elderly Renoir, in a visit arranged by the indispensable Zborowski, advised Modi to paint lovingly, as if stroking the backside of his nudes. "But Monsieur," replied Modi, annoyed, "I do not like backsides."[59] Among Modi's two minor exceptions to the front-facing rule, one is a failed experiment in Cubist style, where the prominent backside may express Modi's feelings

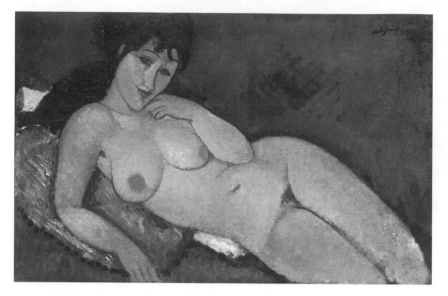

FIGURE 5.5. Amedeo Modigliani. *Nude on a Blue Cushion*. 1917.
Chester Dale Collection. National Gallery of Art, Washington, DC.

about Cubism—or about Picasso. The other backside nude, painted with
an unusual bright, hard, smooth surface, exaggerates the buttocks in a
derogatory allusion to Ingres's *La Grande Odalisque* (1841)—greatly criticized for the added low-back vertebrae that, according to novelist
George Sand, gave the woman the look of a bloodsucker. Beyond expressing his taste in body parts, Modi's two buttocks-facing nudes may
well signify inversion, eros upended, fantasy wrong-side out, dreams gone
awry, less a rejection of eros than an acknowledgement of its built-in limits
and discontents. Significantly, Modi refuses to pursue eros into macabre
lusts or unspeakable cruelties, but his two rear-facing nudes suggest how
nakedness can turn anti-erotic: eros dreaming its own failures or disen-
chantments. The two backside nudes at least confirm that his typical
front-facing posture is a deliberate choice, with affirmative implications
and erotic connections to the inner life. Even Modi's self-portraits, as Cocteau wrote, "are not the reflection of his external observation, but of his
internal vision."[60]

"If anyone wants to understand the drama of Modigliani," Ilya Ehrenburg wrote from his post–World War II stance as among the most famous and prolific authors of the Soviet Union, "let him remember, not

hashish, but the gas chamber; let him think of Europe lost and frozen, of the devious paths of the century, of the fate of any of Modigliani's models around whom the iron ring was already closing."[61] Medical eros may seem to some a powerless and irrelevant alternative to medical logos, but the affirmations of eros carry significant weight. The nakedness of Modigliani's nudes casts a revealing light on the antiseptic removal of clothing that so often signals the start of a medical examination. "Eroticism," as Bataille had asserted, "is assenting to life up to the point of death." The great nudes, whose power reaches far beyond the milieu of Modigliani's life span, suggest that patients, doctors, and everyone touched at some point by serious illness might find in eros and its affirmations—right up to the point of death—both strong medicine and quiet refuge, even a source of resistance, as they confront personal pain, social suffering, and the numberless modes of contemporary violence, soft or hard, from toxic dumps to genocide and so-called holy wars. Medical logos has enough biological calamity to deal with that it does not need to reject the assistance—in related dramas of the inner life—available for the asking from medical eros.

The series of great nudes may claim their least obvious kinship, finally, with the "great odes" of Keats, which similarly emerge from a remarkable creative burst while the poet was dying of tuberculosis. Minus the "great odes" Keats is a promising minor poet, and Romanticism minus Keats has lost its heart. The "great odes" redefine Keats and reshape Romantic poetry. The nudes of Modigliani, created in the era of the Great War, unfold in a bittersweet Keatsian drama of love and death that both redefines Modigliani's lifework and, in so doing, reshapes an understanding of Modernism. Mass death on an unprecedented scale and his own lingering fatal illness provide a context within which the great nudes offer a testament to the power of eros, an affirmation of life, accessible to anyone, in pain, out of pain, or living in the lucky interval before pain strikes, as it almost surely will, once again.

CHAPTER SIX

The Infinite Faces of Pain:
Eros and Ethics

I went to a concert upstairs in Town Hall. The composer whose works
were being performed had provided program notes. One of these notes
was to the effect that there is too much pain in the world. After the concert I was walking along with the composer and he was telling me
how the performances had not been quite up to snuff. So I said, "Well,
I enjoyed the music, but I didn't agree with that program note about
there being too much pain in the world." He said, "What? Don't you
think there's enough?" I said, "I think there's just the right amount."

JOHN CAGE, "GRACE AND CLARITY" (1944)

*J*ust *the right amount of pain?* In his curious, unsettling remark,
John Cage perhaps intends his koan-like paradox to reorient a musical companion whom he regards as overinvested in rational judgments
and in computational thought. The sum total of world pain is unknowable—who can say what is *too much* or *just the right amount?*—and Cage,
steeped in Zen Buddhist teachings, no doubt understood pain as
embedded in a larger account of suffering, or *dukkha*, radically at odds
with concepts of a computational, mind-based, reason-directed ego.[1]

Cage encountered enough destitution as he scraped by as an impoverished composer in postwar New York City to distance his paradox from
flippant denials of real-world misery. The first Noble Truth (and a foundation of Buddhist thought) is the maxim that *suffering exists*. Suffering
and pain are not identical, of course; a stubbed toe is painful, momentarily, but not usually a source of suffering. Pain, no doubt, is often intertwined with suffering, even a direct cause of suffering, but for John Cage
an affirmation of life does not depend upon the global reduction of pain.
"Our intention is to affirm this life," he wrote in 1944, "not to bring
order out of chaos nor to suggest improvements in creation, but simply
to wake up to the very life we're living, which is so excellent once one
gets one's mind and one's desires out of its way and lets it act of its own
accord."[2] Waking up is a traditional philosophical image for sudden
inner illumination, a mind-altering transformation, and for Cage awakening implies both fully experiencing the world as it is and fully letting
go of ego-based, computational rationalities that presume to measure,
say, which of two musical performances is *better*—or just how much
world pain is *too much* pain.

"Pain is a universal experience," so begins the blue-ribbon Institute
of Medicine report *Relieving Pain in America* (2011), before, in a reflex
basic to medical logos, instantly shifting to computational thought:
"Common chronic pain conditions affect at least 116 million U.S. adults
at a cost of $560–635 billion annually in direct medical treatment costs
and lost productivity."[3] The report is correct, of course, and the computational thinking basic to medical logos has a valid point to make. Meanwhile, however, no new drug, no social program, nothing, has managed
to sweep back the rising tide of new pain that daily washes up on the
shores of biomedicine. A recent survey from the National Institutes of
Health (not prepared to let go of computational thought) estimates that
23.4 million American adults—a huge 10.3 percent of the current
population—experience "a lot" of pain.[4] What, in the face of such
mounting, unrelieved, bottomless distress, does the Institute of Medicine's blue-ribbon panel recommend? The understanding and treatment of pain in America, according to these very distinguished specialists, requires nothing short of a "cultural transformation."[5] A *cultural*

transformation in the understanding and treatment of pain may not require sudden illumination, or waking up the very life we're leading, but it certainly could use a little help from medical eros.

The Institute of Medicine report—recognizing the limits of medical logos—challenges doctors and therapists with a radical new and transformative agenda: to "promote and enable *self-management* of pain." Self-management, as a deliberate practice, seeks to enlist patients and nonpatients in moving beyond a molecular gaze trained on genes, nerves, tissue damage, and neurotransmitters. It needs patients and nonpatients to understand and to personalize the current recognition within medicine that sociocultural contexts significantly influence chronic pain.[6] Jobs, families, and substance abuse are the sociocultural trio that most often provides the focus for current clinical interventions, but pain engages far wider personal and cultural aspects of human lives, from spirituality and social media to poverty, exercise, and nutrition. Cultural transformations cannot occur without a sufficient buildup of personal transformations. Medical eros has a key role to play in extending the sociocultural discourse on pain and in encouraging the personal inflections of desire that actively promote and enable strategies of self-management.

Desire, as a personal, emotional force, is something that John Cage mostly wanted to get out of the way of, or to reduce to the status of an observable phenomenon, like a preference for vanilla ice cream. A practicing Buddhist may perhaps succeed in the eradication of craving. Many patients, however, weary of shuttling among specialists, are ready for a program of self-management that respects their desire to get off the biomedical drug-taking treadmill. They are ready to participate actively in reducing their personal burdens of pain. Such self-management, however, will fail without an approach that mobilizes desire. Medical eros can contribute toward the necessary cultural transformation, then, not only by circulating new success stories of self-management, helpful in engaging individual desire for change, but also by engaging patients and nonpatients in understanding the role that narrative can play in the individual experience of pain. In particular, as a contribution toward self-management, I want to ask an eros-related question (with far-reaching implications) that respects the harsh reality of personal suffering. *Might the self-management of pain—beyond biomedical reason, analysis, and*

computation—depend far less on finding the right medication than on under-
standing and responding to pain (both our own pain and the pain of
others) much as we might understand and respond to a story?

The *Inexpressibility* Topos: Pain and Language

The *inexpressibility topos* refers to the claim "that a particular experience, person, or object, is beyond verbal description."[7] This ancient claim is a standard feature in eighteenth-century aesthetic theories of "the sublime," and readers of Elaine Scarry's important book *The Body in Pain* (1985) often conclude that pain too is inexpressible. It is a claim open to question. Scarry begins *The Body in Pain* with a section titled "The Inexpressibility of Physical Pain," followed immediately by a section titled "The Political Consequences of Pain's Inexpressibility." Inexpressibility thus provides the origin for a fascinating and original discussion of pain-related topics, ranging from torture to patent law.

It is important to notice, however, both Scarry's modifying comments and her shifts of emphasis. Her "overt subject," Scarry writes, in the opening section, is "the difficulty of expressing physical pain."[8] *Difficulty* of expression, of course, is not identical with absolute *inexpressibility*, and Scarry herself notes how this *difficulty* may be overcome, imperfectly, by verbal means.[9] *Resistance*, like difficulty, is another modifying term used to soften the claims of absolute inexpressibility. Scarry is certainly right that pain resists language. She goes further, however, in citing the passage from *On Being Ill* in which Virginia Woolf imagines a sufferer trying to describe a pain to a doctor ("language at once runs dry").[10] This instantaneous running-dry of language is "more radically true," Scarry writes, of the severe and prolonged pain that may accompany cancer, burns, stroke, or phantom limb. "Physical pain," she concludes in a very broad generalization, "does not simply resist language but actively destroys it."

There is good reason to emphasize that pain *resists* expression, as Scarry does, but the absolute destruction of language by pain and the absolute inexpressibility of pain are not exactly Woolf's point. Woolf is not offering a theory of pain but rather employing the illustrative example of a sufferer with "a pain in his head" in order to support her main argument that illness has been underdescribed in literature. Her description of language running "dry," further, does not imply that pain is absolutely inexpressible. Rather, Woolf wants to replace the neglect of illness in literature—presumably, the literary neglect of pain too—with a whole new verbal discourse: a language "more primitive, more sensual, more obscene." If language can run dry, writers and cultures have the power to renew language: creek beds may refill. Pain, especially chronic pain, whatever its fate in literature, is not doomed or fated to absolute inexpressibility. Language and narrative hold a crucial place in any future cultural transformations focused on self-management.

Intense pain certainly resists language and introduces major difficulties of expression. At its absolute upper limit, it can blot out consciousness and defeat any utterance beyond a scream. David Biro, shortly after finishing his medical residency, experienced pain so severe during a bone-marrow transplant that, as he writes, "it literally strangled my vocal cords." "All I wanted to do," he adds, "was to crawl inside a hole and shut my eyes until it, or I, just went away."[11] Suicide is an extreme but, sadly, not uncommon response to unremitting intense pain. Biro, returning to clinical work as a physician, looked for ways to break into the silences of pain, to insert the wedge of language and of metaphor into moments when pain has released its absolute stranglehold. In *The Language of Pain* (2010) Biro both acknowledges his debt to Scarry's work and undertakes to describe various means of teasing pain, at least in its less intense versions, into expression. When pain takes on its more familiar forms of, say, carpal tunnel syndrome or fibromyalgia, even visual analogue scales (rating degrees of intensity) give a modest voice to pain; such numerical data prove important and telling enough to be required now in hospital charts. Pain also, in less statistical formulations, obliquely infiltrates multiple modes of verbal and visual expression, from infant cries (which a parent quickly learns to read in their varying intonations) to sexual whispers, oral speech, writing, cinema, and the visual arts. In its porous social existence, pain has regularly absorbed a variety of religious and cultural meanings. Our personal beliefs *about* pain can directly affect the pain we *feel*, so there is urgent value in bringing such beliefs into expression. Pain itself—if we regard it as a noun in search of a content—may remain as mysterious as love: irreducible to neurobiological correlates. Eros, in many cases, is entangled with pain: both partake of not-knowing. As a state of being that calls for self-management, however, pain is also subject to continuous clarifications that owe much to the research methods of medical logos. Most important among these clarifying insights is the crucial distinction—clinical rather than philosophical—between *acute pain* and *chronic pain.*

Medical logos, in its pragmatic distinction between acute pain and chronic pain, does more than add a new system of classification. Biomedicine has become adept at controlling acute pain, as in postoperative recovery. Major hospitals have acute-pain teams trained to treat especially intense short-term episodes that may occur in cancer, for example, or in stroke. The very rare cases of excruciating, intractable, untreatable acute pain may require drastic means to short-circuit consciousness, but such instances offer a poor model for what happens in chronic pain. Chronic pain—with its immense costs to individuals and to the national gross domestic product—is often defined as pain lasting for more than six months, with or without an observable lesion. Although frequently less intense than acute pain, chronic pain produces measurable changes in the brain, which may make the pain self-perpetuating, more intense, and almost untreatable. Inexpressibility is not the main dilemma that faces many chronic-pain patients. Instead, the dilemma lies in finding people, inside or outside medicine, who will truly listen to what they are saying—not tune them out—and lend assistance. Dying patients, we might assume, will receive the necessary attention to relieve pain. A prominent study, however, showed that 50 percent of dying hospitalized patients spent at least half their time in moderate to severe pain.[12] A follow-up study, after six months spent emphasizing practical remedies, found no improvement at all.

Medical eros would contend that the goal in self-management is precisely to talk more effectively and openly about pain—to improve the discourse and to oppose institutional or personal impediments—in ways that ultimately benefit patients. In this aim, medical logos and medical eros not only share common cause but have incentive and opportunity to collaborate.

Pain, whether chronic or acute, is often (but not always) located in a specific area of the body, but, whether local or unlocalizable, it is always an event of consciousness. "The brain," as neurosurgeon and pain specialist John D. Loeser writes, "is the organ responsible for all pain." "All sensory phenomena," he adds, "including nociception, can be altered by conscious and unconscious mental activity."[13] Loeser is past president of both the American Pain Society and the International Association for the Study of Pain; he is well-known in the wide world of medical logos; and his statement reflects years of firsthand work with pain patients. Nociception is the technical term for the processes of neurotransmission that occur, say, if you hit your thumb with a hammer; but hammer-blows bear little relation to chronic pain, and Loeser insists that the activity of sensory neurons does not constitute pain. Human pain is an event of consciousness, a subjective product of the brain, where intricate neural networks link sensation with perception, cognition, memory, and emotion. It orchestrates such an instantaneous interrelation between body and mind that the common terms *physical pain* and *mental pain* misrepresent the central role of consciousness. The terms, an outmoded legacy of the philosophical split between material bodies and immaterial minds, ignore the biological mind/body interactions that make pain, like eros, both *always mental* and *always physical*. Consciousness or inner life is where chronic pain, with or without an observable lesion, plays out its baleful and often self-defeating narratives.

The International Association for the Study of Pain—the most prestigious worldwide organization of scientists, physicians, and therapists dealing with pain—opens the door to a narrative approach when it insists, in its official *Classification of Chronic Pain*, that pain is "always subjective" and "always a psychological state."[14] Pain, especially chronic pain, resists the reduction to a direct one-to-one relationship with tissue damage. Lesions are often undetectable, so the primary object of study if you are studying human pain (as distinct from counting laboratory tail-flicks) is not an object at all but rather a subjective state. Even tissue damage as measurable as a prolapsed lumbar disk does not necessarily result in pain. The self-management of pain—as a mind/body state centered in consciousness—thus would seem to require a new model that integrates a microlevel molecular gaze with macrolevel personal, psychological, sociocultural accounts that inevitably affect human consciousness.

An Integrative ("Zoom") Model of Pain

An Integrative Model of Pain—or, in reference to the zoom-in / zoom-out function on computer screens, a Zoom Model—seeks to acknowledge the shifting interplay among the multiple levels of mind / body relations that underlie and participate in the human experience of pain: from micro-level cellular processes to macrolevel individual beliefs, social practices, and even oral or silent narrative frames and reframing. One version might look something like Figure 6.1.

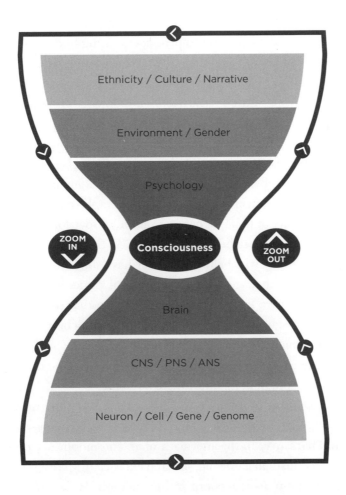

FIGURE 6.1. An Integrative ("Zoom") Model of Pain. David B. Morris.

There is no pain to consider when consciousness is shut down. A consciousness-centered integrative Zoom Model, however, allows us to understand how different levels of explanation might best match up with biomedical treatments or with patient self-management. Some types of chronic pain, for example, respond less well to drugs than to psychosocial therapies and to treatments based on a cognitive-behavioral approach. Chronic pain with a single identifiable lesion, on the other hand, might call for an aggressive approach using opiates or surgical intervention. Some pain seems produced almost *wholly* by the brain. In one study, researchers attached volunteers to an electrical stimulator and told them that its current might possibly produce a headache. Volunteers were not told that the stimulator was set to produce nothing beyond a low humming sound. The result? Half the volunteers reported pain.[15]

A model of pain consistent with interacting microlevels and macrolevels finds important support in the rich biomedical literature on *pain beliefs*. Researchers show that specific beliefs affect the pain we experience, especially beliefs about cause, control, duration, outcome, and blame. Such beliefs affect not only chronic pain but also acute pain and postoperative pain. Beliefs about pain, moreover, often maintain a direct link with emotions: anger toward a negligent employer, for example, or fear of catastrophe, or hope for compensation, or love for a spouse. Specific pain beliefs even predict pain intensity. As this research shows, patients function better who believe that they have some control over their pain, who believe that medical services are of value, who believe that family members care for them, and who believe that pain has not left them severely disabled. In one study, specific pain beliefs correlated directly with treatment outcomes.[16] If you believe that your pain is disabling or that you have no means of control, for example, this internal narrative of belief already predicts an unfortunate outcome.

Self-management of pain, consistent with a new integrative Zoom Model, cannot ignore the beliefs that we almost unknowingly embed in speech and narrative. In the aftermath of an automobile accident, Lous Heshusius, a Canadian academic, suffered excruciating chronic pain, and she offers a first-person account in her memoir *Inside Chronic Pain* (2009).[17] She tallies up 27,000 hours of chronic pain over an eleven-year period (*ICP* 7). She also lists some two hundred and forty appointments with doctors and specialists, nearly five hundred appointments with alternative professionals, a dozen appointments for tests and assessments, and countless hours spent keeping track of prescriptions, bills, and insurance. Finding a photograph taken before the accident, she encounters her own image as almost unrecognizable: "I had become someone else," she writes. "'A crumbled woman,' is how one of my daughters described me. A strange shadow of my former self" (*ICP* 26). *Crumbled* is also the word that Heshusius uses to describe the twisted steel beams of her accident-demolished car: she, too, in her own mind, is wreckage. Human damage, unlike bent metal, leads to what she calls a "tormenting journey" (*ICP* xxv). She singles out several doctors for warm praise, but mostly she records her general and tormented dismay at the medical establishment. Her language proves as instructive as her indictment. "In this book I show as clearly as I can," she writes, "what happens when a life that is going along just fine takes that sudden turn into the hell that is chronic pain" (*ICP* xxiv).

Heshusius's metaphoric description (*the hell that is chronic pain*) seems more than a casual figure of speech, since it reappears in several versions during her account. She imagines pain as "a devil with raked horns" (*ICP* 33), and she regards her book as a form of revenge in which "I rise to Pain's devilish power" (*ICP* 13). Her words powerfully illustrate how various beliefs, metaphors, and miniature fragmentary narratives so often accompany or infiltrate illness. They do not allow me to make clinical judgments about her pain, and I refuse to do so, but her words can prompt two general thoughts relevant to the self-management of pain. First, some pain beliefs cause direct harm, and among the most harmful are pain beliefs that contribute to the mental-emotional state known as *catastrophizing*: "characterizations of pain as awful, horrible and unbearable."[18] Pain sometimes surely *is* god-awful, but effective self-management depends on knowing that we can also make our pain worse if we catastrophize. Second, the process of "story-editing" that psychologist Timothy D. Wilson recommends—a conscious *reframing* of the harmful stories we may tell ourselves—can have significant beneficial outcomes.[19] The harmful stories may proceed at a nonconscious level expressed only in metaphors and images—but, once identified, harmful stories can be reframed, Wilson shows, in ways that would permit helpful self-management. Two distinguished pain specialists recently discussed disappointing clinical results that seem directly related to the microlevel, cellular understanding of pain pursued in medical school curricula. They ask if it is time to "flip" the pain curriculum.[20] Patients will benefit, they argue, when medical students focus less on the microlevel cellular neurobiology of pain and more on its macrolevel and sociocultural dimensions. Patients, too, in the interests of self-management, may need to flip their own implicit or internalized biomedical pain curriculum.

Pain, like cancer, is plural, and so are the narratives of pain that self-managers need to take into account. There are many types of cancer and many types of pain, from the stabbing pain of postherpetic neuralgia, say, or the queasy pain of migraine, to the dull ache of deep muscle pain or the burning pain of a skin abrasion. Macrolevel environmental influences, however, also weave around and through whatever cellular processes underlie consciousness. A young mother in a happy, stable marriage may experience the pain of childbirth differently from an isolated, impoverished, stigmatized rape victim. Anger and sadness, in laboratory experiments, correlate with increased pain intensity, and the social emotions of guilt and blame play a role in the undertreated pain of HIV/AIDS patients. Persistent undertreatment in medical settings is a cultural or environmental fact that directly influences pain. Ethnicity, race, and gender also influence pain in a complex biological and cultural mix. Chronic low back pain patients in Japan, for example, proved less impaired in psychological, social, vocational, and avocational function than similar patients in America.[21] Pain, in short, is irreversibly porous, open to modifying influences from cultures and beliefs. The good news is that consciousness, as rooted in the hubbub of human social and psychic life, holds the power to modify and to ameliorate pain through its influence over thoughts and feelings, unlike the crude neural mechanism that Descartes compared to ringing a bell by pulling on the attached rope, as if pain were no more than a mindless alarm signifying tissue damage. The placebo effect is well-documented, as when a toothache disappears as soon as we catch sight of the dentist, but the nocebo effect (as in voodoo death), too, demonstrates the power of the mind in combination with explicit or implicit cultural narratives to add or subtract pain.

"Find things to give you pleasure in life," advises Sean Mackey, chief of the division of pain management at Stanford University, "whether it be through the one you love or going and listening to great music or reading a good book." Such activities, he suggests, will activate the brain's reward system and reduce pain. It is Mackey's laboratory that published the finding that simply looking at the picture of a romantic partner reduced moderate pain by 40 percent.[22] Pleasure is among the home-brewed analgesics available with the cultural transformations implicit in a new Zoom Model. Medical eros would endorse Mackey's view that narrative pleasures—from books to film—constitute a potent resource in the self-management of pain.

Replacing Yourself: Narrative, Pleasure, and Ethics

Human brains, whether we like it or not, manufacture narratives. Our ancestors told stories about the gods, including Eros, and we fill seats at the local cinema courtesy of the same inborn narrative drive. Jill Bolte Taylor, a brain neuro-anatomist, suffered a massive stroke that impaired the language-processing areas in the left hemisphere of her brain. As cognitive function gradually returned, she observed with a scientist's objectivity (but also with the bemusement of a recovering patient) that her left brain, as if operating under its own power and command, "enthusiastically manufactured stories that it promoted as the truth."[23] Taylor came to describe her left brain, almost fondly, as "my storyteller," and she recognized its power to lead her astray. "I learned that I need to be very wary of my storyteller's potential for stirring up drama and trauma." *Confabulation* is the medical term for pathological versions of this unwilled narrative stream of brain fiction.[24] Paralyzed patients after a stroke, for example, sometimes deny their paralysis and confabulate bogus stories to account for their limitations. (Doctor: "Why can't you lift your arm?" Patient: "I've got arthritis in my shoulder.") Such patients are not lying or engaging in deceit. Stories, when we need an explanation, are simply what our brains *can't help* producing. We *tell* stories, even to ourselves, much as birds build nests. Why? As Joan Didion puts it, *we tell ourselves stories in order to live.* A life devoid of enjoyments would strike many people as not worth living. Perhaps we are also drawn to stories—or stories draw us—through the same life-enhancing force that inclines us to hear a joke, to read a book, or to see a film: the expectation of pleasure.

Pleasure suffers from a mild case of disrespect today, as if it is insufficiently serious or has been trivialized by jet-set plutocrats, but medical eros rejects the view that pleasure is inherently frivolous. Ancient philosophers agreed. Pleasure in the classical world occupied a central position in discussions of human moral life. Plato devoted an entire dialogue (*Phaedrus*) to pleasure, and, if little else, this ancient respect might incline us to question the modern cultural contradictions that both glorify mindless pleasure (girls gone wild) and suggest its triviality in comparison to (the correct answer) world peace. Classical pleasure, as a moral state, has somehow dwindled into amoral fun—if it feels good, do it—and we are forever looking for something better. The cultural transformations needed in the understanding and treatment of pain include a sense that pain raises important ethical questions. An ethics of pain, in turn, depends on recognizing its almost paradoxical relation with narrative pleasure.

Narrative, in order to claim standing within the citadel of medical logos, has to make a serious claim to knowledge. Rita Charon, in her bold *JAMA* article "Narrative Medicine," argues that competence in understanding narrative produces a distinctive form of knowledge: *narrative knowledge*. *JAMA*, of course, issues from the headquarters of biomedicine, and thus there is strategic value in a focus on narrative knowledge, as Charon expertly explains how such narrative knowledge serves as a complement to logico-scientific understanding. Narrative pleasure, however, from the perspective of medical logos, is almost as objectionable as not-knowing. Pleasure does hold one minor and almost negligible niche within biomedicine. Laughter has been shown to stimulate endogenous opiates and to relieve pain, so comic narratives presumably have therapeutic value if they excite laughter (rather than smiles). That's about all. Medical logos, if accepting of narrative at all, prefers to focus on the knowledge that narrative might yield rather than on its possibilities for pleasure.

Medical eros has no headquarters, but it has allies who recognize the importance of narrative pleasure. In *The Pleasure of the Text* (1973), theorist Roland Barthes characterizes the two main reader responses to narrative as *plaisir* and *jouissance*. Pleasure belongs to the everyday novels and entertainments that don't strain our capacities. *Jouissance*, or the pleasure that Barthes associates with complex, code-breaking texts, covers in French both bliss in general and, in particular, sexual orgasm.[25] Stories in effect constitute little engines of pleasure. They draw us less from a sense of duty than from off-duty desires, up to and including sexual desire. Virginia Woolf valued poetry because it gives invalids access to the sensuousness of sound, music, and nonsense, where pleasure is enough, and such pleasures certainly extend to escapist narratives such as her tale of Lady Waterford. Medical eros, in asserting the validity of narrative pleasure, would defend its role as complement to analytical knowledge and rational competence. Eros, in addition, offers a somewhat scandalous opportunity to circumvent the knowledge-seeking mind-set keyed to thinking *about* stories, as if stories could be reduced without loss to objects of study. Instead, it insinuates both the primacy of pleasure and the benefits that flow, if indirectly, from an emotion-rich, subjective thinking *with* stories.

Thinking *with* stories is a concept that I borrow from the sociologist, cancer survivor, and pioneer scholar of illness narratives Arthur W. Frank, and it refers to a process very different from the operations of analytical reason common to medical logos.[26] Frank focuses far less on the hermeneutics of narrative (what stories *mean*) than on its pragmatics (what stories *do*). The pragmatics of thinking *with* stories always involves an element of reason—thought can't be wholly irrational or it ceases to be thought—but it also invokes a pleasurable collaboration with feeling. Thinking *about* stories turns narrative into an *object* of thought. Thinking *with* stories is a process in which we do not so much work on narrative, analyzing it objectively, as take a radical step back and (giving free play to pleasure) allow narrative *to work on us*.

"That story is working on you now," a young male Apache tells anthropologist Keith Basso about a particular Native American narrative. "That story is working on you now," he repeats. "You keep thinking about it. That story is changing you now, making you want to live right. That story is making you want to replace yourself."[27] Basso's purpose is to show how the western Apache people still live in a local landscape richly endowed with narrative meaning. Even a passing allusion to identifiable

places, such as Line-of-White-Rocks or Red-Ridge-with-Alder-Trees, instantly evokes for tribal listeners traditional tales of what happened
there. In a culture that scrupulously avoids direct rebuke, such allusions
evoke the moral stories associated with a particular place and thus provide unobtrusive and indirect but steady moral guidance. Such stories almost literally get under your skin. Basso shows, in effect, how thinking
with stories enlists narrative pleasure in the stealth service of ethics.

Medical eros might invoke the stunning concept of stories that make
you want to replace yourself in order to underwrite a new *affective* bioethics of narrative; this bioethics, as we will see, has direct relevance to
the understanding and management of pain. Such an affective bioethics
provides a complement and (at times) a rival to the traditional principle-
driven bioethics endorsed by medical logos. From this new ethical and
affective perspective, stories are not entertainments or trivial fictions but
experiences that incur an obligation on the listener.[28] They exert a "call."
The moral call of stories—as psychologist Robert Coles describes this
narrative power—is not restricted to indigenous peoples in remote locations.[29] Coles tells how stories exercise a moral force among his patients
and students in Boston. A respectable minority tradition in philosophy,
from Aristotle to Iris Murdoch, has staked a claim for stories as engaging
what the philosopher Mark Johnson calls *the moral imagination.* "No
moral theory can be adequate," he writes, "if it does not take into account
the narrative character of our experience."[30]

Today, across disciplines, a substantial scholarly literature is beginning
to focus on so-called narrative ethics.[31] Narrative now holds an established
place within the indispensable medical subfield of bioethics, although
bioethics still prefers to keep narrative pleasure at arm's length. Good
precedent thus exists for rejecting a dismissive view of stories as merely
disposable products of the entertainment industry or as artifacts so inherently indeterminate as to produce endless wrangling over interpretations.
Medical eros, by enlisting narrative pleasure in service of bioethics, can
offer practical help both in the patient's self-management of pain and in
the self-understanding of physicians charged with managing the pain of
others. Patients and doctors will both benefit from understanding how
the stories we tell about pain and the painful narrative situations we encounter regularly include an emotional resonance that, even if appar-

ently far removed from pleasure, can work on us more effectively than medicolegal arguments and (if we let it) show us what to do.

Pain and Narrative Ethics: Three Probes

Medical eros, while it has a special affinity for narrative and pleasure, shares less evident common ground with pain. "Pain," wrote Emily Dickinson, "has an Element of Blank."[32] The blankness of pain—only one "Element," but crucial and intrinsic—enfolds a not-knowing fundamental to eros. Pain for Dickinson, which she personifies as if it were a super-human being endowed with blankness, does not know its own origin and when (or if) it will end. This inherent not-knowing means that pain always contains an excess or surplus that remains forever inaccessible to reason and to analysis. The blankness of pain, on the other hand, in its overlap with the native terrain of medical eros, offers an opportunity to explore how thinking *with* stories (instead of thinking *about* stories) helps illuminate issues in ethics where eros comes into play. Three probes are enough to begin an exploration of the relationship among pain, ethics, and eros.

Probe one concerns a medical school symposium on the topic of pain and ethics. It took place in the early 1990s, but the impact on me was unforgettable, and the key issues have not appreciably changed. The typical procession of speakers concluded with the chair of anesthesiology. He spoke in convincing detail about the burdens on his budget and staff, citing recent university cutbacks in funding and new state directives about mandatory care for the poor. His measured tones and what struck me as his visible personal integrity left me unprepared for the sweeping ethical conclusion. When it comes to the treatment of pain in his department, he stated as a blunt matter of fact, "it is no longer possible to do the right thing."

This chilling conclusion, which I suspect could be repeated today (less openly) in many medical specialties, offers a narrative glimpse into the ethics of postmodern pain. The dilemma is not postmodern in its embrace of doubt or contingency—the speaker assumes, with refreshing certainty, that he knows what constitutes *the right thing* to do. He also knows, with equal certainty, that ethical action—*doing* the right thing—is now no

longer possible. Reason, principle, and moral agency all seem at an un-
decidable impasse: the postmodern showdown where action collapses in
endless talk. The impersonal construction *"it is no longer possible"* suggests that this new dilemma does not concern the moral failure of specific individuals—anesthesiologists, administrators, legislators—but
rather it concerns the insignificance of individual action. The moral failure
apparently lies with systems and institutions that make personal choices
irrelevant. An ethics responsive to such distinctive postmodern dilemmas
may require tools as unfamiliar to medical logos as inquiries into narrative point of view. It may require thinking in which moral action has less
to do with reason or fixed principles than with the stories we tell and the
emotions we feel—or deny.

Probe two concerns a journalistic story reported in the *New York
Times* in 1999 about a California Medicaid patient, Mrs. Ozzie Chavez.[33]
The ethical issues remain timely, although the relevant background requires a brief comment on medical insurance and on narrative structure.
Narrative often embeds basic and familiar structural patterns: boy meets
girl, boy loses girl, boy gets girl. (The names and details are fungible.)
Medical insurance, which is now often systematically intertwined with
pain, embeds its own mininarrative structure: you are insured, you get
hurt, you get compensation. This mininarrative structure is not innocent. It is not free from social implications, but rather entails built-in social
and personal costs. Compensation may sustain and possibly even create
pain. Developed nations, for example, face rapidly mounting claims for
pain associated with automobile accidents, but in Lithuania (where
drivers had no recourse to medical insurance) studies showed no significant difference between accident victims and a control group in reports
of headache and neck pain.[34] The implication? The head and neck pain
of chronic whiplash syndrome is, in developed nations, in part an arti-
fact of compensation narratives. It is not necessary to assume fraud. It
appears that disability payments for chronic pain actively impede medical
treatment if compensation serves as an incentive for patients to retain
pain.[35] The issues at stake here, as regards pain, are not entirely economic
or medical but ethical.

Narrative bioethics may demonstrate its value precisely in illuminating
the conflicts native to every local world where moral action is no longer

strictly an individual Hercules-type choice between virtue or vice but rather concerns shifting points of contact where powerful social or institutional narratives intersect with personal narrative identities and individual life stories. A prestigious task force studied rising claims for workers' compensation payments associated with chronic pain and found that, in many cases, the chronic pain could not be correlated with an organic lesion. The task force concluded that chronic pain *in the absence of an organic lesion* should not qualify as a medical disability—eligible for compensation—but should be reclassified as "activity intolerance."[36] *Activity intolerance*, hardly an official biomedical diagnosis, reframes the dominant sociomedical narrative (in which chronic pain merits disability insurance) as a tone-deaf counternarrative of personal inadequacy. The personal pain narratives that we live out today increasingly come into conflict with powerful if invisible sociomedical narratives that, in some cases, may establish trajectories for chronic pain patients that are as damaging on ethical grounds as nineteenth-century narratives of hysteria.

Mrs. Ozzie Chavez—back to probe two, where the emotions are less veiled—met the income threshold at which the California Medicaid program covered obstetrical expenses, and the birth of her child thus belonged within an established social compensation narrative. The dilemma: the anesthesiologist refused Mrs. Chavez a standard form of anesthesia in labor because she did not pay an additional (illegal) fee demanded in advance. "I'm not a wimp when it comes to pain," Mrs. Chavez told the *Times* reporter. "But it was a very painful delivery." Demands for additional payment, as it happened, were not rare because of California's well-known substandard Medicaid reimbursement policies, so this encounter is more than a typical "horror story" (another narrative subgenre) about uncaring doctors. Mrs. Chavez had her own narrative point of view, however, and it is chilling. The anesthesiologist wouldn't even come into the room until she got her money," Mrs. Chavez explained. "I was lying there having contractions, and they wouldn't give me an epidural. I felt like an animal."

Narrative bioethics will not get to the bottom of this event and expose the bedrock truth about what really happened—who was right, and who was wrong. A narrative approach, however, helps to illuminate the conflicting forces that define her experience. Bioethicist Tod Chambers's reminder that there are no artless narrations certainly helps expose the rhetorical strategies implicit in the unofficial comments and official stories issued in response to Mrs. Chavez's dilemma. The American Society of Anesthesiologists in its newsletter ran an account that printed one member's particularly unsympathetic argument: "Poor people can't expect to drive a Rolls Royce or to eat in a fine French restaurant, so why should they expect to receive the Cadillac of analgesics for free?" As if to head off a looming public relations disaster, the president of the ASA deftly steered the discourse away from economics and particularly far away from Cadillacs and fine restaurants, to refocus directly on ethical issues and principles. "It's unethical," John B. Neeld Jr. asserted, invoking a hallowed pillar of bioethical principlism, "to withhold services because of reimbursement." End of story?

A narrative bioethics—attentive to situations and emotions—would not regard the case closed when one character invokes a hallowed principle. A *narrative situation*, to invoke Rita Charon, is always part of the relevant data. Who invokes the principle? Why? Whose interest does it serve? Narrative bioethics helps illuminate the hidden conflicts and reminds us that all stories include gaps: no narrative tells *everything*. What *don't we know* about Mrs. Chavez, John Neeld, and the unnamed anesthesiologist? Not-knowing, that is, matters as much in ethics as in law, and medical eros, at home in non-knowing, can also ask what is left *unsaid*. John Neeld doesn't say (perhaps it is *unsayable*?) that pain relief is withheld in America every day—and not just for inability to pay. Medical undertreatment for pain has been well-known for over fifty years, but its ethical implications have gone largely ignored, even among bioethicists.[37] Narrative bioethics is not fixed on assigning blame but rather focuses on elucidating the stories (both told and untold) in ways that—with all voices heard and with even *the unsaid* adequately accounted for—we are likelier to know what the right thing *is*.

The right thing to do, regrettably, grows even harder to determine because we live in an era marked by the massive overprescription of opiate painkillers. The results are deadly, and only medical logos holds the prescription pad. Hydrocodone and oxycodone products (currently the most popular prescription painkillers) kill more people than heroin or cocaine, and the United States consumes 99 percent of the world's hydrocodone, much of it illegally.[38] The Centers for Disease Control and Prevention calls heroin use in the United States an epidemic: more than 8,200 people died of heroin overdoses in 2013 alone, while 45 percent of those who used heroin were also addicted to prescription opioid painkillers.[39] Doctors are caught in a no-win situation as social debates and medical research almost monthly change the landscape. Researchers have discovered that in rats morphine paradoxically spurs a "cascade" of reactions in the brain and spinal cord that actually prolong chronic pain.[40]

The self-management of chronic pain with opioids is a tricky business—dangerous, too—especially when doctors disagree, but when discussion turns to ethics it is important to observe that prescription practices in the United States were strongly influenced by the massive campaign for the promotion and marketing of OxyContin, an oxycodone preparation created by Purdue Pharma. "From 1996 to 2001," as physician Art Van Zee explains, "Purdue conducted more than 40 national pain-management and speaker training conferences at resorts in Florida, Arizona, and California. More than 5000 physicians, pharmacists, and nurses attended these all-expenses-paid symposia, where they were recruited and trained for Purdue's national speaker bureau."[41] This type of drug company symposium, he adds, has been well documented to influence physicians' prescription practices, even though physicians attending these symposia—I would add, no doubt with narratives of their own to tell—deny any influence.

Medical eros, through its affinity for narrative, has a surprisingly important role in the ethical management of pain, as the experience of Mrs. Chavez indicates, and no role is more important than its power, as we have seen, to expose potentially harmful narratives. Such harm is particularly evident in the commonplace *Us/Them* narratives that divide people into hardened opposing camps, with one group often demonized, depending on whose side tells the story.[42] Such Us/Them narratives may often reflect rather than create divisions, but they are devilishly effective in perpetuating and intensifying conflict. They sustain racial, ethnic, national, and religious stereotypes, with stigmatized groups and marginalized individuals at special risk for harm. It is no coincidence that Mrs. Chavez is poor, Hispanic, and female.

Race and ethnicity, which often overlap with lower socioeconomic status, have a direct relation to the undertreatment of pain.[43] The pain of people identified with marginalized groups is often disregarded, as in the once (and perhaps still) "dramatically undertreated" pain of AIDS patients.[44] Raymond C. Tait coauthored a study of workers' compensation data showing that African Americans with job-related lower back injuries were treated differently from whites, incurring lower costs, fewer compensated work absences, shorter claim periods, lower disability ratings, and smaller settlements. As Tait explained to a reporter: "Our data pretty clearly say it's a race issue."[45] African Americans in the United States face a "disproportionate burden" of worse outcomes for pain. White skin can be more important than traumatic injury in predicting the likelihood of receiving opioid analgesics in the emergency department.[46] Sickle-cell disease in the United States, for example, affects mainly African Americans, whose urgent emergency room requests for pain medication intersect with powerful social narratives about drug-seeking behavior. In New York City, pharmacies in white neighborhoods are three times likelier than pharmacies in minority neighborhoods to carry adequate supplies of opioid analgesics. Patients in the developing world routinely fail to receive adequate pain medication, while third-world pain gets indirectly enfolded within the well-publicized American "war" on drugs.[47] Wars often create a need for new narratives that implicitly justify, excuse, ignore, or deny the pain of enemy combatants, and noncombatants who are badly injured often have their pain reclassified and bureaucratically abstracted, in the newly militarized narratives, as mere collateral damage.

A narrative ethics of pain needs to pay special attention to stigmatized groups and to individuals whose voices, overwhelmed by dominant social narratives and power structures, often go unheard or unheeded. Pain is bad enough, but dying patients and the elderly frequently drop from sight, much like children, as if their status erases the need for pain relief. Even well-researched differences between women and men in pain sensitivity—a measure subject to biological and psychosocial variables—easily blend with stereotypes characterizing women as hyperemotional, as if their pain were somehow less deserving of attention. Barroom brawls erupt over failures to understand that pain sensitivity differs by gender, but men and women appear equal in their ability to tolerate pain intensity. (Dentists already have taken note that true redheads carry variants of the *MC1R* gene affecting pain receptors in the brain, which makes them resistant to subcutaneous local anesthetics.)[48] The questions for narrative ethics are less about data, principles, and logic as grounds for moral action than about who controls the stories, about identifying and reframing harmful narratives, and about truly hearing what is said and recognizing what is left unsaid. Speech is action—as charged with ethical significance at times as a father's curse. Medical eros would observe that Mrs. Chavez (who insisted it was a painful delivery) didn't complain about feeling pain. Her exact words were that she felt *like an animal.*

Probe Three: The Infinity of the Face

Medical eros, in its focus on narrative, views pain in its social structure as always concerning at least two inner lives. There is, first, the person in pain; but pain also, most often, involves a second person: the person who observes the pain of the other. The physician occupies this second-person role, but its structural position is also occupied by caregivers, family members, friends, or strangers. The question for the second-person observer—ethical as much as medical—is, What *call* does pain make? What response or obligation does pain incur in the person who occupies the position where a response is called for, where even turning away or doing nothing is an implicit response? This is the urgent question that Susan Sontag posed in *Regarding the Pain of Others* (2003), and it is a question of major concern for medicine, where the pain of others is a daily presence and entails its own professional *call*. It is also the question addressed by the writer-director Preston Sturges in his 1944 biopic *The Great Moment*, the nonfiction story of William Morton and the invention of surgical anesthesia.[49] The narrative pleasures of cinema, fraught with ethical implications, often place the film audience in the second-person role of observing the pain of the other.

Medical logos would seem to be the moving spirit behind *The Great Moment*—a title that almost predicts a celebration of scientific achievement—and the film is loosely based on René Fülöp-Miller's historical novel describing the invention of surgical anesthesia, *Triumph over Pain* (1938). Morton—a dentist too poor to afford medical school—conducts the self-experimental tests with ether that lead directly to the discovery of surgical anesthesia. For the next fifty years Massachusetts General Hospital celebrated this anniversary—October 16, 1846—as Ether Day. On that momentous day, at Mass General, chief surgeon John Collins Warren performed the first successful public demonstration of pain-free surgery; patients thereafter no longer faced the monstrous pain and lethal aftermath of operations performed without anesthesia. Surgery blossomed with the option of slower, more intricate procedures.

Morton's achievement certainly warranted scientific honor and financial reward. However, as in the Darwin–Wallace controversy over the theory of evolution, counterclaims soon embroiled Morton in dispute. The film begins with a flash-forward showing Morton as an old man, unrecognized and unrewarded, worn out with poverty, frustration, and setbacks. The film gains emotional power, then, from our knowledge that Morton will die a ruined man as the result of a fateful act that he performs—his truly "great moment"—to save one patient from harrowing pain.

The Great Moment recounts Morton's story as a conflict between abstract principles and a higher emotion-based or eros-driven ethics. It is also a drama in which competing desires collide: while excited crowds throng outside Mass General in anticipation of the groundbreaking operation, delegates from the Massachusetts Medical Society meet behind closed doors to stop the surgery. They, rightly, cite the Hippocratic principle of do no harm (*non-maleficence* in modern principlism), arguing that physicians are forbidden on ethical grounds from using medicines with unknown ingredients, which was a valuable protection against quack potions. Morton's dilemma is that he can't patent ether, a natural substance, so his only sure source of financial reward will come from a still-unpatented ether inhaler. Meanwhile, he has disguised his chemical discovery under the pseudonym *Letheon*. If Morton's desire for gain is less than saintly, the upper-crust delegates of the medical society (the word *snob* springs to mind) are far from spotless, desiring mainly to keep a lowly dentist in his place. All power resides with the delegates, and Morton thus faces a stark ethical choice. His fortune depends on temporarily maintaining the secret of Letheon, but secrecy means that an unknown patient will undergo a harrowing, fully conscious, unanesthetized leg amputation performed (as Warren says dryly) "in the old way."

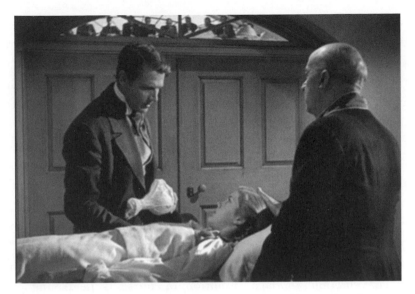

FIGURE 6.2. Operation scene from *The Great Moment* (1944),
directed by Preston Sturges, with Joel McCrea as William Morton.
Paramount Pictures.

The conflict now moves to a new level as Warren yields to his medical society colleagues and prepares to operate. The camera follows Morton down a long hallway in a lingering portrait of his isolation and indecision. *Ave Maria* plays softly on the soundtrack while a priest attends to a young girl on a stretcher outside the operating room; the unknown patient has acquired an age, gender, and body. Morton ends his long walk at the stretcher. Above his head, the film puts viewers in the second-person position as we glimpse the crowded amphitheater in which the girl's awful ordeal is about to begin. She assumes almost the role of sacrificial victim as Morton mumbles a few words of gentle concern (Figure 6.2).

The girl—nameless—knows nothing of the medical dispute about principles. With one prominent tear glistening on her cheek, she responds to Morton, saying that "a gentleman" has made a new discovery and that the operation "doesn't hurt anymore." The dramatic ironies turn bitter as Morton and the audience recognize his complicity in her upcoming ordeal. Narrative ethics throws light on dramatic choices and actions. What will Morton *do*?

"Not to relieve pain optimally," writes the revered bioethicist Edmund Pellegrino in a 1998 *JAMA* essay on palliative care, "is tantamount to moral and legal malpractice."[50] The decision for Morton, without the benefit of an essay on bioethics, is instantaneous. Looking into the girl's eyes, as if seized with a sudden epiphany, he acts. Simultaneously—this is still Hollywood—the doors of the operating theater fling open with a near-celestial flood of light. A musical crescendo assures viewers that the girl is spared. As distinct from the just-celebrated medical event, the film's *great moment* is Morton's private moment of truth: an ethical decision. It is not entirely a happy ending because viewers already know, via the opening flash-forward, that Morton's act of moral courage will mean the ruin of all his worldly hopes.

The concept of thinking *with* stories, so basic to medical eros, offers a chance to reflect on how the second-person position (as regarding the pain of others) entangles ethics with two apparently unrelated phenomena: emotions and faces. Emotion, of course, is the driving force in Morton's ethical decision. The film represents moral action not as a product of rational analysis—sifting evidence, analyzing arguments, weighing principles—but as an almost spontaneous emotional impulse. Morton, unlike the chair of anesthesiology, both knows what the right thing to do *is* . . . and he also *does* it, spontaneously. Emotion, in this exploratory *thinking-with* stories, emerges as necessary for moral action. Neuroscientist Antonio R. Damasio describes a patient with a localized brain injury that impaired the ability to feel emotion while leaving intact the ability to reason. Significantly, this emotionless reasoner performed well on tests of moral judgment but had lost the power to make decisions.[51] Emotion, in short, proves indispensable to an ethics that not only *knows* what is right but also *acts rightly*. Put differently: medical logos, as if blind to its own blindness, quarantines emotion in ethical decisions only at the certain risk of an ethics hamstrung by an inability to choose and to act.

"The ethic under which I toiled," Rafael Campo writes about his days in medical school, "was that anyone who had time to write about his feelings certainly was not spending enough time searching the medical literature for relevant articles and memorizing the data."[52] The personal transformation for Campo came as he gazed into the face of his suddenly debilitated patient Aurora. *The Great Moment* highlights a similar occasion when Morton stands beside the girl on the stretcher—holding his unpatented ether inhaler like a wounded bird—and gazes into her face. The face has much to suggest about an emotion-rich ethics of pain. Although human brains possess a facial recognition network, the face as an ethical concept holds a different status in the work of philosopher Emmanuel Levinas, and we cannot leave the second-person ethics of pain without a brief conversation with Levinas.

Ethics for Levinas—one of the major continental philosophers of the modern era—is where philosophy begins. Ethics, as he puts it, is "first philosophy." If philosophy can't get ethics right, Levinas considers it useless, so the job of philosophy is to *start* with ethics. Ethics, in turn, starts with the face. The face, as Levinas argues, is more than an anatomical or biological feature: it *represents* the otherness of the other person. It signifies the inherent, ineradicable, inexhaustible *differences* that make each person irreducible to any knowledge that might summarize or "contain" them. The face cannot be reduced to an object of knowledge or even to an object of vision because, for Levinas, the other person—in his or her unknowable otherness—cannot be objectified. The face, instead, evokes an *experience*: an experience of not-knowing. It is a not-knowing that differs from ignorance or lack of biomedical data. The face evokes a personal experience of the uncontainable, untotalizable, incommunicable *infinitude* of the other person—which is to say, of everyone.

Levinas, in his thinking about the infinitude of the face, drew on his experience during World War II imprisoned in a German stalag reserved for Jewish prisoners of war. (His mother, father, and two brothers in Lithuania were machine-gunned by Nazi soldiers.) He noted that the stalag guards gave no sign of seeing anything human in their prisoners. War, however, is only the most extreme instance of a dehumanizing gaze. The infinitude of the other person is a concept that—given the ease with which we ignore it—deserves a second thought. Doctors look into the faces of patients every day, in the act of delivering medical care. Do they ever recognize the *infinitude* of the patient? Does a patient ever look into a doctor's face and recognize an unknowable *infinitude*? Recognition suggests a cognitive state, but for Levinas the face makes an immediate emotional rather than cognitive or reflective claim. Our relation to the face, as he puts it, is "straightaway" (*d'emblée*) ethical.[53] This straightaway ethics depends on an emotional contact that Levinas describes as a "shuddering" (*frémissement*), a word translating the term (as he explains in a learned annotation) that Socrates uses to describe the force of eros.

An erotic, face-to-face "shuddering," even without its classical allusion, taps into emotional strata more primitive than reason, and it might well describe what happens to William Morton as he gazes into the face of the young girl. "The face," as Levinas writes of the precognitive, emotional shudder, "opens the primordial discourse whose first word is obligation."[54] Medical eros may find Levinasian philosophy a bit thick and solemn for everyday use—reading Levinas is definitely slow-going—but Morton's gaze into the face of the young patient certainly initiates a discourse of obligation: "Are you the girl, the girl for the operation?" he asks. Her unthinkable imminent pain hangs in the balance between them. The shudder of emotion implicit in their face-to-face contact, which Sturges signals with a full orchestral score, is not the opposite of reason, not a trite, frenzied juice squeezed out of the limbic system, even if it is also quite different both from cognition and from pity. *The Great Moment*, with all the limitations of narrative, nonetheless shows how pain constitutes the occasion for an emotional shudder of understanding in which we grasp the infinity of the other person and act upon a concern that is "straight-away ethical."

Skeptics may interpret Morton's ethics of the face as coinciding too neatly with cinematic displays of male virtue that regularly depend on displays of female helplessness. Or they may contextualize his action and reflect that *The Great Moment* speaks to a World War II audience that exalts male self-sacrifice: a performance called forth by an attractive girl with no name and no history, who might almost serve as an icon of national innocence. No matter. Skepticism has slipped us back into thinking *about* rather than *with* stories. The ethical call of pain and the face of the other, moreover, contain useful suggestions for the self-management of pain. The person in pain needs to recognize that institutions are impersonal not solely as a by-product of size, complexity, or convenience; rather, institutions cultivate and deploy, as to their direct advantage, a stone wall of bureaucratic facelessness, like phone trees or Web sites engineered to eliminate human contact. Neglect of the face takes on new meaning when physicians spend an entire hospital-room visit peering into their laptop screens. *The Great Moment* deploys the pleasures of narrative, as if on behalf of medical eros, in an implicit critique of absent faces: committee decisions made on abstract principle, distributed by memo, and enacted by rotating teams of employees as uncommunicative as their nametags. Self-management needs to look elsewhere.

Medical eros, in its role as contrary and complement to medical logos, reminds us of the ethical implications of pain that reason alone and principles alone cannot convey. The goal is not to steer decisions in a specific direction but rather to get the stories into the open, to sift their competing values, to discuss any conflicts, and to explore their power to work on *us*. I cannot imagine the audience that would endorse a conclusion to *The Great Moment* in which Morton glances at the girl, shrugs his shoulders, and strolls away. Sturges crafts a narrative in which a face-to-face encounter and the prospect of imminent traumatic pain prompt a straightaway ethics that makes it impossible (short of self-betrayal or a perverse fall into evil) for Morton *not* to do the right thing. If we agree with Morton's decision, we, too, share in a straightaway ethics with its erotic shuddering. The self-management of pain will be far more difficult without a respect for the role of eros, emotion, and desire. A truly desirable transformation in the understanding and treatment of pain might well begin with new macrolevel narratives that give as much respect to the face of the other—which is our own face as if seen in a mirror—as to the pharmaceutical compounds and to the microlevel cellular structures that occupy medical logos and the molecular gaze.

Part Three

The Dilemmas

CHAPTER SEVEN

Black Swan Syndrome: Probable Improbabilities

The essence of life is statistical improbability on a colossal scale.

RICHARD DAWKINS, *THE BLIND WATCHMAKER* (1986)

*P*AIN IS THE archetype of a probable event. Almost everyone experiences it at some time, and it is the number one complaint among older Americans. There is a dilemma, however, concealed within the biomedical emphasis on probabilities. *When you hear hoofbeats*, so goes the orthodox medical school advice, *don't think zebras!* Symptoms in medicine constitute the hoofbeat event that sends patients to doctors and that sends the physician in search of a probable cause. It even underlies the concept of patienthood. "May I never see in the patient anything but a fellow creature in pain": the oath of Maimonides, sometimes recited by graduating medical students, takes the probability of pain as an unspoken assumption, as if to be a patient means being in pain.[1] A life entirely without pain constitutes an improbability of the highest order; congenital insensitivity is rare, thankfully, because it is no gift, and people born fully pain-free most often die young. Medical logos and the molecular gaze, which depend upon rational calculation, statistical data, and the orderly law-like discoveries of laboratory science, greatly increase the clinical reliance on probabilities. The generation of probable knowledge is almost synonymous with health care and is regarded as a self-evident good. "The aim of all medical research," writes the clinician and researcher Guy B. Faquet, "is to accrue scientific knowledge to the medical database, and in so doing, provide the foundation for ultimately improving health care."[2]

The probabilistic knowledge accrued to the medical database leads to innumerable practical quandaries, however, such as how to weigh the risks versus benefits of mammograms for women under fifty. Statistical probabilities are notoriously hard for all but statisticians to wrap our minds around. (It remains a puzzle to me why twenty-five "tails" in succession don't increase the odds for "heads" on coin flip twenty-six—they don't, but I'd bet heads anyway.) Probabilities, although they seem anchored in statistics and in the nature of things, are also a product of the pattern-seeking human brain. Early hunter-gatherers no doubt carefully observed annual herd migrations to detect probable patterns, but in its statistical form probabilistic thinking has an almost pinpoint origin in the so-called Age of Reason. "The decade around 1660," Ian Hacking writes, "is the birthtime of probability."[3] Ever since, patterns extracted from actuarial data underwrite the insurance industry, patterns extracted from epidemiological data underwrite public health policies, and patterns extracted from our online choices underwrite what annoying ads will pop up on our computer screens.

Probabilities, in short, sweep across our lives in ways that invisibly construct our everyday world. Take risk, for example. Statistical probabilities encourage us to view risk less as the threat of a future event than as a virtual reality: we are *already* at risk, if the numbers say so. The award-winning actress and human-rights activist Angelina Jolie, at age 38, opted for a preventive double mastectomy after learning that she carries the *BRCA1* gene and faced an 87 percent risk of developing breast cancer. "Once I knew that this was my reality," she said, in words suggesting how far statistics reshape not only our bodies and our health but also our sense of what's real, "I decided to be proactive and to minimize the risk as much as I could."[4]

Statistical discourses of probability proliferate ever new dilemmas as they mesh with other features of biomedical thought. Jolie faces still more preventive surgeries. "I started with the breasts," she continues, in the objectifying language of biomedicine, "as my risk of breast cancer is higher than my risk of ovarian cancer, and the surgery is more complex." Thus, two years after her double mastectomy and facing a 50 percent risk of ovarian cancer, Jolie elected to have her ovaries removed.[5] As a wife and mother, she explains, what motivates her preemptive surgeries is concern for her family. If *logos* provides the risk assessment, *eros* drives the decisions. Eros has its own slant interest in probabilities. Traditions of romantic love, that is, emphasize the one-in-a-million unique individual—the single soul mate in a universe of also-rans—who emerges when two strangers lock eyes across a crowded room. Suppose your singular soul mate, however, is an Ashkenazi Jew. After undergoing eight rounds of maximum-dose chemotherapy, Elizabeth Wurtzel (author of the 1994 autobiography *Prozac Nation*) contends that all Ashkenazi Jewish women should have the BRAC test because they are ten times more likely than other women to test positive.[6] Modern love, it appears, now cannot work its magic free from statistical probabilities. Our bodies are already tattooed with invisible numbers whose acceptable range is keyed to probabilities: cholesterol counts, heart rates, blood pressure, fat-to-muscle ratios, and daily step targets. The question for medical eros is how far, in giving our lives over to a calculus of probabilities, we ignore the improbabilities, singularities, coincidences, and anomalies that make falling in love a welcome adventure, but also hold hidden risks far worse than romantic breakups or predictable divorce rates. The perils turn catastrophic if the one big improbability we ignore is the deadly *black swan*.

Improbabilities and the Black Swan

A key dilemma at the heart of medical logos might be expressed as a paradox: how to reason about fringe experiences that reason can't make sense of. Absolute irrationality poses a less daunting challenge to biomedicine than do shadowy events that fall just short of unreason and evoke the dark regions that medical eros is at home in, including the native habitat of the Black Swan. The Black Swan is a metaphoric figure—the invention of a former Wall Street trader, Nassim Nicholas Taleb—standing for any improbable event that causes massive consequences.[7] Improbability is the key trait of the Black Swan, but not just any unforeseen improbability: the improbable event must entail great damage (or great benefit). A sudden unforeseen crash of world financial markets, for example, would count as a Black Swan, and the example is at least appropriate. Black Swans as financial events certainly reflect Taleb's practical experience as a high-stakes broker in an arena where fortunes are lost and won; but Black Swan catastrophes do not belong solely to financial markets. It is even possible to benefit from Black Swan events, as Taleb did, having taken appropriate precautions to ride out a sudden, unpredictable market collapse. The invisible Black Swan, in any case, is a fact of everyday life, and it also inhabits the databases of biomedicine, with their accrual of scientific knowledge, where lethal anomalies can emerge with blinding suddenness, like Barbara Rosenblum's breast cancer. The Black Swan takes us by surprise and confronts us at our weakest point with an irruption of what had seemed safely excluded from our mental construction of a probable world: the improbable, the not-known, and the unknowable.

We mostly operate like our hunter-gatherer ancestors with brain systems evolved to promote survival by locating patterns of probabilities: probable food, probable shelter, and probable reproductive success. Thus, for Taleb it is crucial to recognize—because it goes against the grain of human evolution—how far our pursuit of probabilities blinds us to the shadow of the improbable Black Swan. The Black Swan, even deadlier because we ignore it, is the opposite of an abstraction. It is a real-life menace that raises practical and ethical questions, as well as thorny, unresolvable dilemmas, about how to live and what to do.

Taleb doesn't mind coming across as a maverick. He has spent his entire financial career bucking trends with notable success, and he relishes the role of self-taught rebel whose personal passions and intellectual pursuits will strike many, he knows, as eccentric. He prefers Marcus Aurelius and Montaigne to current academic favorites, and such intellectual preferences reinforce his native temperament, which (raised to the level of a philosophical outlook) he calls skeptical empiricism. *Skeptical empiricism* embraces the respect for hard empirical facts over abstract theories that drives Taleb's distrust of systems, but it is a paradoxical respect—tempered by his equally strong belief that the facts are never sufficient. Hard facts are the best we have, but they are not good enough because we cannot possess *all* the facts, because facts are inherently *fragmentary*, and because *previously unknown* facts keep emerging to undermine previous fact-based theories and practices.

Faithful readers of the Tuesday science section of the *New York Times* know the feeling that any week now coffee may be declared either good or bad for your health, or both. Taleb's brand of skeptical empiricism does not extend to a distrust of reason as inherently flawed. Facts, for Taleb, are the best raw materials for reasoning, and reasoning is our best tool for thinking; but, nonetheless, facts and reason remain unreliable. The facts are always changing; reasoning is error-prone; and fact-based probabilities are always at risk from an irruption of the improbable. The danger, for Taleb, is that our statistically-based probabilistic thinking tends to shut down an openness to anomalies, which by definition are inaccessible to fact-based, reason-driven, statistical powers to predict or even to anticipate their appearances.

The Black Swan is an emblem of singularities: one-time, unpredictable, and perhaps unrepeatable events. Taleb, during the bull market years of Bill Clinton's presidency, had a front row seat for observing singularities and Black Swan events. As fresh young traders arrive on Wall Street, they rack up huge profits by predicting market fluctuations with computerized algorithms that possess an almost instantaneous capacity for calculation, data processing, and automated reasoning. Their success takes on material shape in the form of the condo in Manhattan, the Mercedes, the country house in Connecticut. Until, one fine day, something unpredictable and improbable happens, and they lose everything: the collapse of the Soviet Union, the burst of the tech bubble, the mortgage meltdown, the global recession. An unforeseen event occurs, a gigantic singularity, and the financial markets go haywire. The bright young traders with their condos, cars, and country houses, in the cold insider lingo of Wall Street, just "blow up."

For Taleb, the everyday world, like Wall Street, proves stranger and more dangerous than most people (embedded in a network of probabilities) assume. Assumptions based on probabilistic thinking are, for Taleb, a self-set trap unwittingly designed to ensnare us. He views the everyday not as a stable, familiar residence—not even as a benign refuge where philosophers who give up on the claims of reason can find solace in common practices and daily forms of life—but rather as the haunt of the Black Swan: a site of radical uncertainty, instability, and catastrophic reversals even more perilous precisely because everyday life, ordinarily, appears so benign. The ordinariness of everyday life is, in his view, utterly deceptive; it's a smokescreen concealing unknown, unsuspected, singular dangers, as if the sweet, quiet couple next door practices satanic rituals and infant blood sacrifice.

Born into a Greco-Syrian community in Lebanon, Taleb declines the descriptor *Lebanese* because national borders strike him as one more slick empirical deception, as slippery new facts force out slippery old facts, and the lines of nationhood change. He saw his homeland, which he viewed as a cosmopolitan, almost paradisiacal crossroads, where for some thirteen centuries Muslims and Christians had lived together in peace, suddenly unravel in a fifteen-year civil and religious war that left over 100,000 dead. He saw his grandfather, a deputy minister, live out his last days as a political exile in a shabby Athens apartment. As Taleb summarized the awful transformation: "a Black Swan, coming out of nowhere, transformed the place from heaven to hell."[8]

The dilemma for Taleb is plain: the everyday empirical world cannot be adequately understood either through facts or through reasoning dependent on facts. Observable facts are inherently unreliable, and thus we certainly can't rely on the logic or reasoning that they support. It was once believed—so firmly as to underwrite the standard example of a logical syllogism—that all swans are white. The syllogistic chain of logic is impervious: all swans are white, X is a swan, therefore X is white. Logical syllogisms constitute a machine for generating valid conclusions, but the validity of logic depends on the validity of the facts or statements fed into the logic machine. The Black Swan stands as a caution—rooted in history—against a reliance upon empirical facts and their logic machines. The historical assumption that swans are white, based (reasonably enough) on the empirical observation of white swans, suddenly unraveled into the conceptual equivalent of smoking wreckage when astonished nineteenth-century travelers to Australia encountered a swan that is ac-

tually black: *Cygnus atratus.* Syllogisms and reason are little help when
new facts emerge and old facts have heart attacks. The Black Swan—not
the name of a system but a cautionary metaphor against systems—reflects
Taleb's experience with the fact-based experience that you never see
coming: singularities, anomalies, and unexpected catastrophic events. It
imagines unseen, unknowable disaster already nested within the everyday
probable world that we construct out of gossamer facts and reason.

Probabilities, Taleb's nemesis, are visible everywhere today in the
world of Big Data. They underlie police work—the acronym Crush
stands for Criminal Reduction Utilizing Statistical History, or, in plain
English, predictive policing—and they power the algorithms behind dating
Web sites, online retail sales, and the U.S. National Security Agency.
Electronic medical records can now become, in effect, "disease surveillance tools," as a recent medical study explains in proposing an algorithm to identify criteria predictive of coronary and heart failure events.[9]
Probability, in its disrespect for accident, whim, and irrationalism, is
almost an anti-eros. We invoke it to describe both supposedly objective
laws of chance and subjective degrees of belief.[10] That is, probability
refers to subjective claims with fluctuating degrees of credibility (by
midnight, there is a high probability I will be asleep) and to objective
law-like regularities (the next coin flip has a fifty-fifty probability of
landing "heads"). Clinical medicine relies on both objective and subjective senses as a basis for its prognostic claims, employing so-called *Bayesian*
probability, which combines objective experimental data with subjective
expert knowledge. (The patient, presumably no expert, adds nothing to
this formula.) The specialists who informed Angelina Jolie about her
87 percent risk of breast cancer put her in possession of probable knowledge. The knowledge also possessed her. She chose to have her breasts
surgically removed not to *treat* disease but to lower her 87 percent *probability* of disease to a less alarming, if still uncertain, statistical level. It
was a brave and difficult choice. We all dwell, like Jolie, amid statistical
probabilities, and, right or wrong, we make life-changing choices based
on what we regard as the most probable outcome. The Black Swan reminds us that, no matter how good the statistics and probabilities are,
we also live in a world of unreasonable, anomalous, improbable, singular events that no one can foresee. These bolts out of the blue can

bring massive sudden catastrophes as real as breast cancer, heart attack, or the collapse of world financial markets.

Black Swans and Magical Thinking

"Life changes fast": Joan Didion's stark opening observation in *The Year of Magical Thinking* (2005) describes, in general terms, the Black Swan moment when her husband, fellow writer, and daily companion of forty years, John Gregory Dunne, as he sat by the fire in their Manhattan apartment nursing his usual predinner scotch, suddenly pitched forward and hit the carpet face-first. *"Life changes in the instant,"* Didion continues. *"You sit down to dinner and life as you know it ends."*[11]

The power of the Black Swan to expose the strangeness of the everyday—the total demented otherness nested within what looks so ordinary and benign—finds a perfect image in the picture of a devoted couple, comfortably well-off and well past middle age, preparing to sit down to dinner once again, as they've done for the last forty-some years. Nothing to notice, no novelistic detail worth lingering over, as their daily domestic ritual unfolds. Then, abruptly, the fabric of everydayness— stitched together through 10,000 probabilities—opens up, rips, unravels, and exposes the hidden strangeness that was always there, unseen, waiting for its moment to emerge and to change everything. Are the details of a forty-year marriage medically relevant data? Not with John Gregory Dunne face down, dead, on the carpet. Medical logos springs into action as the emergency medical technicians and emergency room doctors seek to revive an elderly white male with no vital signs who suffered an apparent myocardial infarction. There is no happy ending. Medical eros, occupying a perspective that differs from the ground-level urgencies facing the EMT crew, would observe that John Gregory Dunne's fatal heart attack changed all the facts. It continued to change all the facts in the world of Joan Didion. Patienthood does not stop—only shifts its shape—at the legal border signified by a death certificate. "Grief has no distance," Didion writes of her new reality, as if trapped in an all-surrounding, battering surf. "Grief comes in waves, paroxysms, sudden apprehensions that weaken the knees and blind the eyes and obliterate the dailiness of life."[12]

The *obliteration of dailiness* under the assault of the Black Swan is what deserves special emphasis here. Dailiness belongs to the land of probabilities, and it can vanish along with the reassuring probabilities that help define an individual life-world. Didion's previous sense of "dailiness" doesn't just vanish, however, as if irreversibly gone. She chooses an arresting image—a vortex—to describe the weirdly interruptive, multileveled state of being that she now inhabits, at least in her inner life. The obliteration of dailiness, that is, remains incomplete; it is punctuated, like grief; its odd, jumpy, epileptic, back-and-forth movement resembles what might happen if everydayness suddenly opened up, as a whirlpool opens up within a flowing stream, with a circling, centripetal inward and downward draw. Something like this vortex-effect suction draws Didion down into an unknown dimension far beneath the everyday surface where, remarkably, she continues to function, carrying on with her social duties as widow, mother, friend, writer, and public figure. The vortex, however, remains a new feature of an altered life-world, as unfathomable as grief, and her steady flow of new dailiness is now punctured with strangeness. The extended period when the vortex operates at full force she calls her year of *magical thinking*.

Where have I met this punctuated vortex effect? Then I recall. The shift into magical thinking reminds me of anthropologist David Lewis-Williams and his theory of Paleolithic cave painting.[13] A shaman leads the torch-lit ritual descent into a pitch-black, subterranean cave: the interior of the sacred earth mother. As they proceed farther into the cavernous darkness, the smoky flickering torches suddenly light up images of bison and of antelope, whose outlined contours take on a three-dimensional kinetic life as they merge with the rough, irregular cavern walls. This prehistoric and truly otherworldly ritual descent, as Lewis-Williams argues, opens up for the stunned participants an "intensified spectrum" of consciousness.

For Didion, the descent of the Black Swan may produce something like a similar split in consciousness, as grief pulls her down in a battering vortex effect, opening onto an intensified magical dimension far removed from the probabilities and rationalities of dailiness. Some psychiatrists now use the term "complicated grief" to describe an ongoing heightened state of mourning that prevents healing, but it does not apply to Didion. Is her mental state an aberration treatable with psychotropic drugs? It was a psychotropic drug that impaired my wife Ruth's vision and broke her leg at the hip. For Joan Didion, Black Swan trauma exposed her everyday consciousness to an influx of forgotten, undiagnosable, irrational otherness that may well belong to our ancestral birthright: a primal dimension of not-knowing well known, as it happens, to medical eros.

William James, a founder of modern psychology and the only American philosopher with a degree in medicine, puts the matter succinctly: "our normal waking consciousness, rational consciousness as we call it, is but one special type of consciousness, whilst all about it, parted from it by the filmiest of screens, there lie potential forms of consciousness entirely different. We may go through life without suspecting their existence; but apply the requisite stimulus, and at a touch they are there."[14] The Black Swan is, for Joan Didion, the requisite stimulus: it parts the filmiest of screens put in place by reason and probabilities, drawing her into a mode of thinking and of being that lies uneasily close to delirium, but also permitting her return as the vortex-effect spins her back toward the everyday world. "On most surface levels," she reports, "I seemed rational. To the average observer I would have appeared to fully understand that death was irreversible."[15] When the surface opens up, however, when the vortex of grief draws her down into the strange, intensified, magical domain, she fully believes that John Gregory Dunne—buried, mourned, memorialized—is nonetheless out there somewhere, just waiting, poised to finish his usual scotch and rejoin her for dinner.

Medical logos, like the financial services industry, is driven by probability, and the focus on probability extends even to such valuable advances as simulated patient interviews using paid actors. "I'm called a standardized patient," writes Leslie Jamison in *The Empathy Exams* (2014), "which means I act toward the norms set for my disorders."[16] Medical *norms*, the probabilistic hoofbeats that medical students learn to recognize, are indispensable in the world of biomedicine and modern health care. Like other indispensable modern enterprises, however, medicine still relies on an instrument for measuring and for creating probabilities devised in the nineteenth century, the so-called Gaussian function or bell-shaped curve. German mathematician Johann Carl Friedrich Gauss (1777–1855) introduced the concept that bears his name and still governs much of modern life. Three standard deviations from

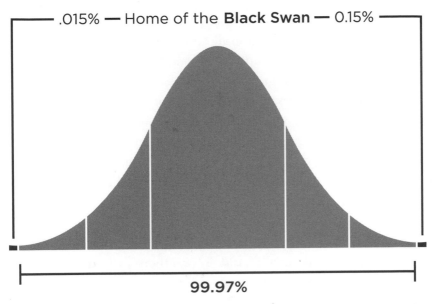

FIGURE 7.1. The Bell-Shaped Curve: Home of the Black Swan. David B. Morris.

the norm—the inescapable, probable *norm*—equal 99.7 percent of any data set. I feel about the bell-shaped curve much as I feel about psychotropic drugs. I suppose they have their uses, but they also set us up for disaster. Disaster, of course, is hidden away in the apparently innocent figure that looks to me less like a bell than, as my brother says, a little hat. The little hat is almost all crown and no brim—as if inviting us to admire its fashionable arch. Taleb is not fooled. The Black Swan nests within those two symmetrical brims (often called *fat-tails* or *long-tails*) that slope away, precipitously, from the third standard deviations. The brims of the little hat—the fat-tails or long-tails—are where the mysterious 0.03 percent of any data set resides in almost complete cognitive darkness, outside the norm; it is easy to forget that those tails exist. Forgetting is easy because life under the bell-shaped curve automatically directs our attention *away* from the almost invisible double 0.015 percent outliers, the bandit hideout of the norm-busting Black Swan (Figure 7.1).

Taleb hates the bell-shaped curve. Not because it is wrong—it has statistical validity and practical uses, especially as we distinguish between high-probability and low-probability events—but because we so often fail to notice its implicit dangers. It creates a descriptive picture that lulls us into a false sense of security. It also allows its descriptive picture to impose predictive patterns. It carves up a classroom of thirty students, say, into a massive central group—whose performance is declared normal—flanked by two miniscule outliers, the rare A+ student and the rare F− student, who are statistically abnormal. Suppose two sets of Mensa triplets register for the class? OK, forget Mensa triplets—how common are they? Taleb's point is that life, which cannot be considered a data set, remains far stranger, far less normal, and far, far more dangerous than the bell-shaped curve leads us to believe. Its so-called norms prove downright perilous when they conceal from us the improbable reality of the Black Swan. A statistical study of the type basic to medical logos shows that random DNA mutations—what one of the study's coauthors calls the "bad luck factor"—are largely responsible for two-thirds of adult cancers.[17] Sudden, improbable events that entail massive personal costs reconfigure our lives perhaps more often than we care to reflect. ("I shut my eyes and saw absolute black.") Hoofbeats don't always mean horses. One September day in 2001, jets over Manhattan didn't mean just another plane full of tourists.

Medical Error and the Logic of Not-Knowing

"Black Swan logic," writes Taleb, "makes *what you don't know* far more relevant than what you do know."[18] Black Swan logic is, in effect, a counterlogic, or an alogic of the improbable: fact-based nontheory against theories. His emphasis on the not-known does not disable Taleb from identifying several distinctive empirical features of the otherwise mostly unseen Black Swan. First, it is an *outlier.* It lies beyond all expectation and outside all probabilities because no observable, factual evidence points to its existence or predicts its arrival. Who knew that Russia would default on its bonds? Second, it carries an *extreme impact.* It doesn't merely disrupt calculations or screw up a theory, but rather it faces real people with real disaster, like the twin towers of the World Trade Center slowly beginning their surreal floor-by-floor implosion. Third, once the Black Swan appears, in defiance of all our calculations and expectations, we feel compelled *to explain it*, usually in ways that sustain our underlying faith in evidence, in reason, and in probability.

Taleb offers no explanations. He proposes no alternate grand narrative. Instead, he argues that it is a mistake to believe that our empirical tools will protect us from the unknown. What we don't know is more relevant, given the Black Swan, than what we know or—worse—what we (wrongly) *think* we know.

The Black Swan, as Taleb describes it, does not contain an erotic dimension, but it certainly plunges its victims into a nightmare of not-knowing. If nothing in our experience—no evidence, no logic, no likelihood—prepares us for the Black Swan, if we are fated to wait until a new, unanticipated, outlier incarnation rips apart our carefully constructed fabric of everydayness, medical eros would ask a fundamental question based, if not on compassion for others, at least on self-love and a desire to avoid complete disaster: Is there anything we can do to protect ourselves?

Yes. Taleb believes there is a limited self-protection available in an awareness of the Black Swan and in a vigilant, proactive, self-protective stance. His almost monomaniacal vision of unpredictable, ruinous threats embedded *within* the everyday flow of financial markets led him to contrive personal investment strategies so conservative that he might as well have stuffed his cash directly under the mattress. He made a fortune, as a result of such strategies, in the unforeseen Black Swan market crash of 1987, a disaster against which he was fully protected. Otherwise, he reveals no temperamental interest in a Bataille-like immersion in the not-known as constituting an erotic destruction of the self-containment basic to his character as he is in his normal life. His advice, to the contrary, is not only that we take practical steps to protect ourselves against the not-known but also that we maximize our exposure to what he calls *positive* Black Swans. For example, if you are lonely, you do not maximize your exposure to *positive* Black Swans—such as the sudden appearance of the one-in-a-million lover—by staying home, eating ice cream, and waiting for the phone to ring. You can go to a bar, lose weight, join an online dating site, or buy a dog. Just remember that these innocuous everyday acts also might, as dating-site veterans know, explode in your face.

Medical eros would join medical logos in emphasizing the need for protections from Black Swan assaults, and not just for patients. It would remind doctors that they, too, live under the shadow of the Black Swan. The

improbable, the unknown, and the unknowable confront physicians
with dangers that are too easily dismissed as coming with the territory.
Unlike the reason-based order and calm of the laboratory, the clinician's
daily workplace proves at times as unpredictable as a combat zone; its
dailiness is subject to rupture, vortex, and obliteration. Health professionals, for example, stand among the first-responders called to help at
inexplicable, unforeseen catastrophes ranging from the earliest cases of
mysterious, deadly infectious diseases such as HIV/AIDS or Ebola to
nuclear meltdowns, radiation sickness, and bioterrorism attacks. Some
threats may be more like grey swans (partly visible, partly predictable)
because true Black Swans cannot be identified or predicted in advance;
but grey swans also emerge from beyond the central dome of probabilities, which means that fully effective precautions and impervious zones of
safety do not exist. There are no best-practice guidelines that offer ironclad protection against unknown pathogens.

Dr. H is the pseudonym for a pediatric surgeon whose error during a
routine heart-valve repair resulted in the death of a two-year-old boy. Malpractice insurance is no shield against error. How many doctors, perhaps type-A, high-achieving, dedicated workaholics, truly believe that
they are at risk for negligent or incompetent acts? A lawsuit followed the
lethal heart-valve error, and the combination resulted in a near total obliteration of Dr. H's daily world. "I couldn't sleep," he explains. "I would
wake up at night. I would sit up at night and my heart was pounding. I
was beside myself with anxiety, fear, guilt. I felt terrible. . . . You go
through the looking glass. It's just a very bizarre world."[19]

The strangeness that can open up within the daily world of biomedicine is not entirely abnormal, as we might wish or imagine, but, as the
response of Dr. H. suggests, it extends far wider than most patients believe. A patient-centered perspective encourages justified alarm at various
statistics that, as we have seen, indicate that doctors and medical errors
in the United States are a leading cause of death.[20] The supra-dyadic relations of illness, however, extend beyond patients and families to include
the doctors who, in the immense majority of instances, pursue their calling
with profound professional skill and personal dedication. Consider, then,
Dr. H's account of an ordinary day on the pediatric surgical ward as he
resumes what looks like professional business as usual following the med-

ical error that swept him through the looking glass. The normal explodes: "Somebody bumped into me in the hall and said 'Hi, how are you doing?' and I just started crying. I mean, I couldn't stop. I think everything had been bottled up. I couldn't even walk, so they sent me home."[21]

Medical error to the individual doctor, despite the cushion of malpractice insurance and formal medical-school lectures and small-group discussions highlighting the topic of medical error, almost always comes with the improbability of a thunderbolt on a cloudless day. Medicine functions best in a bell-shaped and normalized field, with any inherent strangeness subtly denatured, its anomalies and improbabilities squeezed out into the remote scrubland, figured as little brims or fat tails. Medical error thus can prove shattering to doctors whose professional identity and personal self-esteem are so often keyed to the mastery of intricate skills and of esoteric knowledge. A child's death is heartbreaking—even worse if it was preventable. Practical steps toward prevention and (where warranted) professional discipline are necessities. Medical eros would also recognize the heartbreak of Dr. H. What can it mean for a respected surgeon to be sent home from work like a schoolboy? This is a portrait of medical logos at a limit point where the physician implodes. Dr. H has no buffer in his self-accusation, no companionship in his self-exile. There is no reparation, no forgetting, and (perhaps most difficult) no self-forgiveness. The Black Swan has struck, and the statistical probabilities that might estimate the risk-factor of serious medical error in pediatric surgery, in this instance, prove pointless and irrelevant.

Medical logos responds to medical error—even to catastrophes such as Dr. H's medical nightmare—with the resources of logic, reason, and probabilistic thought, and to good purpose. Biomedicine to its credit initiates statistical studies in particular specialties to identify the most common, predictable errors and then takes steps to eliminate these particular errors through system-wide procedural changes: "pre-op checklists, no look-alike medication bottles, computerized ordering to replace handwritten prescriptions, surgery sites marked directly in ink on the patient's body prior to the operation, computerized algorithms for everything from urinary catheters to blood thinners."[22] Taleb, as a high-stakes trader alert to the Black Swan and determined to avoid provoking it, put in place highly rational (but unconventional) financial strategies that allowed him to prosper while less alert investors—trusting to probabilities—watched their 401(k) accounts bubble down the drain. (I did.) Market strategies devised to protect investments, however, are never foolproof, and institutional practices to limit medical error do not offer emotional protection for doctors and for patients whose lives are ripped apart by improbable and deadly Black Swan catastrophes.

There is no certain protection from Black Swan assaults, but at least for certain individuals it is possible to mount an effective response. In 1982 Stephen Jay Gould—the famed Harvard evolutionary biologist and well-known baseball enthusiast—was diagnosed at age forty with abdominal mesothelioma. This rare cancer, according to his quick dive into the medical literature, was regarded as incurable, with a probable median mortality rate, after discovery, of eight months. His immediate dilemma, as Gould saw it through his lens as a scientist, did not lie in the projected mortality rate. The dilemma was how to understand the statistics, and Gould (an "old-style materialist," as he called himself) immediately set to thinking about what the general, probable statistic meant for him in particular. Most patients, given a median mortality of eight months, would most likely conclude *I'm a goner.* Gould, with his knowledge of the bell-shaped curve, knew that *an eight-month median* mortality rate actually meant that half of the patients die in less than eight months, and half live longer than eight months. He decided, calling on his basically upbeat personality, that he would belong to the longer-lived half; he also decided that his age, optimistic outlook, and strong desire to live gave him a good chance of belonging to the minority of survivors who inhabit the farthest limits of the bell curve. "Attitude clearly matters in fighting cancer," he wrote in a magazine article about his approach to illness: a strategy that combined detailed knowledge of statistical probabilities with an emotional commitment to maintain a positive attitude. A gifted teacher, he described the article—a *sui generis* illness narrative—as "a personal story of statistics, properly interpreted, as profoundly nurturant and life-giving."[23]

Gould lived for twenty years after his diagnosis with abdominal cancer. The great value of his personal story of *statistics properly understood* lies in suggesting that medical logos and medical eros together can at least respond to certain Black Swan dilemmas, push back against catastrophe, and allow certain intrepid people to enter into the not-known region of serious illness fortified—in addition to whatever medications prove valuable—with the surplus resistances and affirmations offered by intelligence, strong desire, and a stout heart.

Life beyond the Brim: *Curiouser and Curiouser?*

Jason and Jenny Cairns-Lawrence, a couple from England, were vacationing in New York City on September 11, 2001, when their holiday was interrupted by the terrorist attack on the World Trade Center. Several years later, on July 7, 2005, they happened to be in London when terrorists struck with train and bus bombs that killed fifty-two people. Three years later, in November 2008, they were vacationing in Mumbai when terrorists struck in four days of coordinated shootings and bombings, killing one hundred and sixty-four people.[24] You might think that major world tourist sites would pay the Cairns-Lawrences an annual stipend to stay home. You might also think, because we seem to live surrounded by coincidences large and small, that at least a few scientists or statisticians would take an interest in such well-documented, curious anomalies and want to ask—as the Cairns-Lawrences must at times ask themselves— just what is going on?

Nothing in my experience or research prepared me for the moment, near midnight, when an intense heavy iron globe—an alien, unknown, inexplicable pain—lodged like a small aching cannonball in my upper chest and quickly began to radiate more pain into my left shoulder. Intense pain, it turns out, was not the Black Swan, only its precursor. As the leaden ball of intense pain swelled and spread and intensified, the Black Swan was still out of sight—in this case not hovering, ready to descend, but unidentified and unannounced.

A heart attack—right out of the blue—constituted my personal introduction to the Black Swan. I count it entirely coincidental that the attack occurred in the native home of *Cygnus atratus*, specifically the cowboy/hippie town of Darwin, Australia, about as far north as you can go Down Under without standing in the Sea of Timor. I was in bed when the chest pain started. After a fruitless search for aspirin, I throw on some clothes, ask the night clerk to call a taxi, and, with what now feels like a meteorite in my upper chest, I tell the driver to head for the nearest emergency department. I can't sit upright, so I just sprawl across the back seat, sweating like I'd just run a marathon. As I glimpse the driver in the rearview mirror, I can sense he's already wondering if he'll get paid. I'm wondering, too. Medical friends insist that I should have called an ambulance, with its stock of clot-busting drugs, but I was in no mind to think things through. The Black Swan ushers us into a region of not-knowing that is profoundly foreign to everyday rationalities. Cardiac pain swept me right through the looking glass. Arriving by taxi at the emergency department, however, is a double mistake. I tip the driver handsomely, with everything left in my pockets, and get in line at the admissions window. It is now well after midnight, and a belligerent young woman ahead of me is engaged in a lengthy debate with the attendant about her boyfriend's arm. The normal act of standing in line feels unbearably strange. Am I patiently waiting my turn to die? Politely I say nothing.

I'm not alone, statistically speaking, even though in Australia I'm traveling solo for my first extended trip since Ruth had entered the region of not-knowing in which she no longer knows me and no longer knows whether I'm around. Every year some 515,000 Americans suffer a first heart attack. Another 205,000 Americans suffer a repeat attack.[25] Many, I'm guessing, experience my total shock: *Me?* I am not exactly the poster child for lifestyle illness: my slim list of merits includes regular visits to the gym, a fine primary care doctor, a normal body weight, and a mostly vegetable diet. A heart attack had never crossed my mind, and an unlucky crocodile encounter in the Darwin outback where I planned to look at aboriginal rock art was far more likely. Of course, I had completely forgotten about the accelerated risk facing caregivers; with Ruth safe in her residential facility, I had put aside thoughts of a possible corpselike sleep. Another surprise awaits me. (Do Black Swans come in twos?) After the trauma team controls the pain, stabilizes my symptoms, and dilates my arteries, I am still lying prone on the hospital gurney, my chest swaddled in electrodes, when a well-dressed woman appears. She tells me she's from the business office (the *business office?*) and wants to know what medical insurance I carry. And so it goes: once the Black Swan descends—or arrives by taxi—patients can't avoid such mundane and terrifying questions as *what will it cost* and *who's going to pay?* Other questions roll in like fog. Would I ever get out of there? Was Darwin, Australia, really, truly, the place where I was supposed to die? Then I suddenly realize I am fifteen hours by plane from the West Coast of the United States, with no family or friends within a thousand miles, and now the *business office* is paying a call? The Black Swans just keep on coming . . .

Coincidences, like all statistically improbable events, proceed from beyond the dome of the bell-shaped curve, which helps explain why it is so easy to dismiss them as the anomalies they are. But why are we so quick to dismiss them? Reason—and perhaps the brain, too—finds it easy to shrug off coincidences. The neuroscientist V. S. Ramachandran argues that the human brain *abhors* coincidence because coincidences violate deep evolution-based neural principles favoring probability, regularity, and order. "And your brain," he writes, "always tries to find a plausible alternate, generic interpretation to avoid the coincidence."[26] Maybe that's true. The brains of stroke patients, for instance, can confabulate explanations for why the patients can't move their (paralyzed) limbs. Coincidences, however, also have the power to make us stop and wonder, if only for a few seconds, perhaps giving us a glimpse of the territory that Joan Didion's vortex opened up. Then we pull ourselves together, adjust our uniforms, and go about our normal business of calculating probabilities. We don't need a statistician to tell us that eventually someone will win the lottery; we call the winners *lucky*. Coincidences, on the other hand, often seem to proceed from somewhere beyond luck, and they are memorable enough that almost everyone can recite a few personal examples. Chance or randomness are the terms we use to explain (or explain away) coincidences, when we don't interpret them as acts of God. They confront us with experience that doesn't make sense, that the rational mind has a hard time getting a purchase on—like the idea of the infinite, or like meeting the existentialist philosopher Jean-Paul Sartre at the laundromat.

Do coincidences, if we don't automatically dismiss them as a statistical fluke, have any role in health and illness? "It has been my experience and the experience of many other therapists," reports Rachel Naomi Remen, "that when I am facing a difficult personal issue or a painful decision or am struggling with some recalcitrant and stubborn part of my self, a very peculiar thing will happen. Many of my clients will spontaneously bring in the same issue."[27] Why, I keep wondering, just two days before leaving for Australia and for the first time ever, did I go online on sheer impulse and buy travel medical insurance? The no-nonsense woman from the hospital business office had no intention of leaving without an answer, even at well past 2:00 in the morning; luckily I could pull out my newly minted insurance card and, careful not to dislodge electrodes, hand it over. I was hoping, without great confidence, that it wasn't the product of an Internet scam.

Allure and *wonder* are traits that make coincidences a form of statistical improbability of special interest to medical eros. Not all statistical anomalies generate allure or make us pause and wonder. Allure belongs to the uncanny strangeness that only certain improbable events possess or generate. Allure also shares with eros a power to draw us into mental states intrinsically at odds with reason. Ramachandran argues that the brain resists coincidences because they are unreasonable, but coincidences also possess an allure that draws us to what reason apparently can't explain—their power to attract our attention seems undeniable. There is no attraction, for example, in the statement that Thomas Jefferson died in the same year as the minor German poet Johann Voss. Many people find it amazing, however, that Jefferson died in the same year as John Adams: both were presidents, both were founding fathers of the United States, and both died not only in the same year but on the same day. That day, in fact, was July 4, 1826, the fiftieth anniversary of the signing of the Declaration of Independence. Such radical strangeness is what generates allure and wonder. The rational mind doesn't like what it hears—the improbabilities seem almost monstrous. So our internal statistician marshals all its analytical powers to argue that the strange improbable happening is no more than a blip on the screen, a pesky, meaningless, improbable anomaly. And yet. And yet. It emerges, like the Black Swan, from beyond the dome of the little hat that we place atop the world of facts.

Coincidental events, to the distress of reason, are a regular feature in the literature on identical twins. It is not uncommon to read reports of telepathic episodes when, to cite one instance, an identical twin skiing in the Alps falls and breaks his left leg while the other identical twin, skiing on a different trail, falls at the same time and breaks the same bone in his left leg.[28] Statistical analysis shows that such rare events prove more common when identical twins are raised together or in close proximity, compared with identical twins separated at birth. Most scientists discount such inconclusive data as no more than what information theorists call *noise*—irrelevant, beneath regard. We notice such events, they argue, only because we do not notice the millions of occasions when identical twins fail to break their left legs simultaneously while skiing. In *The Signal and the Noise* (2012), statistician and master of prediction Nate Silver argues that the best forecasters, those who most accurately separate signal from noise, possess a strong grasp of probabilities and pay close attention to detail. This is exactly what reasonable people would expect. Silver adds, however, that the best forecasters also maintain a deep appreciation of uncertainties.[29]

Medical eros can offer to medical logos an appreciation of illness as a condition lived in a state of uncertainties. Uncertainties and improbabilities, like coincidences, may distress the rational mind, but they also evoke, for people not wholly given over to reason and to statistics, the experience of a strangeness embedded within the everyday. Many patients simply do not share the commitment to evidence and reason that is so basic to medical logos. Patients now regularly demonstrate their independence, or their open resistance to biomedicine, by paying large out-of-pocket sums for unproven therapies.[30] P. T. Barnum had a word ("sucker") that he used to describe people whom he regarded as gullible. Gullibility, however, is not the best explanation for what moves patients to explore complementary and alternative therapies. Public desire for such therapies is significant enough that in 1998 the usually slow-footed United States Congress established the National Center for Complementary and Alternative Medicine—later renamed the National Center for Alternative and Integrative Health—with a mandate to explore nontraditional approaches to health and wellness that, it conceded, "the public is using, often without the benefit of rigorous scientific study."[31]

Sceptics might think that legislation creating the NCCAM and NCAIH was designed mainly to rein in demand for unproven therapies, by demystifying their appeal. It certainly identifies the molecular gaze and scientific biomedicine as the arbiters of all therapeutic value. People meanwhile continue to vote with their wallets. Data from a 2007 survey show that 83 million Americans spent $33.9 billion in annual out-of-pocket costs for complementary and alternative therapies—some 1.5 percent of total health-care expenditures.[32] Many patients who pay for unproven therapies continue to consult their primary physicians, without telling their physicians about the parallel nonallopathic health care. Perhaps such patients were quietly and privately negotiating their personal alliances between medical logos and medical eros. What moved them to make substantial cash outlays in nontraditional care was surely less statistical reason (or a calculation of probabilities) than the individual psychodynamics of hope and desire.

One-third of the U.S. population notices coincidences with "some frequency" and tends to make important decisions based on coincidental events that they interpret as signs.[33] Is such attentiveness unreasonable? In retrospect, in the early stages of Ruth's illness, I missed all the signs. Or, worse, dismissed them. I reasoned that they were meaningless blips. I reasoned that Ruth was simply being, in her own delightful ways, not normal. Yes, I had noticed the unusual displays of temper, which simply made me angry in return—another way of not paying attention. Ruth said at times that her brain felt "fuzzy," but I didn't have a clue what to make of the statement. I passed off such episodes as random events that were not worth noticing. Ruth did seek medical assistance, and her doctors prescribed antidepressants, which simply added sexual dysfunction as a predictable side effect. I don't fault her physicians; they had no reason to suspect Alzheimer's disease in a healthy woman in her mid-fifties who was holding down a professional job while working at night on her doctoral dissertation. Even if they had suspected, they had no treatments to offer. The Black Swan strikes out of the blue, and the New Mexico sky overhead looked cloudless.

Probabilistic thinking, I've decided, can actively impair our ability to recognize patterns or even the elements of patterns when the pattern is unfamiliar, incomplete, or bizarre. I would have done far better for Ruth if I had attended carefully to improbabilities. The signs were there, in retrospect, including one truly serious domestic trauma, but in truth I simply missed them. I not only failed to connect the dots, but I failed to recognize the dots. In short, given a mind-set keyed to probabilities, I regarded the evidence as anomalies, or I passed it off as coincidence. The dots were fragmentary, episodic, and low profile, certainly nothing as attention-grabbing as Adams and Jefferson both dying on the fiftieth anniversary of the Declaration of Independence. But the dots were visible, if only I hadn't discounted them, if only I had attended to singularities, if only I hadn't blocked the allure of strangeness. *If only:* the lament of the caregiver immersed in a strange, wild sea of improbabilities.

Improbabilities, as I now believe, were a prominent feature of Ruth's illness. The strangeness was not simply bizarre but statistically inexplicable. With my focus on reason and with my ignorance of the Black Swan, I simply didn't recognize the hard facts right before my eyes. I saw only gradual, minor changes in behavior that failed to add up, as far as I could calculate, to a significant conclusion. I blended them into the crowd of slightly odd or edgy events that pass for daily living. Meanwhile, the Black Swan was overhead, steadily circling.

The Black Swan, as I might add to Taleb's account, strikes not only in sudden spectacular calamities but also in slow-motion unravelings, like the almost invisible day-by-day mental attrition that often marks Alzheimer's disease. Ruth's illness, as it gradually eroded her once powerful reason-based, fact-driven, probabilistic powers of decision making, for a time put us both in the same semiblinded position, blind on blind. It also eroded her power to resist the illness. I have met highly successful people who say that they would commit suicide rather than continue to live with Alzheimer's disease. Well, on which day? Alzheimer's disease, in eroding the power to choose, takes away even the power to choose to end your own life. Suicide, if it is more than a sudden impulse, requires a firm decision. For William Styron, it required elaborate, ritualized preparations. Alzheimer's disease wholly unraveled Ruth's decision-making power.

Brain damage showed me that I had much to learn. I learned that it didn't matter if Ruth wanted to wear six blouses. So what? It didn't matter if it took Ruth forty-five minutes instead of five to sort through her closet in the morning. (I learned to change my schedule to wait until she was finished.) I learned that it didn't matter if the discarded clothes were left scattered all over the bedroom. (I'd pick them up later.) "If I must drool," writes Jean-Do Bauby from within locked-in syndrome, "I may as well drool on cashmere."[34] Illness teaches acceptance. Medical logos deals with uncertainties by utilizing its chosen tools of reason, statistics, and probabilities; medical eros mostly just plunges right in to not-knowing. If desire says to drool on cashmere, then drool on cashmere. If desire says to wear six blouses, then go right ahead. Desire, as we know, can serve us poorly, but it also can serve us well, especially in calamities when reason offers little beyond a calculus for adding up the awful costs. At best, desire offers the insights and feel of full-body immersion in a strange realm of alternate truths, a realm of improbabilities that lovers, too, know well and that they sometimes navigate successfully. "In matters of the heart," as the Swiss-born French novelist Madame de Staël (1766–1817) wrote very wisely, "nothing is true except the improbable."[35]

Nebulous Factors: Flash! Bam! Alakazam!

Probable improbabilities is an oxymoron, like hot ice, offering a koan-like poetic challenge to prose logic. In his authoritative studies, the sociologist and organizational theorist Charles Perrow prefers the phrase "normal accidents."[36] He means that today we have created systems so complex, so interactive, and so open to catastrophe—think of a space shuttle launch—that "we cannot anticipate all the possible interactions or the inevitable failures." If such failure is inevitable, it constitutes in Perrow's view a "normal" risk. We cannot exclude the Black Swan from our increasingly complex and interactive systems, both biological and social, and thus its improbable assaults would seem to constitute, in effect, a *normal* catastrophe.

Terrorist killings happen now with such frequency as to suggest that we have entered a new era of *normal catastrophe*. What constitutes the norm is of course partly a matter of perspective. I experienced a sudden heart attack as an improbable catastrophe, while to biomedicine it was just a normal night in the Darwin emergency department. The cardiac care unit is already staffed, supplied, and set to receive a new patient. I am a direct beneficiary of this statistic-based, data-driven rationality that predicts that someone in, say, Darwin, Australia, will experience a heart attack, and it just happened to be me. Still, normal can be a lot weirder than we normally assume. The near million heart attacks annually in the United States include many silent or unrecognized heart attacks.[37] We never see the Black Swan coming, and sometimes we don't even recognize it when it arrives.

The practical problem facing medical logos involves the paradox of preparing for risks that are not only unknown but also unknowable. The risk management department in medical centers is usually staffed by lawyers hired to protect the institution against the predictable risk of malpractice suits. Risks in biomedicine, however, are everywhere, and sometimes probabilities and predictions can get in the way. One lone, smart, infectious disease specialist figured out, at the last minute, that the life-threatening crisis that brought a friend of mine to the hospital had little to do with complications from chemotherapy. What had put her perilously close to death? *Ehrlichiosis.* In 2010 this tick-borne bacterial infection had an annual incidence of 2.5 cases per million, but it can prove fatal in patients with compromised immune systems.[38] For my friend, the hoofbeats did not mean horses or even zebras—the culprit, most likely, was an eight-legged insect the size of a baby aspirin. The two tiny brims of the bell-shaped curve hide dangers and improbabilities far worse than the brown dog tick. Oedipus, who fled Thebes to elude the prophecy that he would kill his father, kills a stranger at the crossroads—who is, of course, his father in disguise. Fate? Coincidence? Noise? Why, I keep wondering even now, did I purchase that medical insurance at the last minute for my Australian adventure?

The practical problem I faced was how to get out of the Darwin cardiac care unit. Once black-swanned, if I may put it that way, I discovered the strange and invisible laser beams of officialdom that crisscrossed my path like a museum security system. It was a *minimum* security system—I wasn't in chains, after all—but I wasn't quite free either. We patients, it turns out, are never entirely free agents, not once we enter the medical system, no more than the physicians are, for whom hospital privileges are not automatic. My exit was not automatic. Only a required angiogram and echo-stress test would determine whether I would receive official permission to fly home. If I failed the tests, the Australian medical system would send me, at my expense, four hours south by plane for a five-day stent procedure, or possibly for an even longer coronary bypass operation. Or, if I failed but they deemed me stable enough to fly, they would first fly a nurse from Los Angeles to accompany me home, again at my expense. It was carefully explained that if I departed without permission, I would be charged the full cost of diverting a jumbo jet should my heart condition require an emergency turnaround. Swimming home seemed a preferable choice of ruin. I soon realized that I was caught up in a little melodrama of soft biopower from which not even my good-luck medical insurance—its upper limit fast running out—conferred reliable protection.

Eros likes to find or invent a transgressive comic side, especially when logos is firmly in control. I wore dark glasses on the operating table for the angiogram, determined (if need be) to go out cool, and I ran the treadmill test in gym shorts, invoking Yankee gods of sport and fitness. Happily, I won my official release, despite the questionable style choices, escaping to the airport within an hour, en route to Sydney and then to Los Angeles. My seatmate heard an audible sigh—no turnaround—when our plane passed midpoint across the Pacific.

The inescapable strangeness of the everyday is in many ways just too unscientific for medical logos. Medical logos has an official acronym, MUS, for medically unexplained *symptoms*, but it has no acronym for medically unexplained *cures*—for enigmatic, improbable, astonishing recoveries. Remissions from cancer occur in one out of every 60,000 to 100,000 patients, although the true rate is likely higher due to underreporting.[39] Andrew Weill, the telegenic founder of Integrative Medicine, includes in his book *Spontaneous Healing* (1995) numerous reports that count as medically unexplained cures, and Jacalyn Duffin scoured the Vatican Secret Archives examining the records of some 1,400 unexplained recoveries.[40] Should we ignore them, or pretend that they don't exist? Theology calls them miracles, defined as an event beyond human or natural cause, but unexplained cures do not require belief in a supernatural power, only a belief in the limits of probabilistic thinking and in the positive Black Swans tucked away, lurking, in the brims of the bell-shaped curve.

Medical eros, because it is at home with improbabilities, might ask medical logos to explain one particularly awkward statistical dilemma. Biomedicine specializes in best-practice guidelines, it circulates the latest facts almost instantaneously, and medical staffs are similarly well educated. Reason predicts, then, that all specialized treatment centers should have roughly similar outcomes. But they don't. Why not? The surgeon and author Atul Gawande posed this question after examining specialized treatment centers for cystic fibrosis. He found that, yes, outcomes for most centers fell into a broad midrange dome, as predicted by the bell-shaped curve. A few treatment centers, however, showed far better results, some truly exceptional. "We are used to thinking," Gawande writes, "that a doctor's ability depends mainly on science and skill." Science and skill, he allows, may constitute "the easiest parts" of medical care, but they don't guarantee good results. "Even doctors with great knowledge and technical skill," he continues, puzzled, "can have mediocre results; more nebulous factors like aggressiveness and consistency and ingenuity can matter enormously."[41]

Nebulous factors. We are thrust back into dilemmas of the not-known. Is there a loophole or improbable role here for medical eros? For desire? It turns out that the physicians in Gawande's study who got consistently exceptional outcomes were, as he says, unusually *passionate* about their work and unusually *devoted* to their patients. "I was walking along minding my business," as the old song goes, "When love came and hit me in the eye / Flash! bam! alakazam! / Out of an orange-colored sky."[42] *Nebulous factors?* The phrase offers a weird placeholder for nonrational, alakazam-like, probability-busting forces that so often seem linked with individual desire, passion, and devotion: the marks of eros. These are the unruly forces that lie just beyond the reach of reason, beyond algorithms and statistical data, where empirical research, bench science, and the entire evidence-based armamentarium of medical logos cannot yet find the means to reduce them, once and for all, to stable, compliant objects of knowledge.

CHAPTER EIGHT

Light as Environment: How *Not* to Love Nature

All-beauteous Nature! By thy boundless charms
Oppressed, O where shall I begin thy praise,
Where turn th'ecstatic eye, how ease my breast
That pants with wild astonishment and love!

JOSEPH WARTON, "THE ENTHUSIAST, OR
THE LOVER OF NATURE" (1744)

O NCE UPON A time—well, in 1744 to be exact—it was possible to fall in love with nature. Love affairs do not always end well, however, and desire can lead us badly astray. Unhappy endings and erroneous choices, so basic to eros, dominate entertainment news sites when the participants are celebrities, but it also plays out—in quieter ways, on a larger scale, with truly devastating consequences—in the human relationship with nature. The figure of Mother Nature can be traced as far back as Linear B syllabic script, an early form of writing that survives from some twelve or thirteen centuries BCE, and nature (a nurturing, fertile, maternal force) has long been revered as a goddess and personified as female. Goddesses can turn vengeful, however, as Psyche learned the hard way, and even earth mothers can breed monster storms. A 2016 headline in the West Virginia *Lafayette Tribune* reports, "Thousands Affected by 'Once-in-a-Millennium' Flooding."[1] Isn't it at least somewhat surprising, given such increasingly regular disastrous reports, that so many people (from weekend gardeners to wilderness trekkers) still profess an unalterable love of nature?

Nature, as a concept and even as a locus of human experience, is in rapid retreat. It requires entire books to describe the changing philosophical and cultural ideas about the natural world in different societies and eras, but the familiar attribution of gender to the natural world took a significant turn at the dawn of the scientific revolution, when Adam's biblical "dominion" over the animals became a license for portraying humankind, in the language of Descartes, as the "masters and possessors" of nature.[2] The ancient gendered figure of nature as female, in a newly industrialized culture, was easily enlisted to support a transformative geo-sexual politics in which dominion turned into male-domination and male-domination turned into exploitation. The first steam engines were already pumping water from British mines—the dark urban mills and factories humming—when the young English poet Joseph Warton, barely turned twenty, published "The Enthusiast, Or The Lover of Nature" (1744). The poem speaks in the voice of a paramour who addresses nature as his beloved, a beautiful woman whose "charms" enrapture him with ecstasy and love. The love professed by Warton's *enthusiast* is no dried-up metaphor. It indicates, through its use of traditional romantic language in order to address nature as his beloved, the arrival of an innovative, full-blooded erotic passion.

Fast-forward 250 years. "Earth. Rock. Desert. I am walking barefoot on sandstone, flesh responding to flesh. It is hot, so hot the rock threatens to burn through the calloused soles of my feet. I must quicken my pace, paying attention to where I step." So begins *Desert Quartet: An Erotic Landscape* (1995), in which Terry Tempest Williams—writer, naturalist, and advocate for women's health—describes her solitary trek into the remote canyons of southern Utah.[3] Paying careful attention to where she steps, for Williams, is more than a sound strategy for traveling barefoot over hot sandstone. A heightened sensuous awareness of the desert environment belongs also to an elemental journey that strips away the buffers and filters that normally separate us from the natural world, exposing a neglected or hidden truth (that we ignore in our preoccupations and social roles) about the ultimately loving human relationship to nature. Earth, air, sea, and sky are not just classical elements, more than occasional objects of affection: they call to us, permanently, in too often unheard siren songs of the spirit. As Williams writes elsewhere, in a passage that helps explain her barefoot hike, "It is time for us to take off our masks, to step out from behind our personas—whatever they might be: educators, activists, biologists, geologists, writers, farmers, ranchers, and bureaucrats—and admit we are lovers, engaged in an erotics of place."[4]

An *erotics of place*, as it turns out, cannot entirely disentangle us from the dilemmas implicit in eros. The hot desert sandstone soon yields to a contrasting sensation as Williams finally enters a cleft in the canyon wall and leans her body against the dark, cool stone. Through an overhead gap she momentarily gazes up at a slice of blue sky, but then looks away. "I surrender. I close my eyes," she recounts in a prelude to sensual dissolve. "The arousal of my breath rises in me like music, like love, as the possessive muscles between my legs tighten and release. I come to the rock in a moment of stillness, giving and receiving, where there is no partition between my body and the body of Earth."[5] This amorous contact between earth and flesh reflects larger connections that Williams explores between the natural and human spheres, which include her marriage and her Mormon faith. It is her closed eyes, however, that hold my attention. Darkness is the native ground of eros—whose mysteries Psyche violates with a drop of hot candle wax—and, while I admire Williams's commitment to a passionate, nonexploitative relation to the earth, I am concerned by what an *erotics of place* may ignore, what troubles lie as if embedded in the hot sandstone or shut out by her closed eyes. Place is often politically reconfigured as territory, homeland, or hood, fought over in rival claims of ownership. People daily profess a love of nature, but nature is no longer nature. Some scholars drop the term *nature* altogether in preference for talk of environments, webs, or ecosystems; and, while we continue to *say* we love nature, the relationship seems nonreciprocal. Does nature really love *us*? Most important: above and beyond Williams's barefoot, elemental, erotic, desert journey looms the ever-burning sun.

Light Lite: A Thumbnail Guide to Illumination

The creation of light could be said to initiate the entire Judeo-Christian tradition and to unlock a world of troubles. "Let there be light, and there was light." Light and the divine Word, as theologians never tire of explaining, emerge together and united: "And God called the light Day, and the darkness he called Night. And the evening and the morning were the first day" (Genesis 1:3–5). Modern sunbathers soaking up rays at the beach perhaps seldom reflect that light once was considered sacred. The first-day scene of creation in which God utters the *fiat lux* of Genesis is, at least to a nonbiblical mind, eerily unimaginable: there is no earth and no sun. The sun appears only on day four. The light of *fiat lux* thus shines into an utter void. The biblical mentality that could keep light and the sun in separate categories in effect imagined a cosmos in which light abides directly *with* God. Light is the direct emanation of Deity.

The holiness of light, however, is not unique to Hebrew and Christian scriptures. Ancient Egyptians worshipped the sun as the eye of the mighty god Ra, and light thus constitutes their direct, unmediated contact with sacred power. At the first light of day, obelisks tipped with gold suddenly dazzle with divine presence. Its builders constructed the temple at Abu Simbel so that, twice yearly, a shaft of light penetrates two hundred feet through the open door to illuminate a statue of the pharaoh Rameses II: a god-king whose image stands between the sun gods Ra and Amnon.[6] A divine architecture of light extends to medieval cathedrals, with their dim interior spaces designed to permit strategic bursts of light and color.[7] Early Church fathers made the theological foundation of such feats explicit in the formula *God is Light*. Light, for centuries, carries a trace or faint imprint of its sacred origin.

The subsequent secular history of light is no less full of mysteries. "For the rest of my life," Albert Einstein is reported as saying, "I will reflect on what light is!"[8] Einstein makes me feel a little better that I don't really understand light, even after much thought and many books, not in the way I understand other natural phenomena such as rain or snow. The near immateriality of light—no more than a photon in mass—makes a pool of light far different from a pool of water or a snowball. One physicist describes the notorious wave/particle duality of light in an elegant aphorism:

"light travels as a wave but departs and arrives as a particle."[9] What can *depart* and *arrive* even mean, I wonder, when a photon of light circles the earth *seven times each second?* Color is equally puzzling. Do colors exist in the pitch dark, or are they a function of exposure to light? Sir Isaac Newton's prism experiment—dividing white sunlight into its spectrum of multiple colors—set off a whole new poetics of light (as well as a running quarrel between scientists and poets). What *is* light? What is light made of? What are its possible relations to health and illness? Light, although employed as a nearly universal image of mental illumination and of spiritual enlightenment, makes it very easy to feel confused.

Physicists explain that light is electromagnetic radiation, which unfortunately doesn't help me much.[10] We apparently live within surrounding fields of radiation mostly without recognizing it, like fish in water. We don't recognize it largely because most radiation is invisible, although it carries our favorite television shows, cell phone conversations, or just random impulses from deep space. Natural light, as radiation continuously pulsing from the sun, constitutes a specific band range of the electromagnetic spectrum. Visible light, the light we see or see with, is bundled closely on this spectrum with two flanking but invisible bands of radiation, *infrared* light and *ultraviolet* light, so that we generally refer to all three together when nonscientists talk about light.

Infrared light we perceive as heat. The earth absorbs infrared light during the day, warming the air, seas, and soil; at night, the earth radiates infrared light back into space, cooling soil, seas, and air. As a health hazard, the same infrared beams produce both heat exhaustion and sunstroke. *Ultraviolet* light, its partner, is the specific band of the electromagnetic spectrum responsible for the metabolic changes in the skin that produce suntans. It penetrates even dense clouds, which explains why we can get third-degree burns on a cloudy day. Light, then, however puzzling its physics, already merits notice because inattentiveness to infrared and to ultraviolet light can send us to the hospital.

Light holds a firm place in traditions where spiritual well-being provides a segue or passage to individual health and to social enlightenment. The English word *health* shares a root with the word *holiness*. "There is a light within a man of light," says Jesus in the Gnostic Gospel of Thomas, "and it lights up the whole world."[11] Oil-burning "slipper lamps" used by

Christians in Palestine during the Byzantine period (AD 313–638) commonly bear a Greek inscription that reads, "The light of Christ shines for all," a statement of social as well as spiritual inclusion.[12] From medieval mystics to patristic scholars, religious truth often takes the figure of an intense light with direct and indirect impact on the social world. Protestant dissenters in seventeenth-century England, for example, expressed the directness of their personal relation to God through the concept of "inner light": an *enthusiasm*, or, god-within, that supported radical social and political change (up to and including the execution of Charles I). Warton's *enthusiast* appropriates this same religious language to spiritualize, mildly, his new passion for nature. Deists and philosophers in the European Enlightenment chose light as the emblem of universal reason, which they put immediately into the service of social reform, while the nineteenth-century colonial metaphor of carrying light into dark places soon served as a pretext for varieties of mercantile exploitation. Light, in short, evoked values so crucial that to forget light was like forgetting goodness, truth, or money.

Our distinctive modern forgetting owes much to the industrialization of light in the nineteenth century, an event of historic importance.[13] A traditional Navajo dwelling, for example, always faces east, and a traditional Navajo woman begins each day with ritual homage to the sun. Our inattentiveness to light, except as a convenience, indicates how far we organize our lives around different principles. Light now floods our houses at the flick of a switch, night or day, following cables back to our indispensable power companies, which sell us light, or at least the electric current that produces light, as an industrial product. With light on demand, we no longer depend on natural cycles but structure our time as we please. Night is now an extension of day. Casinos, lit artificially and open for business at all hours, deliberately erase the natural cycles of darkness and light, much like hospitals, operating 24/7 in a field of nonstop, human-made illumination where it never *isn't* light.

We did not simply forget about light; we came to live within it and to take it for granted. The new industrial capacity to mass-produce light dazzled nineteenth-century consumers, for whom improvements in lighting were a visible symbol of progress, as gaslights in the 1820s and electric bulbs in the 1880s replaced smoky oil lamps. Soon fireplaces and candles joined other relics of a nostalgic past, transformed from necessities into luxuries, while incandescent streetlamps remade Paris into the world-famous "City of Light."

Meanwhile, a posttheological imagination found new uses for light. Dawn and sunset for Thoreau are not simply natural facts but summarizing symbols of spiritual progress, while a century later military planners gave light a new mission, transformed into laser-weapon systems. Light as weapon returns us to the field of health and illness: the nuclear blasts over Hiroshima and Nagasaki lit up the skies like a false sun, shredding flesh and raining down lethal radiation sickness, forever stripping light of its holiness, while the less-well-remembered 1945 firebombing of Tokyo incinerated some 100,000 people. Still, we remain creatures of light, however negligent. The same force that can destroy incoming missiles also illuminates urban sidewalks at night and floods vacant parking lots with safety.

During the seven years when I lived in New Mexico, in a pueblo-style adobe house on a bluff facing east, every morning I watched the sun emerge with a sudden rush over the topmost peaks of the Sandia Mountains. Light organized my day not with prayer but with sunblock, dark glasses, and a wide-brimmed western hat worn for skin protection. The sun was a daily adversary, stripping the varnish from my woodwork, bleaching the paint on my car, turning my morning drive into a visor-flipping struggle. I learned that light can blind you and kill you if you wander lost too long, unprotected, in the desert sun. Without a passion for barefoot hikes, I live instead acclimated to light as a commodity, available everywhere, on demand and in excess, like Times Square blazing with colorful high-definition noontime ads. I tend to like all-night diners, round-the-clock malls, strobe lights, and Jumbotrons pumping up the wattage at rock concerts. Then I remember Georgia O'Keeffe's famous "Cow Skull with Calico Roses" (1932), which was once featured as cover art for the journal *Emerging Infectious Diseases*. Nature is roses but also microbes, pathogens, and desiccated cow skulls. Is all this surplus light—somewhere a television always on—really what we desire? Or, I begin to wonder, is an unseen force perhaps desiring it *for* us—desiring us to desire it, even to our lasting harm?

Medical Logos and the Biology of Light

Light is the basis of all life on earth. Water, air, soil are necessary, of course, but without light, the blue-green planet we call home is no more than an icy midsize spinning space cinder. Light, as medical logos and the molecular gaze can confirm, stimulates the chloroplasts in green plants to drive the photosynthetic processes on which all earthly life depends. Sightless fish in pitch-black caves, living in total darkness, cannot survive without the light-dependent food chain seeding the water with nutrients, nor can the 285 species of subterranean mammals who, like moles, live in lightless burrows.[14] The earth's primordial atmosphere of carbon dioxide could not sustain human life until photosynthesis generated the oxygen on which we continue to depend.

Much as green plants transform ultraviolet sunlight into the stored energy at the base of the food pyramid, humans convert this light-based stored energy into power for health and for healthy function. What would happen in a total absence of light? No nighttime stars, no fireflies, no laptop glow, no visual directions up or down: total disorientation for the last person standing on a planet otherwise officially declared dead. Driving the last miles home, in the artificial tunnel of my headlamps, I feel a satisfying relief as I turn into my driveway and the security lights automatically snap on. The biology of light is crucial not only because light is what makes earth habitable for humans but also because light, among its contributions, is inseparably linked to our well-being—and to our illnesses.

Consider rickets. Light turned out to be the secret turning point in the flesh-and-blood mystery of a crippling childhood bone disease. The disease arrived in Europe with the suddenness of plague. Rickets, first described by Francis Glisson in *De Rachitide* (1650), ravaged the grim overcrowded factory towns of preindustrial England with such speed and ferocity that it was called "the English disease." It was so common that it spawned an all-purpose slang term for debilitation: *rickety*. Rickets attacked children in the first years of life, softening and twisting the bones, leaving their bodies sickly and disabled. As late as 1922, the same year when T. S. Eliot published "The Waste Land," London physician J. Lawson Dick portrayed the typical rachitic child as dull and heavy,

suffering from malformed bones, wasted muscles, and marked by defor-
mities of the skull, spine, and pelvis. "The disease is partially recovered
from," Dick wrote, "but there is apt to be a permanent arrest or perversion
of the growth and development of the brain itself." Rickets, he wrote, is
"the commonest disease of children in our large towns, and at the present
day it is probably the most serious factor interfering with the efficiency of
the nation."[15] Like AIDS in Africa, rickets was a disease that not only
afflicted individuals but could also impair whole regions and countries.

Nobody knew what caused rickets. A few clues generated controversial theories. Some theories focused on climate, bad housing, and socioeconomic status—because rickets took such a high toll among the urban
working-class poor. The disease is a general product of industrialism,
Dick concluded, adding that it was as difficult to imagine a town without
slums as to imagine children free from the threat of rickets. But why?
Other theorists invoked heritable disorders, infectious disease, or nutri-
tional deficiency. An experiment in 1918 showed that puppies developed
rickets on diets lacking a fat-soluble nutrient described, nebulously, as the
"antirachitic factor." Not every child with a fat-poor diet, however, got
rickets. Could the culprit be endocrine glands? Lack of exercise? Rickets
as an enigmatic crippling disease of childhood evoked the anxieties associated in 1950s America with polio.

Then—thanks to medical logos—a breakthrough! Between 1922 and
1930, researchers in England and in America showed that the cause of
rickets is a deficiency of vitamin D. Vitamin D was the vague "antirachitic
factor" that had mysteriously protected Icelanders and Greenlanders,
who, unlike the light-deprived urban poor, ate a diet rich in cod. Cod liver
oil is a very good source of vitamin D, but so, too, researchers soon demonstrated, is sunlight.

The biology underlying such straightforward observations took years
to understand, earning at least one Nobel Prize in chemistry, and we now
know that human skin produces vitamin D in the presence of ultraviolet
light. Sunlight too weak in ultraviolet rays may not produce the necessary quantities of vitamin D, and the famous pea-soup smog in Sherlock
Holmes's industrial London—so thick and toxic that in 1952 it killed
12,000 Londoners in just four days—guaranteed a deficiency in ultraviolet light. The mud, rain, and snow of English winters also meant that

infants born in October likely spent their first six months in dark rooms. Once doctors understood the biology of rickets, mothers in light-poor slums—and elsewhere—were quick to grasp the extra protection offered by fish-liver oils. Good access to the sun, however, still provides an inexpensive source of vitamin D, and rickets thus offers a striking instance of how human health is linked directly to the biology of light.[16]

Light, as medical logos soon discovered, is responsible for far more than the healthy bones of infants and children. Rickets showed that humans evolved with a biological need for light. Specialized skin cells, called *melanocytes*, both absorb ultraviolet radiation and produce the pigmented substance (*melanin*) that protects the skin from excessive exposure. Moreover, inherited differences in the production of melanocytes are largely responsible for differences in skin color.[17] Skin color, of course, is related to ongoing social conflict, often stoked by passions over ethnicity or race. The biology of light indirectly provides a basis for color-based racial stereotypes responsible both for incalculable injuries and deaths and also for quite well-documented and measurable disparities in minority health care, exacerbated by huge disparities in income. (A more equitable health-care system may evolve when societies understand that there is more genetic diversity within so-called races than across them.)[18] The social and political attitudes that result in substandard health care for black patients in the United States, for example, begin, although it is only a beginning, with evolutionary melanocyte responses to a light-drenched planet that completes one full rotation on its axis some 365.26 times in its annual twelve-month orbit around the sun.

Circadian rhythm is the technical name for biological variations that repeat in twenty-four hour cycles. Although scientists now think that the human cycle is closer to twenty-five hours, humans and hamsters alike share internal circadian clocks timed to the earth's cycles of light and darkness, a primal rhythm that determines the nighttime hunting of lions as well as the crescendo of early morning bird calls. Proper functioning of these internal biological clocks is essential to health, and disruption of our circadian rhythms can result in various illnesses.[19]

The two main properties of circadian rhythms that affect health and illness are simply stated. They are generated within the body, and, ordinarily, they synchronize to light-dark cycles by means of photoreceptors.[20]

This bodily adaptation is significant for health because circadian rhythms prove important to such basic biological processes as aging, mental performance, blood pressure, kidney excretion, immune functions, cell growth, cardiovascular activity, and brain neurotransmission.[21] Not all human biological cycles are circadian—there are seven-day and monthly cycles, too—but circadian rhythms are now well recognized, and doctors remain on alert for disorders of the circadian timing system. For example, light triggers the production of *melatonin*, a hormone affecting crucial health-related processes from ovulation to sleep.[22] Melatonin levels, moreover, contribute to a variety of circadian rhythm disorders, such as jet lag.[23] NASA shift-workers, compared with subjects in a control group, reported better sleep, better performance, and better physical and emotional well-being after receiving a week of light treatments.[24] Astronauts on a Mars voyage would doubtless approve if the shift-workers at mission control slipped in a few extra light treatments.

Light, in its circadian patterns, may also underlie biological processes implicated in emotional and psychological well-being. A seasonal pattern for depressive episodes, quickly publicized as *seasonal affective disorder*, with the catchy acronym SAD, made news starting in 1984.[25] Circadian rhythms keyed to seasonal alterations in light seemed a possible cause of SAD, but after decades of research the data remain inconclusive and at times contradictory.[26] A 2013 review article in the *American Journal of Psychiatry* offers what is probably a safe summary of the current state of research: "A wide range of studies have demonstrated the efficacy of light treatment for SAD and have minimized the possibility that light treatment works by a placebo effect."[27] Mild seasonal diminishment of mood and energy, as research shows, is common in the northern hemisphere, even among people who do not qualify for a diagnosis of major depression.

One surprise: the antidepressant effects of light are not mediated solely through photoreceptors in the eye. An organ-based, nonvisual system of light-sensitive molecules—often involving a photoactive pigment called *melanopsin*—also seems capable of driving the circadian system. Ruth, raised in sunny Los Angeles, wilted during our winter sojourns in the Midwest, when arctic air over Lake Michigan generated cloud-cover thick as a mattress. Two sun-filled winter weeks in Key West had therapeutic benefits. Outdoor bars, roaming chickens, and palm trees may augment the health benefits of light, my informal research suggests. In a psychiatric inpatient unit, patients in sunny rooms had an average stay almost three days shorter than did patients in nonsunny rooms.[28] Light in moderate doses somewhere with outdoor live bands is doubtless a fine all-purpose tonic.

Medical logos has expressed enough interest in light to generate a new subspecialty called photomedicine, which occupies the border between basic science and clinical practice. Dermatologists, for example, use ultraviolet light (especially UV-B) as therapy for a number of skin diseases, including psoriasis and vitiligo. Meanwhile, light has indirectly contributed to health care when concentrated in lasers. Lasers create a monochromatic, intense, narrow beam of light that proves invaluable in performing various quasi-medical tasks, from melting material for dental fillings to bleaching tattoos, but their truly remarkable use lies in surgery. With its power to seal off small blood vessels, the laser permits surgery with almost no bleeding, which is especially advantageous for tissues rich in blood vessels. It is also ideal for microsurgeries in areas too confined or delicate for a scalpel, such as the throat or eye. In the detached retina procedure, a laser can accomplish what a scalpel can't: weld the retina back to the eyeball.[29] Surgeons now use lasers together with fiber-optic endoscopes to shine precision surgical light into the once-total darkness of interior organs.

Light offers medical logos a medium for endlessly inventive uses, even as the newest means to store and to transport medical records. Photons are so far superior to electrons in carrying information that they have given rise to a whole new medically-related discipline, *photonics*, which specializes in technologies that shoot laser-generated photons through glass-lined fibers. Medical data whiz by at nearly the speed of light. Photonics has recently joined forces with an even newer biotechnology, *optogenetics*, which employs genes encoding light-sensitive proteins. The genes (introduced into specific cells of a host organism) can then direct the synthesis of the light-sensitive protein—providing an internal, organic, self-replicating surveillance system for studying such multinetworked, elusive human functions as memory and pain.[30] Light, then, in ways unrelated to environmental experiments with solar power, is emerging as a raw material that medical logos can inventively work up to employ in the service of health.

XP: Light Is Not Our Friend

Light, in its shiftiness, includes a potential for inflicting significant harm. Periodic darkness, through its link with the circadian system, is as crucial to health as light is, and too much light breeds irreparable damage. Researchers at Leiden University Medical Center in the Netherlands tracked the health of rats exposed to 24 weeks of continuous light and compared them with a control group exposed to alternating 12-hour cycles of light and darkness. The light-saturated rats showed not only reduced circadian rhythmicity but also reduced skeletal muscle function and bone deterioration. They got fatter, had higher blood glucose levels, and gave evidence of immune system damage.[31] If you are a rat, which is as far as the Leiden research allows us to conclude, you will be far healthier with periodic exposure to darkness. If you are a human being and sleep in darkness, sleep "resets" brain connections crucial for memory and for learning.[32] For the unlucky few born with the genetic disorder xeroderma pigmentosum, however, sleep and periodic darkness do not help. Exposure to light leads ultimately to suffering and early death.

Xeroderma pigmentosum, or XP, is a rare genetic condition that, in its awful damage, offers a haunting confirmation that evolution has gifted us with built-in protections against light. Lacking these genetic protections, the skin of patients with XP is so sensitive to daylight that exposure to the sun can cause life-threatening burns. Skin cancers often begin before children reach age ten. Ultraviolet radiation leads to malignant changes in the eye as mucous membranes dry out and eyelids atrophy.[33] In extreme cases, parents keep children sheltered from daylight or, for rare outdoor excursions, bundle them up like mummies. Despite such precautions, children with XP tend to die at an early age. While rickets assures us that human health depends on light, especially during childhood, XP tells us that our health depends not only on proper exposure to light but also on genetic protections that prevent the damage caused by excess light. Without the proper function of these protective genes, children with XP who do not die early live impaired and painful lives. Their fate serves as a grim reminder that—even with our current genetic protections intact—humans will suffer irreparable damage if the atmospheric shields that protect us from excessive light ever fail.

In the United States, XP counts as a Black Swan. The probability of being born with XP is one in a million, sort of like the odds of finding your soul mate. The genetic diversity within a mobile, multiethnic population makes XP about as worrisome as the odds of a major earthquake occurring on the Hayward fault in the next fifty minutes. In southwest Brazil, however, more than twenty people in the small sundried rural community of Araras, population 800, suffer from XP. At age 38, Djalma Antonio Jardim has undergone more than fifty surgeries to remove skin tumors, not to mention the skin he lost as the disease eats away at his lips, nose, and cheeks. About one in three individuals with XP will develop progressive neurological abnormalities—seizures, hearing loss, difficulty swallowing, poor coordination, loss of intellectual function—and such problems tend to worsen over time.[34] Gleice Francisca Machado, a village teacher in Araras whose son has XP, says simply, "The sun is our biggest enemy and those affected must change day for night in order to live longer." She adds, evoking our ancient kinship with the sun, "Unfortunately, that is not possible."[35]

XP is the extreme case that exposes what happens, almost beneath notice, as the human body encounters sunlight. And it's not only human bodies: ultraviolet exposure damages the immune system of nonhuman animals and even affects the mutation rate of plants. The everyday human example of sun damage is, of course, skin cancer.[36] It may seem odd that equatorial populations (despite the increased exposure to ultraviolet radiation) suffer far less skin cancer than do northern populations. The explanation is that, as protection, they evolved dark skin and a surplus production of melanocytes. Northern populations, who have a decreased exposure to sunlight, evolved pale skin that produces more vitamin D, but at the cost of increased risk for skin cancers.

The atmospheric ozone layer offers us vital protection from solar damage, and thus it caused deep concern when scientists discovered a massive hole opening up, annually, over both poles. This ozone depletion—due largely to the use of industrial chlorofluorocarbons (CFCs)—occurs when chlorine molecules come into contact with sunlight. Happily, climate scientists now say that the ozone layer is "healing"—their term—thanks mainly to the phasing out of CFCs under the 1987 Montreal Protocol.[37] Nations still affected by the ozone loss, particularly Australia, meanwhile have seen large increases in skin cancer. Both melanoma and non-melanoma skin cancers are escalating worldwide. The most important risk factor for nonmelanoma skin cancers is ultraviolet light exposure, most often from the sun.[38] Melanomas occur also in protected areas of the body *not* exposed to the sun, such as the stomach, but the worldwide increased rates of lethal cutaneous melanoma and alarming increases in the rate of skin cancers raise important cultural as well as strictly medical issues about sun-related illness. Medical logos mostly acts as the designated skin-cancer cleanup squad.

It is absurd to ask biomedicine to take on full responsibility for a dilemma whose source is in part cultural and environmental. Rickets and XP remind us that humans evolved in a taut relation with light. Medical logos possesses the knowledge to intervene when the absence of light (as in rickets) proves damaging or when the excess of light (as in skin cancer) proves damaging, but such medical interventions often help individuals without addressing the wider cultural issues behind such damage. If the source of urban gunfire is cultural, not medical, then medicine with all its technical skills and biochemical knowledge cannot address the problem at its root. Medical logos, in this sense, can patch up the victims of Chicago gun violence, but it is at present powerless to stop urban gang warfare. Human health is hard to dissociate from human desires. Biomedicine and medical eros need each other, they depend on each other, and their ideal relationship may well resemble a dance of contraries.

Medical eros, in an ideal health-related dance of contraries, is well-positioned to address the contributions that human desire makes to the problems of light damage. Sun worship has changed its meaning and its purpose since the time of the ancient Egyptians. Humans have not always lathered up with suntan oil for a day at the beach. Soaking up rays in a thong is a distinctively modern, erotic relation to light. Modern trends in fashion, often with an erotic subtext, celebrate the exposure of athletic bodies in muscle shirts, cutoff jeans, and less. Three erudite books discuss the relation of eros to sport, but without an interest in light, even though Olympic competition originated outdoors, under the sun.

The far more than three learned discussions of eros and film usually ignore the role of light, even though lighting is crucial for on-screen ambience as well as for the semidark erotic ambience of the cinema.[39] If rickets
was the representative disease of the industrial age, when factory workers
raised sun-starved children with soft, twisted bones, skin cancer may
be its counterpart for the postindustrial democratic age of the ozone hole
and the tank top.

Medical eros occupies a strategic position from which to reverse or mitigate damage directly or indirectly caused by human desire and wrapped
up in our own changed relation to light. Medical logos can suggest preventive strategies, such as large floppy hats; it can enlist its knowledge to
support treaties and regulations aimed to reduce damage to the ozone
layer. However, this is exactly the point, given all we have learned from
photomedicine and from the science of light, where medical logos needs
assistance from medical eros. What we need, in addition to floppy hats
and smart treaties, is a well-considered culture-wide redirection of desire.

Daisyworld: Light and Global Climate Change

Global climate change is for authorities ranging from Nobel laureates to
Pope Francis the most extraordinary dilemma that we confront in the
twenty-first century. Its impact will reach far into future generations. After
some initial skirmishing over how to name it, global climate change is now
securely locked into our political and journalistic lexicons, and the damage
is as well documented and alarming as seas without fish. (In the last fifty
years, fish species utilized by humans have declined by half.)[40] We know
that humans are driving pelagic species into collapse through overfishing,
and the international scientific community agrees that humans, mainly
through burning carbon-based fuels, are warming the air, seas, and earth,
driving global climate change. Controversies muddy the issue of cause,
and the geological record shows fluctuation in world climate, as the earth
cycles in and out of ice ages with no humans present to add or subtract a
degree of temperature.

Healing in the ozone layer indicates that humans can undo and reverse
damage that humans cause, if we accept responsibility. The alternative
is alarming. The World Wildlife Fund predicts that coral reefs will

disappear by 2050 if sea temperatures continue to warm at current rates. Authoritative forecasts of a 10- to 32-inch rise in sea levels by 2100 will put Miami and New Orleans (as well as coastal villages in the developing world) under water.[41] These are not Black Swans. They constitute a slow-motion, approaching catastrophe that human desire can either escalate in speed and scale or possibly reduce. Light and desire are two key players in this high-risk game of planetwide climate change, and both are related to the prospects for human health and illness. A visit to Daisyworld can offer some clarification.

Daisyworld is the optimistic theme-park name of a simplified computer model that British geophysiologist James Lovelock constructed to illustrate how the earth—somewhat like a gigantic creature—might incorporate periodic climate change within a larger, fluctuating homeostasis. Light, as an engine of global climate change, could stand as a symbol or logo for Lovelock's vision of planet Earth (constituted by multiple interlocking ecosystems) that he introduced under the name Gaia Theory. Lovelock's Gaia Theory postulates that living organisms are "tightly coupled" with the environment. In later revisions, he came to describe Gaia—the earth with its tightly coupled living organisms, human inhabitants, and interlocking ecosystems—as "a self-organizing superorganism."[42] Although Lovelock does not single it out explicitly, light is the central, indispensable feature that governs the self-organizing properties of Gaia. "The self-regulation of the system," he writes, almost in passing, "is an active process driven by the free energy available from sunlight."[43]

Here is how Daisyworld works. As a virtual planet, simplified for the purposes of computer analysis, it consists entirely of white daisies and dark daisies. Lovelock then changes the planetary temperature by adding more or less solar radiation. His point is that, despite changes in surface temperature, Daisyworld as a self-organizing superorganism always maintains a stable climate favorable to life. The dark daisies prefer the cold and absorb light, while the white daisies prefer warmth and reflect light. As Daisyworld gets colder, dark daisies flourish, which would seem a dangerous imbalance, but then as the dark daisies multiply and absorb more light, Daisyworld gets increasingly warmer, at which point, of course, the white daisies stage a comeback. Lovelock's core idea is that Daisyworld offers a model of the earth as a complex biotic system that self-corrects for its own imbalances. In failing to call attention to the central importance of light, however, Lovelock also fails to explore how light (tightly coupled, in its effects, with human desire) holds the power to bring this beautiful and intricate planetary self-organizing superorganism—over many eons, not just temporarily—to wrack and ruin.

Daisyworld, as a simple sunlight-driven model, is a pretty peaceful joint. Lovelock, as manager or steward, supplies the correct quantum of sunlight free energy used to test the system, and his system runs as designed. (Too much sunlight will fry everything.) Suppose, however, that we introduce into Lovelock's simplified and stable model little humanoid creatures who reproduce like daisy-loving rabbits—8 billion and counting. These little humanoid figures, when not reproducing, like to fight. They cut down rain forests, frack for shale oil, melt polar ice caps, and release tons of hothouse gases. While they are admiring photos showing the bright lights visible from outer space, the sea levels rise, coastal populations move inland, and even more fighting breaks out (over scarce food, contested territory, and dwindling resources). The white and dark daisies didn't hate each other. They didn't hire lawyers, blow up mosques and churches, create international drug cartels, or stockpile nuclear weapons. Unlike the inhabitants of New York City, they did not produce 12,000 tons of residential waste daily. At some unknown tipping point, isn't it probable that Daisyworld's elegant self-organizing light-driven, desire-inflected system—white daisies, dark daisies, little humanoid figures, the whole shebang—will collapse into a fished-out, clear-cut, pumped-dry planetary chaos?

Planet Earth and its damaged ecosystems will survive and self-regulate over many millions of years. Humans, on a shorter timeline for survival, may not be so lucky. It is thus important to recognize how Daisyworld inadvertently repeats the lesson that light (too much light) is not our friend. Solar radiation takes no interest in us, but we should take an interest in it. Too much trapped solar energy will make our lives miserable. Global climate change, described in a document produced by the U.S. Environmental Protection Agency, promises a grim watch-list of dangers to human health. Young children, older adults, people with medical conditions, and the poor are most vulnerable to heat-related illnesses. Climate-related

flooding that devastates infrastructure will produce thousands of evac-
uees, many suffering from afflictions ranging from intestinal illness
and depression to post-traumatic stress disorder. Increased airborne
carbon dioxide has already multiplied pollen in some ragweed varieties
60 to 90 percent, creating epidemic-level allergies, while warmer temperatures add more days when ground-level ozone hits unhealthy levels.
Ticks carrying Lyme disease have extended their range northward; in
2002 a new strain of warm-weather West Nile virus emerged in the United
States. We already see a large increase in skin cancers and in potentially
fatal melanomas. Nowhere does the EPA, in discussing threats from climate change, mention the crucial link between light and human health.[44]

Medical eros would insist that light cannot be reduced to photons, melanocytes, and bands on the electromagnetic spectrum. Light as a
natural force can be redirected by the twists and turns of human desire,
for better or for worse, and desire as a planetary force finds a striking correlate in the celebrated NASA composite photo (Figure 8.1) that shows
the earth, as viewed from outer space, lit up like an incandescent geopolitical pinball machine.

Light on demand, beginning with the domestication of fire, is among
the most significant human inventions, transforming nighttime darkness
and extending human vision, with far-reaching effects that extend all the
way, circa 2015, to forty-six well-lit megacities with populations over 10
million and growing. Light in the nighttime NASA image not only indicates concentrated areas of human activity but also reflects the technological skills and relative affluence required to fire up the night sky such
that it can be viewed from space. Such nighttime photos of the illuminated
earth are often offered as a tribute to human progress: a visual erotics
of light, as if the entire planet pulsed out its burning affection and admiration. The glowing traces of human habitation visible from space, however, also convey a less congratulatory suggestion: they expose the
world-changing effect of human desire (aided and abetted by science,
technology, and commerce) as we tirelessly mine the coal, strip the
forests, and pump the oil needed to convert fossil fuels into electric current. This alarming turn in human desire is a relatively recent cultural
event, and it finds almost joyous celebration in a philosophical text (at

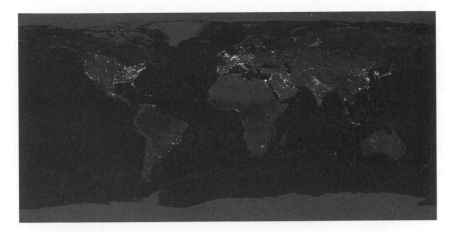

FIGURE 8.1. NASA Earth Observatory image by Robert Simmon.
Data provided courtesy of Chris Elvidge (NOAA National Geophysical
Data Center). Composite photograph. 2012.

the heart of the American enterprise) that bears the resonant one-word title *Nature* (1836).

"Nature is thoroughly mediate," writes Ralph Waldo Emerson. "It is made to serve. It receives the dominion of man as meekly as the ass on which the Saviour rode. It offers all its kingdoms to man as the raw material which he may mould [*sic*] into what is useful. Man is never weary of working it up."[45] Emerson is usually understood as a prophet of the spirit. He writes about the material world as the sign of an ideal or transcendental reality beyond mere matter, and this spiritual bent carries over in his allusion to Genesis 1:26, where God gives Adam "dominion" over all living creatures. Emerson's quasi-religious view of nature as "thoroughly mediate," however, should come with a large red banner reading *Beware!* His view of nature in this passage is far less sacramental than *instrumental*. Humans—if we extend Emerson's concept of nature as thoroughly mediate—not only *work up* nature into products for human use but also today presume to *manage* nature in a self-appointed (if biblically authorized) role as stewards. Can we manage nature if we can't manage ourselves? In Beijing, which ranks as only the ninth worst polluted city in China, simply breathing the air is equivalent to smoking a pack of cigarettes daily. Still, there is room for managerial skill. Chicago, a leader in reducing migration casualties, now boasts 90 to 95 percent compliance from skyscrapers in turning off lights between midnight and dawn, slowing the nocturnal carnage of birds. Even environmental success stories, however, given the interconnections we can't always recognize, may conceal trouble. Artificial light, even if wisely managed to protect birds, depends largely on the consumption of fossil fuels, which helps drive global climate change. Natural sunlight, moreover, is what (as in Daisyworld) supplies the ultimate driving force for a planetary climate change: change revved up by human desire in a twisted understanding of nature as "made to serve." The result, if not catastrophic extinctions and vanishing biodiversity, is certain to be a swollen global burden of human misery and illness.

This is what Emerson does not tell us. Sunlight has a primary role in regulating global climate via solar radiation, but here, too, human desires intervene. The usual culprits are so-called greenhouse gases—particularly carbon dioxide and methane—but even though they are produced mainly by human activities, they are no more than accomplices. The mastermind is solar radiation, as light orchestrates a three-step, real-world collusion. First, greenhouse gases accumulating in the atmosphere prevent daytime solar radiation from bouncing back into space at night, so the trapped solar radiation directly increases surface temperatures. Second, as temperatures rise, the air and seas also grow warmer, reducing the global snow cover (that ordinarily repels solar radiation) and melting polar ice. As a result, surface temperatures rise further, especially in the all-important ocean currents, which directly affect major air masses. Third, as ice caps melt and as sea levels rise, the increasing heat creates atmospheric turbulence and monster storms that batter heavily populated coastal areas, while fertile inland areas suffer drought and famine. The impact on human health is already visible as tropical pathogens move north and as violent storms create social havoc. In the New Orleans floods that followed Hurricane Katrina, local police fled and the public order almost collapsed.

Light is far too important to environmental health to be left inexplicit, taken for granted, or just plain absent from the discussion. Interest in light has mainly focused on solar energy as a source of clean, inexpensive power to underwrite our current lifestyles. Innovations such as solar heating, solar architecture, solar cars, solar phones, and even a space-age invention called artificial photosynthesis all promise positive changes. The

International Energy Agency declared in 2011 that "the development of affordable, inexhaustible and clean solar energy technologies will have huge longer-term benefits. It will increase countries' energy security through reliance on an indigenous, inexhaustible and mostly import-independent resource, enhance sustainability, reduce pollution, lower the costs of mitigating climate change, and keep fossil fuel prices lower than otherwise."[46] This list of global advantages, it is interesting to observe, does not envision any possible Black Swan downsides. It does not mention the close and often dangerous relation between light and health.

The World Health Organization takes a different perspective on the immediate future of solar radiation. It estimates that climate change, in the two decades from 2030 to 2050, will cause an additional 250,000 deaths per year. Most of the people who die as an indirect but clear result of climate change will perish from malaria, diarrhea, heat exposure, and malnutrition.[47]

Light and its impact on human health will take the largest toll precisely where the promising global advantages of solar energy are hardest to realize: in the developing world. The picture is not pretty. Chaos tends to multiply in a complex network of interlocking systems, and social suffering is likely to increase fastest—with multiplier effects—in developing nations that lack effective public-health infrastructures. Drought and floods will threaten already precarious food supplies just when warmer temperatures favor the spread of infectious disease and when unsanitary conditions breed disease-bearing waterborne parasites. As disease levels increase, the breakdown in social order will undermine local and national governments, with dire consequences for economic activity, trade, immigration, and other large-scale social patterns, with an extreme impact on individual health. One sure lesson of the HIV / AIDS epidemic: any new, cunning virus constitutes an international peril. There is no eco-paradise or nearby planet to run to.

The most dangerously underestimated threat that light poses to life on earth—not just to human beings but to the biodiverse web of life on which we depend—concerns the warming of the oceans. Water makes up some 71 percent of the earth's surface and offers a vast absorbent medium for the reception of light. Most of the water (96.5 percent) is contained in the oceans, with the rest distributed among lakes and glaciers. The International

Union for the Conservation of Nature, in a report based on the work of eighty scientists from a dozen countries, depicts an alarming future when warming ocean temperatures will unlock billions of tons of frozen methane from the seabed, baking the surface of the planet. This light-driven warming is even now having its greatest impact upon such building blocks of life as phytoplankton, zooplankton, and krill, with effects rippling up through the food chain. Environmental activist and longtime defender of marine wildlife, Paul Watson, describes the human stakes with stark conditional logic: "If the oceans die, we all die!"[48]

Medical eros alone can't resolve interconnected global crises, but a focus on the health-related impact of human desire has a significant role to play. While medical logos can anticipate the dangers and prepare first responders, medical eros can help redirect individual and social desires in ways that maximize protection and minimize threats in the long term. The stakes are serious, and not for humans alone. The mile-high Sandia Mountains frame the southwestern city of Albuquerque, which grew after World War II (in a paradigm of urban sprawl) from a small desert town to a postmodern metropolis of one hundred and eighty-seven square miles. Today more than half of the world's population dwells in urban areas, and in the next generation the number will be almost 70 percent. New residents to Albuquerque are attracted by a dry climate that boasts a whopping 280 sunny days annually. Above the high-desert city, on the peaks of the Sandia Mountains, you can find sedimentary rocks with the fossilized imprint of trilobites, brachiopods, and other ancient marine invertebrates that once thrived in a prehuman, prehistoric sea covering almost all of bone-dry New Mexico. The speeded-up version of climate change possible in Daisyworld, as inflected by human desire, might well see iPods and smartphones mixed among the shards and nautiloid fossils. Medical eros would urge ways of redirecting desire. It would help us turn our desires toward the creation of new, respectful, life-affirming, even truly earth-loving relations to light.

Luminosity: Spirit and Health

"I like to bring light to the place that is much like that in the dream," the artist James Turrell explains, "where you feel it to be something itself, not something with which you illuminate other things, but a celebration of the thingness of light, the material presence, the revelation of light."[49] Turrell has dedicated his career to working with light, light as so basic to human perception that it appears even in our Technicolor dreams, which otherwise would unfold in total darkness. Ezra Pound in his *ABC of Reading* (1960) described artists as the "antennae of the race."[50] Artists such as James Turrell and fellow Californian Robert Irwin may well help advance a healthy culture-wide shift in our relation to light. Such a new, life-affirming contemporary relationship to light is not an impossible fantasy, given the changing history of human attitudes toward light, and it is important that light (in its relations to health and illness) should not emerge mainly as contributing to problematic medical conditions from skin cancer and heatstroke to XP. Turrell's *Roden Crater Project* is a culmination of his lifelong artistic meditation on light: a colossal earthwork decades in creation, carved out of an extinct volcano in Arizona, that invites viewers to experience light in celebration of its dreamlike thingness—almost abstracted from the objects it illuminates—as a sensuous, awe-inspiring, material presence with the power (which Bataille attributed to eros) to take us outside and beyond ourselves.

Turrell's aim is to create, in a natural setting screened from urban haze, an experience that brings the viewer face to face, so to speak, with light. Light pollution obscures true darkness—with its access to nighttime stars—for 80 percent of Europe and North America, which makes us both light-saturated and light-deprived.[51] A restored or renewed experience of light is what matters to Turrell. Planning for the immense project began in 1972, and ever since Turrell has been transforming the desert volcano into a multichambered space for reexperiencing light. Roden Crater, in its focus on light, in effect stands outside the contemporary land-art or earthworks movement associated with Robert Smithson, Walter De Maria, and Michael Heizer, which to some degree liberates art objects from museums by transforming the earth into art. The 600-foot tall cinder cone at Roden Crater, by contrast, is no art object but creates the impression that you are standing inside a gigantic telescope pointed at the open sky. The stars at night, viewed from within the crater-telescope, with no ambient light pollution, look much as they looked to our ancient ancestors. You might discover, Turrell says, that in one chamber you can see your shadow in a pool of water cast solely by the light reflected from the planet Venus. Roden Crater, encouraging such individual reawakenings along with their accompanying emotions, is a kind of antigallery. The work on display is not for sale, almost immaterial, and nothing but light. With its alternating sun-warmed basins and cool, crypt-like dark spaces encased in volcanic rock, the interior is not designed or meant for human inhabitants but rather, in Turrell's words, is a "habitation for light."[52]

Light, reexperienced with the primal intensity and even perhaps with traces of the sacred status that it once held for the ancient Egyptians, offers a unique occasion for the awakenings often associated with spiritual renewal. Turrell's Quaker background, filtered through a modern Zen sensibility, brings with it the enduring Quaker commitment to an "inner light" and to a personal relation with the divine. Roden Crater offers what Turrell calls "a stage where the landscape of our thoughts is united with the infinite."[53] As a light-filled environment that unites thought and infinitude, Roden Crater also has the advantage of a high-desert setting that invokes the awe of elemental forces. It gestures toward traditions of the sublime, whose early theorists (such as Joseph Warton) held that the awe-inspiring powers of the natural world, like panoramic vistas stretching toward infinitude, transport us beyond ourselves and simulate or inspire a personal experience of the divine: a rapt state in which mere human concerns slip away. The one invariable illustration of sublimity that eighteenth-century theorists invoked for well over a century was the omnipotent *fiat lux* of Genesis: *God said, Let there be light, and there was light.*

Roden Crater extends into a sublime dimension his impressive but more modest light-centered installations in museums and in various public buildings, where Turrell in effect brings modern art and its institutions into contact with a quasi-religious vision that begins and perhaps concludes in sensory experience. "We eat light, drink it in through our skins," he observes, perhaps in reference to basic photosynthetic and photobiological processes. This renewed experience of light, even granting its quasi-religious dimension, inescapably approaches the erotic. "Seeing," Turrell insists, "is a very sensuous act—there's a sweet deliciousness to feeling yourself see something."[54] The distinctive experience of light that

Turrell orchestrates in Roden Crater in effect regards the earth as far more than the sum of its interlocked ecosystems and as far more than raw material awaiting its call to be "worked up," as Emerson might say, in the service of humankind. The earth, newly reimagined as a habitation for light, becomes the setting for an art-based experience that is more than aesthetic. Turrell and Roden Crater in this sense belong among a select group of artists and artworks engaged in redefining spiritual experience. Mark Taylor, professor of religion at Columbia University, argues that Roden Crater explores a new vision of spirituality, and Taylor's view is shared by Stuart A. Kauffman in *Reinventing the Sacred* (2008), who examines various contemporary perspectives that seek to reconcile science, reason, and religion.[55] Taylor notes that from Roden Crater spectators can glimpse nearby Hopi villages where light remains a crucial element of ancient spiritual practices. Light, as Turrell reorients our vision, invites viewers to share an almost primal experience of the earth, as if at Roden Crater we were seeing both light and the earth, like Adam, for the first time.

Spirituality, slowly but surely, is gaining a respected place within biomedicine, which had previously relegated it to the hospital chapel. Last rites were almost an implicit sign of failure, a notification that medical logos had nothing left to try—no procedures, no drugs, no cures. Medical planners, turning their attention from the molecular gaze to the bottom line, cannot ignore research showing that a significant majority of patients would like spiritual issues considered as part of their medical care. A number of medical schools now include optional courses on spirituality. Oxford University Press is a reliable indicator of change, and the year 2012 was notable for the publication of the *Oxford Textbook of Spirituality in Healthcare*.[56] Spirituality can be meaningfully distinguished from religion: *spirituality* refers to a personal attribute or inclination, while *religion* refers to a formal and organized theology (with traditional or newfangled dogma, creeds, and rituals).

The key point is that biomedicine has begun to recognize the spiritual as well as religious needs of patients. The absence of such recognition resulted in the destructive cross-cultural conflicts between a Hmong immigrant family and their American doctors recounted in Anne Fadiman's classic *The Spirit Catches You and You Fall Down* (1997). The collision of cultures looked more like a battlefield when medical logos prescribed neuroleptic drugs as the proper treatment for a Hmong child with epileptic seizures. The immigrant parents, who trusted animal sacrifice, saw their child's condition as a spiritual endowment and as a divine gift, and neither doctors nor parents could find common ground.

Spirit is not easy to define—neither is love, which has not impeded poets, artists, lovers, philosophers, and theologians ever since Socrates left off his trademark dialectic reasoning in order to retell a story about eros and about a ladder leading from the love of bodies to a love of ideal form. Later religious traditions, eager to revise and appropriate pagan classical legacies, were quick to notice that Platonic love finds its highest satisfaction on a spiritual plane. Physician-writers such as Richard Selzer, David Hilfiker, and Rafael Campo, without rejecting biomedical knowledge or endorsing particular theological traditions, understand medicine and the act of healing as a calling (a devotion to the care of others) that approaches or includes a dimension that some would call spiritual. Selzer describes a spirit or almost numinous power in certain patients that he compares, indirectly, to classical traditions in which gods temporarily took possession of mortal bodies.

Spirituality in health care, even if largely confined to the patient side of the bed, recognizes a place for desire—expressed openly at times as a desire for God—that is certainly relevant to medical eros. Health in various spiritual traditions is regularly associated with spiritual well-being. The experience of serious illness, as it attacks our health, can also shake us and change us, raising spiritual doubts or questions. The final loss of light and descent of darkness signals the start of an uncertain journey. "Brightness falls from the air," writes Thomas Nashe in his haunting "Litany in Time of Plague" (1592), which continues with the refrain, "I am sick, / I must die. / Lord, have mercy on us!" Nashe may have felt some need of divine forgiveness as the author of an infamous erotic poem, "The Choise of Valentines; or the Merie Ballad of Nash His Dildo," which some call flatly pornographic.[57] A firm belief in God or in an afterlife is not necessary in order to express spiritual longings, or to experience religious doubt, but it is a sign of significant change that family medicine (as a specialty) emphasizes care focused on what it refers to as "the whole person." The words *wholeness* and *holiness* share an entwined history, despite some unruly or dark desires native to the whole person, and family medicine now endorses for physicians a standard questionnaire designed particularly for "spiritual assessment."[58]

"Spiritual needs change with time and circumstances," an editorial in the *British Medical Journal* observes, recommending that "healthcare teams ensure accurate and timely evaluation of spiritual issues through regular assessment."[59] Evaluation and assessment, of course, return us to the domain of medical logos, where even spiritual needs are subject to external observation and rational analysis. Rachel Naomi Remen—drawing upon her background in pediatrics, family medicine, and psychotherapy—reminds the medical students whom she teaches that their institutions stand "in a direct and unbroken lineage" to the temples of Asklepios. "I remind them," she writes, "that for all its technological power, medicine is not a technological enterprise. The practice of medicine is a special kind of love."[60] There is more than one way to acknowledge the spiritual dimensions of health and to enlist the healing force of eros. Love, for ecofeminist Cynthia Moe-Lobeda, is a powerful energy for good with which to mount active opposition to the structural evils built into capitalist economies and into our social hierarchies that despoil the earth, oppose social justice, and, I would add, damage the health of individuals and communities, beginning with the poorest and most vulnerable.[61] The power of eros *to bind* also includes a quasi-spiritual power to unbind: to resist the oppression and injustice that leave certain people not only in need of medical care but also in urgent need of liberation and enlightenment.

Light in its spiritual dimensions always includes a *ricorso* that brings us back to the earth. The Zuñi people traditionally regard the sun as the sacred source of life; the Zuñi word for *daylight* even doubles as the word for *life*. Zuñi pueblo rooms are always dim—with fireplaces for winter heat, but no candles[62]—so there is special significance to the Zuñi ceremony for newborns. On the eighth day, the newborn infant is taken outdoors before dawn. At first light everyone faces east—parents, relatives, friends—and corn meal is sprinkled in reverence to the rising sun. It is a ceremony that reconfirms the bonds of community and that recognizes light as the sacred source that binds the people and their lives to the earth. The prayer begins: "Now this is the day. / Our child, / Into the daylight / You will go out standing. / Preparing for your day, / We have passed our days."[63] Sunlight and daylight are such simple, primal forces, truths of nature, but they are also the beginning of life on earth and indispensable to human health.

My daily desert ritual, at least on weekdays, ultimately led homeward at night to the security lights over my garage, halogen bulbs, and an LED-backlit computer screen: a model of postmodern forgetting. The earth will survive my forgetting, just as it survived the six-mile-wide Chicxulub asteroid, which many scientists believe eradicated the dinosaurs by blocking sunlight with thick clouds from planetary fires and volcanic ash. And not just dinosaurs—this cosmic Black Swan erased 93 percent of all mammal species.[64] It is not humans alone who will pay the price for light-driven global climate change. A new erotics of light appropriate to the *anthropocene*—as scientists now call the era when humans began to alter the earth—is far preferable to another landscape of the dead. Yes, the earth will recover, as it did before we muddled onto the scene in our personas as scientists, capitalists, industrialists, developers, technocrats, systems analysts, and managers, upright cousins to the chimpanzee with whom we share a common ancestor and 98.8 percent of our DNA. Light is not an inappropriate metaphor for the wisdom and compassion that we earthlings need. We might even recall, as an emblem of our mutual solidarity with the earth, especially amid illness or the nearness of death, the purpose served by the once indispensable and now almost archaic lighthouse. It is the nearby lighthouse—"tall, robust, and reassuring"— that Jean-Dominique Bauby sees in his very first wheelchair expedition. "I placed myself at once," he writes, "under the protection of this brotherly symbol, guardian not just of sailors but of the sick—those castaways on the shores of loneliness."[65] The lighthouse with its beam shining into the darkness might serve as a visual reminder that we are all, in a cosmic sense, castaways.

CHAPTER NINE

The Spark of Life:
Appearances / Disappearances

All goes onward and outward . . . and nothing collapses,
And to die is different from what any one supposed, and luckier.

WALT WHITMAN, *LEAVES OF GRASS* (1855)

"**S**HE HAD THE SPARK OF LIFE," says the grieving late-middle-aged husband about his wife, Fiona, in the 2006 film *Away from Her*. Sarah Polley, the Canadian writer-director, preserves the husband's key phrase from Alice Monro's short story on which the film is based about an aging woman who checks herself into a residential Alzheimer's facility.[1] It took several years before I worked up my nerve to watch the film on DVD, but it was worth the wait. The attractive, well-run, homelike residential facility made me think, enviously, that Canada must be a world leader in the compassionate treatment of degenerative neurological diseases. I had to remove Ruth abruptly from her first for-profit facility where residents in packs raided the closets of newcomers. I suspect that the management was more concerned with filling beds than with carefully screening the patients who filled them. *Away from Her* certainly cleaned up the pervasive messiness I remember—life coming apart at the

249

seams and spilling out everywhere—that still wakes me up at night. Ruth, too, had the spark of life. You could see it in her eyes. My eyes are a gambler's mask; they won't give me away, most of the time, and you won't learn much. Ruth's eyes flat-out dazzled with light, and Alzheimer's disease has now snuffed out the spark. Ruth passes her days with blank, unfixed eyes and doesn't recognize me or even look up as I stroke her hair. I gaze into her face, and she has not vanished—she is still here, but she's no longer Ruth. I don't really know who she is. At times her vacant look actually frightens me. I see all the old familiar traces, but daily and gradually, right before my eyes, she is disappearing.

Disappearances now get my interest, especially what I'd call incomplete or in-process disappearances, where you can still see traces of what is about to vanish. The spark of life is infinitely precious not least because it tends to escape our attention before it suddenly goes missing, somewhat like health. "Health," the philosopher Hans-Georg Gadamer writes, "is not something that is revealed through investigation but rather something that manifests itself precisely by virtue of escaping our attention."[2] Health, for Gadamer, remains an "enigma" (*Verborgenheit*), concealed in an un-recognized mystery that differs from the not-knowing of illness because illness, most of the time, tends to *attract* our attention. Gadamer lived past the age of one hundred, despite a medical prognosis that had pre-dicted his early death, so he was certainly acquainted with mysteries that escape the molecular gaze. Health, as Gadamer defines it through an in-herent invisibility, differs from the gym-toned state pursued as a visible goal by the consumers of fitness products, but fitness and health can also both vanish suddenly, as illness plunges us into crises often as sharply defined as a gunshot wound. Medical logos, of course, measures a return to health through, among others, the measurable restoration of function and the reappearance of healthy vital signs. The spark of life has no place in a hospital chart. It belongs to the unofficial archives of medical eros, and it may be most urgently valued, as I have been led to discover, in the process of its own disappearance.

My desire to see Ruth restored, to see the spark of life in her eyes, turns slightly less agitated when I recall Reynolds Price's hard-earned advice to be brutally realistic about your limits and *thankful for air*. Ruth's limits now are obvious; mine aren't. And brutal realism has brutal costs.

Gun violence in the United States is now a serious public health issue in pediatrics, where twenty children and adolescents each day sustain firearm-related injuries that require hospitalization.[3] What playground spark vanishes forever when a child suffers a near-fatal gunshot wound? *Thankful for air* is not how I feel after visits to Ruth. Every day, she once said, she looked for something to make her happy, and she usually found it. Happiness is more than I can manage. I know that disappearances belong to our hidden contract with time and death, and I remain grateful for the days that I shared with Ruth, which have disappeared into the past but not wholly vanished. The main dilemma I face in my new roles as visitor and as behind-the-scenes care manager is not concerned with disease or with happiness. It is about how to understand the disturbing interlock between appearances and disappearances.

One quite personal disappearance—or series of daily disappearances— was the loss of a desire to write, since writing, as I mentioned earlier, was so central to my daily life. The caregiver's dilemma, I found, extends farther than I anticipated. I had expected collateral damage as my own invisible health visibly slipped away, but I had not expected to lose a taste for pleasure. Desire, too, had gone missing. My state of anhedonia never approached clinical depression—I enlisted a psychologist to keep track in case I tipped over the edge—and it never produced absolute writer's block, not completely. I still hit deadlines, but the work took on an unaccustomed dutiful, mechanical feel. *Hypergraphia*, as neurologist Alice W. Flaherty explains, is the medical term for "an overpowering desire to write."[4] This odd condition is correlated with changes in a specific area of the brain. I must have experienced brain changes linked to a near opposite condition. I called it *atrographia*: an overpowering *loss of desire* to write. Imagine that you can walk, but you gradually experience an intense loss of desire to walk. My state exactly: I could write, but writing lacked all pleasure, joy, and desire. Eros loss. Maybe work can go on minus the electrifications of eros—but why? Joyless work, drained of desire, may yield a certain numb bolus of acceptable product, but not much more. Some 15 percent of men and more than twice as many women experience the loss of sexual libido, which merits medical attention. My libido was alive and well. The loss of a desire to write, however, was new and didn't even rise to the quasi-medical level of writer's block. It was

Ruth who bore a medical diagnosis, while (to all appearances) I looked at least not ill. We had both lost our way. Both lost the spark. I could still see the firefly traces, even as they were in the process of disappearing, and recognize the loss, which made it far worse.

Appearances: The Convergence of *Eros* and *Logos*

My claim is that medical eros and medical logos can accomplish more together, as contrary powers and even as edgy disagreeing complements, than either can accomplish alone. Sometimes, together, they are mutual accessories and share overlapping interests. Physical appearances—to which eros seems especially attached—are a case in point.

Appearances, as a daily fact of life, have claimed increasing attention and importance in a media-driven visual culture where looks matter: hair, abs, big butts, tattoos. Medical logos and medical eros both have investments in this trend, which shows no sign of slowing as social media accelerate it with intimate selfies and online postings. Medical logos, especially through cosmetic surgery and pharmacology, has lent its scientific knowledge and technical skill to enterprises far removed from traditional aims and methods for treating disease. Ohio-born Cindy Jackson in the year 2000 became the official Guinness World Records titleholder after recording fifty-two separate cosmetic surgeries. *Lucky Diamond Rich*, as he is known, in 2006 held the Guinness record as "the world's most tattooed person," meaning that he was 100 percent tattooed. Surgeries, unlike tattoos, are medical procedures, and Cindy Jackson's multiple cosmetic surgeries were designed not to correct disfigurements but rather to *reconstruct* her appearance so that it approached, as close as possible, her idea of visual, bodily perfection. If medical logos supplies the knowledge and skill required in this questionable enterprise, then medical eros is surely complicit in whatever personal and cultural desires lead someone to enlist surgeons in such world-record excess.

Desire, as eros draws us toward immoderation, always threatens to spill over social lines of containment. The overflow may reflect artistic as well as cosmetic desires. The French performance artist who goes by the single name Orlan is no Barbie-doll wannabe. "I'm interested in multiple identities, mutant identities, nomad identities," she says, as if reading directly from contemporary French theorists Gilles Deleuze and Felix Guattari. Her multiple surgeries—filmed—are designed to reconstruct her face so that it simulates—eyes, nose, mouth—features borrowed from famous paintings and statues. Her new nomadic identity is thus a deliberate performance of creative self-fashioning focused not on fashion (as outer costume or high couture) but on flesh. As she says, "I give my body to art."[5]

Medical eros and medical logos go hand in hand, even if unknowingly, in the new social drama of altered physical appearances—culpable, laudable, or neutral, depending on the particular situation—but both are inescapably entangled, even when the nonsurgical aim involves simply losing half your body weight. The decorative enhancements of body art, from genital beading to traditional Japanese *irezumi*, are most often harmless (even artistic) expressions of personal and cultural desire, although medical logos may be called in to zap unwanted tattoos or to cure infections. Performance-enhancing drugs, on the other hand, are often illegal or rule-breaking pharmacological products meant to aid in the pursuit of athletic speed, strength, and agility. Improved physical appearance may be a secondary motive for athletes—steroids can produce disfiguring acne, among worse side effects—but desire still rules in the quest for victory or gold. The booming worldwide market for drugs that improve sexual performance offers a more obvious desire-driven confederation of eros and modern medicine. By comparison, whiter smiles, thicker hair, and slimmer waists seem an innocuous, everyday pharmacological pursuit in cultures focused on outward appearances. Medical logos and medical eros regularly join forces, then, in facilitating the pursuit of sexy, youthful, attractive appearances.[6]

The pursuit of attractive appearances might seem merely a personal matter, but the associated dilemmas reach further than questions about whether to buy collagen or Botox injections. Social ills and psychic traumas also attend a media-driven culture in which bodily perfection ("a perfect 10") becomes a plausible standard. Appearances matter, of course, as everyone knows. Pinups and calendar art reflect a Paleolithic neurobiology of reproductive success in which outward traits such as bilateral symmetry and thick hair are signs of health in a prospective mate. Birth defects and disfiguring injuries can bring with them lasting psychological distress, so medical logos merits sincere thanks for the repairs it can offer. Medical eros, too, can point to success stories. In a significant cultural shift, television and new media have developed a respectful openness to people with disabled bodies or marred appearances, from wounded warriors and wheelchair athletes to the victims of terrorist attacks. Alongside the predictable phalanx of good-looking movie stars and charismatic celebrities, the disabled, the disfigured, and the seriously ill are increasingly emerging into public view. Medical eros and medical logos together, in an unscripted and spontaneous coalition, are helping people with disabled, impaired, and less than perfect 10 bodies make their newly visible social appearances.

Appearances often have an undeserved bad name as superficial, trivial, deceiving, false, unreal, or simply fleeting: the binary opposite of everything solid, real, and true. It is high time to give appearances their due. Appearances, we might say, constitute physical realities as genuine as the Earth's shadow cast against the moon. A lunar eclipse captures our attention, and nobody criticizes the shadow as somehow false, deceiving, or unreal. It is, as we take for granted, the appearance of a real shadow. Appearances constitute social realities as significant as Aurora's crimson silk scarf and her three shades of green eyeshadow; her glitzy appearances proved far truer to her personal identity than the staid professional demeanor behind which her still-closeted doctor, Rafael Campo, initially screened his sexual confusions.

Appearances as a social reality hold special importance to people and groups who face discrimination and stigma. Starting in the 1980s, for example, gay rights activists risked injury and death as their protests offered a visible target for hate, but their struggle continued on less visible fronts as well, such as resistance to the stigmatizing images of emaciated gay men on public health posters, which simply reified erroneous cultural beliefs equating homosexuality with disease. Even the psychiatric *Diagnostic and Statistical Manual* had classified homosexuality as a form of mental illness, until—after massed protests at the 1970 meeting of the American Psychiatric Association—the seventh printing of *DSM II* revised the classification to "sexual orientation disturbance." It was not a huge step, but it was a step forward. The social fact of marred, impaired, or wasting appearances, in America as in Africa, carried its own powerful subtexts.

Disability rights activists face similar battles focused on social appearances. Indeed, for decades in the United States the disabled were either invisible, socially speaking, or they were reduced to the sum of their physical appearances, as if each was all (disabled) body. Eros and logos together are responsible for the changes that now welcome images of the disabled body, as in promotions for the Special Olympics. The broken body, the grotesque body, the refugee body, the body in pain, all have made new appearances. Doctors Without Borders and Amnesty International, for example, have brought widespread attention and much-needed medical care to poor, sick, elderly, forgotten, and homeless people who were once invisible.

The new appearance of nonstandard bodies (as a site of medical care and of public respect) is more than an expression of concern for equality or for social justice. It turns appearances—formerly, the agent of a narrow, glamorized ideal—into a freewheeling, liberated carnival of alternate bodies: tattooed, pierced, ripped, androgyn, dreadlocked, shaved, hump-backed, be-gothed, multiracial, obese, or strung-out. Such a vision shifts how we understand both health and illness. I know a woman astonished at discovering that her husband regarded her bald head (the side effect of a harrowing course of chemotherapy) as a complete sexual turn-on. Eros no doubt just smiled—and notched another arrow.

Desire, of course, is regularly ignored by the molecular gaze as *not a medical issue*, and philosophers strongly influenced by neuroscience may regard it as the relic of an obsolete folk psychology. Nowhere is desire more important, however, than as it relates to medical care, not simply for the ill but for the imperfect, diseased, or disabled body. Medical logos alone simply cannot explain why some physicians such as David Hilfiker (no saint, he insists) choose to work almost exclusively among the poor, pursuing what is sometimes called *poverty medicine.*[7] The desires that move physicians may differ widely, from spiritual growth or far-left politics to a passion for community service or a love of family, but reason alone or the worthy goal of adding knowledge to the biomedical database won't account for the long hours that physicians spend caring for

seriously sick and damaged people so desperate for assistance that the
ideals of physical perfection or of perfect health seem laughable. We
may each prefer different objects of desire, and our desires may find
expression in our differing ideas of paradise. I like the counter-ideal expressed by poet Wallace Stevens—the right standard, in my view, for
the era of nonstandard appearances—when he wrote, "The imperfect is
our paradise."[8]

Imperfect appearances—as self-assertion or even as an aggressive act
of public re-education—have already achieved a place among contemporary forms of guerrilla theater: a site of political resistance and
combat. Disability aesthetics, as it is called, may wholly reject traditions
of beauty.[9] Or it may redefine the beautiful in ways incompatible with traditional aesthetic norms. British photographer and educator Jo Spence
(1934–1992), for example, whose working-class politics and opposition to
standard biomedical treatment profoundly shaped her experience of
cancer, crafted photographs that both acknowledge and resist commercial
images of the erotic body. She stages her appearances, like an actor, to
offer a defiant, audacious counterimage that both subverts norms of
female beauty and also asserts a contrary set of values, as seen in the
photograph in Figure 9.1, which features her cancer-damaged breast.

This is not the image of a recovering patient. Spence co-opts the avi-
ator glasses from a tradition of hip glamor—glamor as limiting as the black
rectangles once pasted across the eyes of patients in early medical textbooks—and then, as if asserting the inner privacy of a Modigliani nude,
she directs her shuttered gaze outside or beyond the room that her glasses
reflect. The glasses allude to a standard erotic lexicon while the photo
declares allegiance to a nonstandard, new eroticism. The glasses, in effect, invoke an iconography that she sets out to unravel in order to reconstruct, after her own desires. "I began to reverse the process of the way I
had been constructed as a woman," she explains, "by deconstructing myself visually in an attempt to identify the process by which I had been
'put together.'"[10]

We are all in some sense "put together" by forces that we do not entirely understand or control. We may have put the clothes into our closets,
but who or what put them in the store? Why did we desire them? Bodies
are no less constructed than appearances, although such bodily construc-

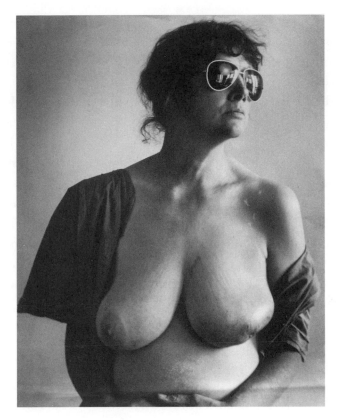

FIGURE 9.1. Jo Spence in collaboration with Terry
Dennett. *A Picture of Health: Heroine.* 1982.
Copyright the Estate of Jo Spence.
Courtesy Richard Saltoun Gallery, London.

tions (inflected by cultural desires) meld uneasily at times with a less mal-
leable biological substrate, as in the preference for insanely small women's
waists, or in the ancient Chinese practice of foot-binding. Jo Spence's self-
portrait offers a political and deconstructive critique of the erotic images
and desires that can deform the female body in the name of beauty—or of
health. She titles her self-portrait, created in collaboration with photographer Terry Dennett, *A Picture of Health: Heroine* (1982). The title, in
conjunction with the image, asserts a new vision of health and of heroism,
but it does more: it explodes outmoded traditions of female beauty (even
as revised in Modigliani nudes) while it reclaims erotic desire as inseparable from her marred, scarred, and fearlessly imperfect appearance.

Appearances matter, then, in their power to affirm or to resist, and health (as more than a state of limbs and fluids) holds close commerce with appearances in their social and political impact. Appearance, on the most obvious level, provides visual evidence crucial to physicians about a person's health or illness, while recovery from illness often includes visual signs that we interpret directly as a healthy appearance. This close relationship grows vexed and harder to interpret, however, when health as an ideal comes to seem as oppressive or limiting as conventional standards of beauty. The World Health Organization, with an annual budget nearing $4 billion, defines health in a formula still in place since 1948 as "a state of complete physical, mental and social well-being and not merely the absence of disease or infirmity."[11] How many people, I wonder, can claim to possess "complete physical, mental and social well-being"? Not me, not millions of refugees, and not many military veterans disabled with injuries. A 2015 study in *The Lancet* contends that over 95 percent of the world's population has health problems, with over a third dealing with *more than five* ailments.[12]

A misguided, almost moral, imperative that drives people to achieve near utopian levels of well-being may actually *increase* the cultural load of illness, which is the paradox behind a collection of essays titled *Against Health* (2010). The authors are not truly against being healthy but rather against the cultural fervor that turns body-monitoring from a psychological trait into almost an ethical duty and a commercial responsibility.[13] *The Lancet* study shows that only one in twenty people (4.3 percent) worldwide had no health problems in 2013. Can't at least some of us—the other 95.7 percent—live relatively healthy lives while also dealing with something less than optimal states of physical, mental, and social well-being?

It might be better, after 1948, to redefine health not as an optimal state of mind, body, and spirit but rather as the subjective estimate of how well we function *despite* our state of imperfection: despite illness, disability, and bodily failures. *Function*—not some impossible optimum state—seems to me what matters, and, on such a view, health is less an appearance (rosy cheeks, average body weight, good posture) than what invisibly disappears into our everyday functions. Everyday function is of course often visible as an appearance, but it does not disappear when we are unseen, and everyday function in an imperfect state at least reconstructs health as a paradoxical appearance that indicates its presence, in Gadamer's words, "by virtue of escaping our attention." Health, in short, is less the visible appearance of well-being than a manifestation of its own disappearances.

Health as everyday function—redefined (abstractly) as the manifestation of a disappearance—needs a concrete example to give it flesh and blood. The AXIS Dance Company, founded in 1987, ranks among the first and most influential professional companies pursuing so-called physically-integrated dance; meaning, it employs dancers both with and without physical disabilities. Its performances offer at least one instance suggesting how disability and bodily impairment might somehow, like health, evaporate before our eyes into everyday function. Whereas Bill T. Jones in *Still/Here* employed able-bodied dancers to *represent* disabled and terminally ill patients, AXIS Dance Company—along with companies from England and Australia to South Africa founded on similar principles—employs in its performances a mixed ensemble of able-bodied and disabled dancers. Their work begins, in effect, by removing disability from a medical context in order to resituate it in a new aesthetic realm, from which its disruptive and transformative energies can flow back into the wider culture. Simultaneously, they challenge conventional aesthetics and especially traditional dance by emphasizing a new inclusiveness. The challenge aims to be subversive, as in modernist avant-garde traditions, but these distinctively postmodern transgressions undercut certain elitist tendencies within modernism that, especially in dance, favor classically trained, beautiful, athletic, graceful, and, yes, thin and muscular bodies. The AXIS Dance Company puts disabled dancers on stage, mixed with able-bodied dancers, in a choreography that sometimes permits embodied disabilities to disappear (or, better, to all-but-disappear) before our eyes.

One visual image is insufficient to indicate how the AXIS Dance Company upends traditional ideas of dance. Eros, of course, is not its main focus, but the dancers moving in choreographed geometries (suggesting mutual attraction and repulsion) are impossible to disentangle from erotic implications. AXIS can even eroticize everyday appliances associated with disability. The wheelchair thus appears on the AXIS stage not as

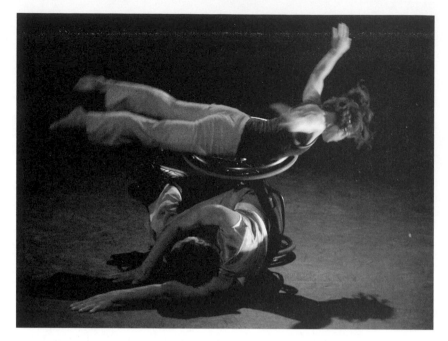

FIGURE 9.2. AXIS Dance Company. Sonsherée Giles and Rodney Bell. Choreographer, Joe Goode. Photographer, Brian Martin.

medical conveyance—not even quite possessing whatever thing-like quali-ties that wheelchairs ordinarily possesses—but rather, through its trans-formation, a platform for the erotic meeting of two bodies, much as AXIS transforms desexualized stereotypes of people with disabilities. Figure 9.2 shows the AXIS Dance Company members Sonsherée Giles and Rodney Bell performing in an award-winning piece from 2008 by pop artist and choreographer Joe Goode.

An overturned wheelchair is usually a sign of trouble; I still cautiously steer Ruth around her indoor facility, fearful of sudden bumps that might pitch her forward out of the chair. The overturned AXIS wheelchair, dis-abled from signifying only disability, now serves to surmount divisions between health and unhealthiness. Less a device to accommodate limitations than a bridge to overcome disconnection, the overturned wheelchair mysteriously links male and female, able-bodied and dis-abled, dancers and (if they respond as I do) audiences. It even bridges usually separate orders of experience, from loss and impairment to ecstasy and transcendence, in a performance that enlists dancers, bodies, and movement in a radical act of erotic or eros-like subversion.

The AXIS Dance Company, while subverting not only conventions of dance but also conventional ways of reading bodies and minds, has received seven Isadora Duncan Dance Awards, and its principles and methods are most significant—beyond a specific focus on eros, on dance, or on health—for inviting audiences to imagine new ways of understanding disabled bodies. Dancers with disabilities not only mingle and switch positions with able-bodied dancers (in ways that blur their differences) but also at times make their differences obvious by appearing on crutches or using prosthetic limbs. Some companies now include dancers who are mentally disabled. The overall effect, in blurring boundaries, is an art that does more than simply *include* the disabled; rather, it *depends* on them. They are *necessary* in the subversion of our conventional ways of reading bodily appearances. Disabled bodies are not enfolded invisibly within the cultural norms that had previously excluded them, like an assimilated minority, but instead they emerge into view precisely to explode oppressive norms and to create a new integrative cultural space where disabled bodies make a valued reappearance—by almost (but not entirely) disappearing. Medical eros might see in such near disappearances the model for a new and nonutopian ideal of health. After all, one in seven people today is disabled, and the Black Swan circles. Meanwhile, I struggle to deal with troubling disappearances—the spark of life, the desire to write—since, despite Gadamer, I am still drawn to traditional images of good health (like rosy cheeks) that resemble solid and reassuring appearances.

Pathologies of Desire: Violence and the Seductions of Reason

Eros in its appearances often seems almost inseparable from violence. A potential for violence is certainly among its least attractive qualities, whether expressed as jealous rage, rough sex, or a fascination with death. Medical eros cannot simply wish away the troubling kinship that links eroticism with violence. Violence likely has biological roots in the fight-or-flight response that humans share with other primates, and the human social order, too, depends on an accommodation with violence, expressed via armies, police, and systems of discipline. Even the sacred, as a category regulated by human desire, relies on violence. As the anthropologist René Girard has argued, religious rituals and the social cohesion that they promote regularly find support in violent acts that range from ceremonial human sacrifice and scapegoat rituals to reenactments of the Crucifixion and religious jihad. Violence and the sacred, he argues, are "one and the same thing."[14]

Are eros and violence, too, one and the same thing? The crucial issue for medical eros is not whether desire can include or incite violence— sometimes it does—but rather how to redirect erotic desire toward beneficial, therapeutic, productive ends. Bataille has documented the bloody dark-side of desire in *The Tears of Eros*, and we have daily evidence of the covert links between death and desire. Eric Trump, writing in the "Modern Love" column of the *New York Times*, describes how his life-threatening kidney failure during his years as a graduate student served as an aphrodisiac to spark a clandestine affair with his much-older, still-married female professor. It was his end-stage renal disease and imminent death, Trump writes, that "seduced us into believing we loved each other."[15] The shadow of approaching death, it appears, can be far more erotic than what Trump calls "the banality of health." (His lurid romance crumbles when a kidney-transplant and antirejection drugs unexpectedly save his life.) Eros can never entirely break free from such dark-side complexities, but Girard offers a helpful clarification in arguing that violence has *a dual nature*: "At times violence appears to man in its most terrifying aspect, wantonly sowing chaos and destruction; at other times it appears in the guise of peacemaker, graciously distributing the fruits of sacrifice."[16]

The dual nature of violence—as peacemaker and warmonger—makes it crucial, Girard argues, for societies to control *harmful* violence while promoting *beneficial* violence, and medicine, although doctors seldom emphasize it, has a place for beneficial violence. Chemotherapy and radiation saved his life, but Reynolds Price suffered unremitting chronic pain and lost the use of his legs as a direct result of life-saving medical treatment. The hard-won diagnosis of diphtheria, in William Carlos Williams's story, comes only after the use of force. Force is not identical with violence, however, and patients occasionally act in ways that are undeniably violent, as when drunks resist doctors in the emergency department, for example, or when dementia patients strike out blindly or uncontrollably at staff members. Ruth's facility disallows the use of physical or chemical restraints, and medical eros must tread cautiously amid hard questions about the rights of patients who are violent, the safety of staff, the protection of fellow patients, and appropriate legal or ethical countermeasures. I would like to raise a different question about harmful violence, no doubt impolite but impossible to dissociate from eros. Is there also a violence inherent in reason?

Doctors, as Atul Gawande claims, tend to have a *fierce commitment* to the rational. Can a *fierce* commitment resemble or turn into a violent passion? The question implies that reason may become less an instrument used in the treatment of illness than the object of medical desire. It is as if—to create personified abstractions—Reason enlisted Desire in the amorous pursuit of Reason. Reason (Narcissus-like) fiercely desires Reason in a circular pursuit that can only end badly. The violence facing contemporary doctors is sometimes in part self-inflicted, from suicide and alcoholism to burnout, and it cannot be traced to a single source. A fierce commitment to reason certainly entailed significant personal and professional harm for Rafael Campo, as he explained, but the relevant issues for medical eros spill out far beyond biomedicine to the wider cultural contradictions in which doctors, patients, and everyone in between find ourselves caught.

Today it is hard to avoid getting caught up in a concealed triangular relationship in which desire is the mediator between consumers and the newest technology. The hyper-rationality embodied in our technological gadgets is a large, if concealed, part of their allure. Even our phones now are "smart"—and we regularly discard the previous, well-functioning phone for a new model that is even smarter. Maybe smartness, as a quality, draws us as much as the material object. For many patients, the newest miracle drugs and high-tech treatments have certainly become objects of desire, and it is hard not to separate the smart-power embodied in the new medical technologies from the doctors authorized to access it. The traditional romantic liaison between doctors and patients takes a new twist today, and erotic metaphors are not entirely far-fetched. "Above all," writes Gadamer, "it is the patients approaching the doctor for help who are so seduced by the astonishing technical means of modern medicine that they see nothing but this aspect and marvel only at the doctor's scientific competence."[17]

The erotic seduction directly invoked in Gadamer's word *verführen* ("seduced") recalls soap-opera plots, but Gadamer identifies a strangely different erotics of medical seduction in which it is patients who seduce themselves. As if engaged in a weird form of self-hypnosis, they dangle before their eyes the gleaming biotechnologies that embody, like the doctor, all the allure of science and reason. Patients, of course, are hardly unique in this one-person dance of self-seduction. Reason and technology exert an openly erotic attraction over consumers in electronics stores, kindling desires for products that we didn't know we wanted because the manufacturers and advertisers make sure that the objects already embody our desires. We are becoming familiar with this new erotics of self-seduction in science-fiction films where a young man falls in love with an attractive female robot or with the throaty voice on his speech-enabled computer. Gadamer recognizes the harm posed by this new reason-driven love affair with biotechnologies: doctors and patients run a great risk of forgetting that "the application of this knowledge is a highly demanding and responsible task of the broadest human and social dimensions."[18]

Biotechnologies are the proper province of medical logos, but medical eros offers an important, complementary perspective for understanding the subtle and complex ways in which biotechnologies engage personal and social desire. The harmful violence of reason is not always self-evident, unlike the violence of brute force; it is more dangerous precisely for being usually concealed within social norms. We remain unaware of its operation, like a worker who feels burned out but does not recognize that burnout may be the result of a punishing work schedule nonetheless considered reasonable. Even the violence of brute force, however, now regularly lies in quasi-concealment—like the laser-guided "smart bombs" that blow up enemy trucks or compounds in little exploding puffs of smoke on a video screen. We are encouraged to forget that there are drivers and passengers inside. The seductive, soft violence of reason—implicit in the technologies that underwrite smart bombs and surveillance systems—certainly makes its appearances inside certain routines and assumptions of everyday medical practice. Patients often assume, consistent with the romance of biomedical science, that almost any punishing therapy must be somehow reasonable. Isn't what happens, then, almost like a romantic betrayal when medical logos has no reasonable explanation to offer for our suffering?

Modern Medicine: Eros and the Planet Mars

There is no greater loss for a parent—no greater personal tragedy—than the death of a child. Perri Klass writes from her experience as a pediatrician about how this cruelest form of harmful violence, even if the causes are natural, also ripples through surrounding lives and distributes its violence in supra-dyadic confusions. Klass ends her collection of short stories *Love and Modern Medicine* (2001) with the story of such a loss: an episode in which, after the death of her six-month-old child, a grief-stricken mother moves in with her half-sister.[19] The grieving mother is Deirdre, and the story is told by her unnamed half-sister, who is both the narrator and, like Klass, a pediatrician. Deirdre's daughter has recently died from the nightmare condition that haunts both parents and pediatrics: sudden infant death syndrome.

Each year in the United States, about 3,500 infants die suddenly of no obvious cause. About half these deaths—*which cannot be explained after investigation*—are classified, retrospectively, as sudden unexpected infant death (SUID) and sudden infant death syndrome (SIDS). Not-knowing and the failure of rational explanations thus become an official requirement for a posthumous diagnosis. In the United States SIDS is the leading cause of death among infants aged one to twelve months, although the overall rate of SIDS has declined since 1990. Further reduction of the risk remains an important public health priority, especially in non-Hispanic black, American Indian, and Alaska Native populations, where the risk is disproportionately high.[20] Deirdre, like many parents, had focused her worries on the supposed dangers of childhood inoculations—she continues to harangue her pediatrician half-sister on this hot topic—but no reasonable risk-assessment could have adequately prepared Deirdre for the sudden death of her healthy six-month-old daughter. It is impossible, as Nassim Nicholas Taleb says, to protect ourselves fully against the Black Swan.

Every death alters the web of relationships that receives it, but the death of a child can drive parents apart and destroy a marriage. It is an ominous sign that we learn nothing about Deirdre's absent software-engineer husband. Deirdre—white, middle-class, glamorous, and financially comfortable—never suspected the violence threatening her daughter from within the brim or fat tail of the bell-shaped curve. Money, glamor, and white, middle-class privilege in effect created an illusion of security; meanwhile, not even the compassion evoked by the death of a child can mend the edgy relationship between the two half-sisters, which has a long history. The pediatrician-narrator never particularly liked her more attractive half-sister, and eros has ratcheted up the sisterly strain. Although they share the same father, Deirdre is the child of the father's favored, younger wife, while the narrator grew up with the older ("difficult") ex-wife. Deirdre now occupies a spare room on the third floor, and—with two children and a radiologist husband to occupy her concern—the narrator has little time and less medical wisdom to offer her grieving half-sister. Why did the child die? Medical logos, in the voice of the narrator, is reduced to a stammer: "No one knows. So many theories. Respiratory. Central nervous system. Persistence of fetal hemoglobin. Nobody knows" (*LMM* 178).

Medical logos runs on knowledge, so when facts and knowledge fail, it is pretty much in the dark. Medical eros, on the other hand, is less handicapped by not-knowing, and it has resources to offer when biomedical knowledge falls short. Rational answers—even when available—may prove less important in medical trauma than explanations that help clarify a surrounding field of emotion. Klass tells a story of absent fathers and of estranged daughters, a story of resentful loss and bitterness that runs generations deep. How deep? Nobody knows. Deirdre moves around the house in her bathrobe like a restless ghost, with a faint odor of herbal tea indicating not so much her presence as where she recently *was*. Life amid absences goes on in the narrator's house regardless, despite Deirdre's tragedy, despite not-knowing. School projects are due, and thus the narrator faces an urgent need for craft store supplies. This annoying, everyday need, she senses, is also what Deirdre and her lost daughter have lost. She knows, too, what an unthinkable moment it would be—awful beyond comprehension—for a mother to reach into the crib one morning and find a corpse. "I cannot walk my mind through it," she reflects. "Love and modern medicine, both useless" (*LMM* 182).

The uselessness of *both* love and modern medicine—eros *and* logos—is a cold truth at the moment when a parent confronts the inexplicable death of an infant; but total futility is not the end point for Klass's narrative. While logos cannot offer a rational answer, eros and the mysteries of not-knowing apparently hold the resources for an eventual repair. Do we really understand how healing works? "Don't ask me why I mount the stairs to knock and invite Deirdre," the narrator says as she prepares to drive with her two children to the crafts shop. "Don't ask me why she comes. We belt ourselves into the front seat; the children click themselves into the back" (*LMM* 180). *Don't ask*, in colloquial conversation, means *there's no rational explanation*. It means, *I don't know why*. It means, in effect, *nobody knows*. So don't ask. Nonetheless something has changed. In the crafts store, one son has selected a pumpkin-sized Styrofoam ball to serve as the planet Mars in his model of the solar system. Deirdre holds the future planet Mars and then, unexpectedly, smiles. The narrator notices: "She is tall and queenly and lovely in the Styrofoam aisle, lovely especially when she smiles." The narrator quotes her half-sister: "'It doesn't weigh anything,' she says" (*LMM* 182).

A weight has lifted, a burden has shifted, a change has occurred, both in Deirdre and in the narrator. The facts have not changed. What has just happened? Nobody knows. Deirdre's smile remains enigmatic, maybe no more than a Mona Lisa trace with unknowable origins, but the narrator's change is more evident. Her dislike for her unwelcome, grief-haunted, glamorous half-sister has altered. The burden of their history of bad feeling and the long drama involving fathers, daughters, and step-daughters—a drama reaching back as far as Greek tragedy and the House of Atreus—at least momentarily lifts its dark shadow. The enigmatic concluding line takes us inside the narrator's consciousness—into the inner life as gently inflected by eros—as she reflects on the statement that for Deirdre was a quite literal remark that the large Styrofoam ball *doesn't weigh anything*: "But it will be a planet," says the narrator, "when we're done with it."

Love doesn't weigh anything either—it has few technologies at its disposal, if you discount sex toys—but it includes, even amid its own history of failures, the possibilities of inexplicable transformations that can repair the damage of harmful violence. Mars, the red planet, named for the god of war, is here no match for Eros.

The inexplicable failures and harm of eros, as unpredictable as the sudden death of an infant child, imply also, as Klass suggests, the possibility of inexplicable benefits. The same, in fairness, must be said for medical logos. Love and modern medicine are both capable of great harms—and great good. Every culture seems to need its doctors as well as its poets. Klass's narrative of family trauma does not lend itself to a summarizing interpretation, as if it contains a hidden moral lesson, but rather it honors the incomprehension, heartbreak, and turmoil that can follow the sudden death of an infant, and it honors, too, the possibilities for inexplicable change: a change as improbable and weightless as a craft store Styrofoam ball transformed into the planet Mars. Not-knowing can be a source of anguish when rational answers are unavailable, but it can also prove a matrix of healing possibilities when eros mysteriously helps *reconstitute* the bonds that eros can also, just as inexplicably, rip apart.

Disappearances: Eros and Loss

Eros specializes in material, sensuous *appearances:* what we can touch, see, or feel, like a lover's caress. Eroticism, even while it deeply engages the inner life, entangles us in a world of surfaces. The dilemma in surface appearances, of course, is that traditions of dualism reaching back to Plato encourage us to believe that surfaces and appearances are inherently deceptive. "I used to believe that truth was found only below the surface of things," writes Terry Tempest Williams. "Underground. I was a disciple of depth. What was hidden was what I desired." Desire, in this effort to probe beneath the surface, seeks its object in what cannot be seen or touched or felt. Then something changed for Williams in her understanding of desire: a change no doubt reflected in her barefoot trek over hot desert sandstone. "I am interested now," she continues, revising her desires in favor of earthly surfaces and of material appearances, "in what my eyes can see, what my fingers can touch, what my hand can know by moving slowly across flesh, or fur, or feathers, or stone."[21]

The problem with appearances—as I make at first daily and then weekly journeys to visit Ruth—is that they bundle so tightly with disappearances. Sensory knowledge (what the eye can see and the hand can know) is not only limited, as a skeptical empiricist such as Taleb will insist, but also favors appearances. Eros is a connoisseur of sensuous appearances, of course. The hand moving slowly across flesh, fur, feathers, or stone does not seek hidden depths or a deferred knowledge, mediated through surfaces, but rather immediate contact: contact that initiates an erotic commerce with the inner life of consciousness. Disappearances, however, are the flip-side of sensuous, tactile, material, earthly appearances. They are the still-visible traces of sensuous appearances on their way out.

All phenomena are, etymologically, appearances. The English words *phenomenon* and *photo* both derive from the Greek root *phainein*, meaning *to show, to shine, to appear*. All material things, all phenomena, viewed through the lens of geological time, are appearances that prove inseparable from their ultimate disappearances. Nothing gold can stay, and nothing not-gold can stay. The linkage with disappearances is also an everyday affair. Pop stars appear, then disappear. An actor appears onstage, then disappears offstage. An infant is born, appears, and then disappears via SIDS. This movement from appearance to disappearance is not linked to dualities of surface and of depth, or of deception and truth. The actor's appearance onstage—playing the role of Abraham Lincoln—is neither true nor false, neither real nor unreal: it simply *is*. So, too, the disappearance offstage. What matters here is the shuttling movement between appearance and disappearance. Whatever appears—flesh, fur, feathers, stone—is equally subject to disappearance. Eros could claim this fact as a primal rule or condition of desire, citing various laws of physics in support. My dilemma arises because, while appearances often bring joy, as expressed in the Zuñi ceremony to welcome the new eight-day infant into the world of daylight, disappearances more often than not bring regret, sadness, grief, or even the deepening hurt that ultimately corrodes body and spirit.

Disappearances can be gradual, lingering, and almost imperceptible—like the slow fade of disappearing ink—or fast and abrupt. Whether fast or slow, abrupt or gradual, the act of disappearing is a process, and at least

to keep my own thoughts and usage from complete unraveling into confusion, I want to distinguish between *disappearance* as a process and *vanishment* as a fait accompli. What has vanished is gone; what disappears
is still in the process of going away. This artificial distinction matters
here because I am not concerned with vanishment but rather with the in-
between state when an appearance (flesh, fur, feathers, stone) enters into
the process of *dis-appearing*. *Dis-appearance* (hyphenated to indicate its
specialized usage) is the often-extended condition in which people, places,
and things (the rich, sensuous world of appearances) enter into the lethal
slow dance toward vanishment, akin to the gradual wearing away of a glacier, which geologists call *ablation*. At some point, ablation ends and the
glacier is gone, replaced by the boulder-strewn rubble it crushed and carried during its slow disappearance into vanishment. The dinosaurs have
vanished; they are no longer dis-appearing. Physicists contend that matter
and energy shuttle endlessly back and forth, minus a small sacrifice to en-
tropy. When people, places, and things vanish, however, an irreversible
loss occurs. No more shuttling back and forth. Dis-appearance, in this
sense, resembles a way station on the fast track to vanishment and irreversible loss. Eros knows all about dis-appearance. I now see Ruth
entering into this extended process of dis-appearing.

As Alzheimer's disease took its awful, gradual toll, its relentless ablation of mind and of body, I never fully grasped what was happening right
before my eyes, in the sensory world of surfaces and of appearances. I
could still touch and feel and see Ruth. She was still there. Then I encountered Anne Carson's strange book *Nox* (2009).[22] *Nox* is Latin for
night, and night in Carson's book is not the counterpart of day but
rather the pagan realm of ultimate darkness into which people, places, and
things—all sensory appearances—ultimately *dis-appear* in their slide
toward irreversible vanishment.

Carson in her writings regularly circles back to eros. *Eros the Bittersweet* (1986), her brilliant first book, explored the triangular geometry of
desire: a three-sided figure comprising the lover, the beloved, and the gap
or obstacle that separates them. She indirectly returns to eros and to the
triangle of desire in her boundary-crossing book *Nox*, if *book* is really the
right word; half the text (each left-hand or verso page) contains her scholarly gloss on each word in a famous elegy by the Roman erotic poet

Catullus. The elegy by Catullus, on the death of his brother, ends with the famous lines *ave atque vale* (hail and farewell). *Nox*, in the recto half of the text, constitutes an extended memorial or "epitaph" (as Carson once calls it) on the death of her brother Michael. *Nox* thus connects two lost brothers in parallel explorations. One exploration resembles fragments assembled from a classical dictionary; the other resembles a scrapbook packed with photos, memorabilia, and brief meditations on loss. *Nox*, with its collage-like shards, occupies a sort of semantic twilight—a no-man's-land of meaning—in which clarities appear and disappear, as new mysteries emerge. It immerses the reader in an experience of not-knowing—in some sense an experience of flickering darkness that almost reverses the situation of visitors to Roden Crater—whereby not-knowing emerges as a more or less steady state that no effort of logic or reason or scholarship can fully overcome. It is the fertile darkness from which basic questions arise. Questions, for the author, about time, desire, history, and writing. For readers, questions may begin with the book's strange and resistant material appearance.

Multiple dis-appearances are what engage Carson inside a book that, as you hold it in your hands, arrives in a grey rectangular box—"the color of a rainy day," as *New York Times* reviewer Ben Ratliff further describes its appearance.[23] The first dis-appearance, once you open the box, is the standard codex form of ordinary books: separate pages bound between hard or soft covers. Instead, inside a box with the look of a small, fat casket the reader encounters a single sheet of stiff continuous accordion-folded paper. (Like a winding sheet?) *Nox*, then, from the moment of its initial appearance, engages in strategies that suggest a book in the process of disappearing. The codex, of course, replaced the classical scrolls on which the poems of Catullus once circulated. Scrolls haven't vanished, but they are fast disappearing outside special collections and religious rituals, much as codex books are now disappearing and may soon survive mainly in niche markets. Digital, electronic publication is now transforming not only the appearance of books but also the social and material environment within which reading occurs—maybe even changing the brain-based neurobiology of reading. The online retail giant Amazon reported in 2010 that its customers were buying bestsellers in e-book form by a ratio of two to one over print.[24] In medicine and science, where timely updates are crucial to research and to treatment, electronic publication is superior to traditional print media. *Nox* makes its appearance in the world as an extremely irregular book, almost a nonbook, a book in which Michael's death is the focus for contemplating other, more public instances of disappearing, and a book that also stages a resistance to the vanishment of books. It simply cannot be duplicated or simulated by a digital version.

Nox resists the vanishment of books especially through a material appearance as sensuous as what the hand encounters moving slowly across flesh, fur, feathers, or stone. Readers must deal with *Nox* as a thing-like object irreducible to its semantic content, which in any case is interruptive and at times deeply obscure, like an ancient manuscript riddled with lacunae. The single accordion-folded sheet seems to put up resistance just leaving its box, and we encounter a book so strangely resistant that, by design, it is permanently *unopenable*. You can open up the box, that is, but the text and its meaning defeat the normal processes of opening up. Although we have learned how to "scroll up" and "scroll down" virtual pages on e-readers, in a forgotten reference to classical scrolls, nothing is smooth or familiar about reading *Nox*. *Nox* reshapes the experience of reading as a jagged process of radical estrangement. The reassurances of linear form disappear like the chain bookstores that once seemed a sure-bet growth stock. The estrangement gets even stranger as readers unfold the accordion-pleated text and encounter the photo-facsimile of an original scrapbook that Carson, presumably, once put together with her own hands. Narrative threads emerge, vanish, reappear. Images blur. Pictures block text. Data turns indecipherable. It is easy to get lost. *Nox* in its dense material appearance transforms the act of reading into a continuous negotiation with dis-appearances of meaning, dis-appearances of narrative, and dis-appearances of what once looked like solid facts.

Carson is a specialist in dis-appearances, and dis-appearances are a state that she invests with almost philosophical significance, albeit rooted in everyday experience. Think of a lover watching the taillights disappear as the beloved drives off into the night, forever. Dis-appearance marks a transitional moment—fast or slow—in the passage from presence to absence. It is similar to the state that Carson elsewhere calls "unlost," a coinage that she applies to an ancient individual known today (in a brief epitaph written by Simonides of Keos) as Spinther. "Spinther," Carson observes, "would have vanished utterly save for a single Simonidean line of verse."[25] *Total* vanishment—gone without a trace—is oblivion, with not even a buried dinosaur fossil to let us know they were here. Dis-appearance, by contrast, stays *just this side* of vanishment, identified mainly by the traces that it leaves in its passage toward nothingness. The survival of the unlost is about as thin as appearances can get, but it is not nothing. It encompasses the twilight remains of Spinther (a name you can grow fond of) or the extended moments when a long marriage breaks apart. Dis-appearance always traffics with the border where, not far off, you can glimpse the black night of vanishment. The lost brother of Catullus remains a total blank, as Carson explains in *Nox*; without even a name, he is completely unknown except that Catullus addresses him once (as "brother") in a poem that almost miraculously survived the destruction of multiple ancient manuscripts. Her deceased brother Michael faces a realistic prospect of vanishment but for whatever resistance his intellectual writer / sister (whom he called "pinhead") can mount in fending off oblivion.

"Every time a poet writes a poem," according to Carson, "he is asking the question, Do words hold good: And the answer *has to be yes*."[26] Carson, herself a poet, must ask if *her* words "hold good"—but what does the question mean? The idiom "holding good" implies that something remains valid, true, or in force, like a promise made yesterday that *holds good* today. Illness, like other forms of trauma, can drain words of their currency. "What my mother and I shared were words," writes David Rieff, acknowledging their kinship as writers, "and yet now they felt all but valueless—like Confederate dollars or Soviet roubles."[27] Words, like currencies, can fail to hold good; words, too, are subject to dis-appearance.

Dis-appearance, as theorist Paul Virilio argues, takes on special significance in modern societies with their radical new emphasis on speed. The universe holds nothing faster than a photon—which is fast replacing ink as the medium of literary production—and Virilio argues that some change occurs so rapidly that we experience it without knowing. Hundreds of dis-appearances occur daily, he writes, and "most often pass completely unnoticed."[28] Who has time or desire to mourn the dis-appearance of typewriters, letters home, virginity until marriage, drive-in theaters, eight-track tape decks, smallpox, nation states, 1956 Chevys,

Fred Astaire movies, or the young Elvis Presley? The loss happens—loss accelerated by the planned obsolescence incorporated into the design of modern commodities—but minus the knowledge and the emotional experience of loss. It thus creates what Virilio calls our "epileptic consciousness": the jolting, modern experience of things dis-appearing right before our eyes—chain stores and national brands, former lovers, online postings, old friends moved off the grid or dead—minus a conscious *experience* of loss. Like Carson's brother, Michael. Just gone.

Death is a dis-appearance but not necessarily, for Carson, total vanishment. *Nox*—a title just three letters short of vanishment—confronts death and loss without the consolation typical in elegies. Her title recalls another famous poem by Catullus in which night signifies the bleak nothingness that follows death: *nox est perpetua una dormienda. Dormienda* (from *dormire*, to sleep) means not just a sleeping but a future-perfect sleep that *must be slept.* Death for Catullus is no gentle good-night. It is a pagan, endless night that must be slept all the way through. *Nox*, similarly, is no Tennysonian journey through loss and grief to a wild-bells Christmas recovery. It is a sober nonelegiac struggle against vanishment carried out in an improbable ragtag mosaic-like boxed memorial constructed of verbal scraps and visual shards. Its saving grace, beyond a resistance to vanishment, is the indirect presence of eros.

"What is erotic about reading (or writing)," as Carson puts it in a literary version of the geometry of desire, "is the play of imagination called forth in the space between you and your object of knowledge."[29] Eros, in Carson's work, carries readers into a space where they are immersed in the fertile darkness of not-knowing, where imagination can play its creative role and from which resolutions may emerge, much as in the woods outside Athens. Eros thrives precisely in the gaps and absences of not-knowing where reason flounders, where desire enlists multiple cognitive and emotional powers—not analytical reason alone—to bear upon experience that cannot always be quantified and measured, like the death of a brother. The power of eros can be jolting, difficult, or even heartbreaking, much like the epileptic consciousness of continuous dis-appearances, but eros also inhabits regions of the inner life where meanings and knowledge matter less than imaginative intensities and emotions. The free play of imagination that reading calls forth can offer the same erotic solace—far distant from sexual transport—that others may find in a network of supportive friends or in the fellowship of a local church congregation. Such networks, research shows, are often crucial to the health and long-term survival of individuals who pass through traumatic loss. Reading puts us in contact, at the very least, with the voices of writers and fictional characters. My mother, in the months after my father died of congestive heart failure, consumed books—sometimes as many as one book per day—as if they were the only sustenance that kept her inner life from wasting away into nothingness.

Eros for Carson—a writer of formidable intelligence—is inseparable from reading and from thought. Socrates, after all, represents her ideal of what she calls the passionate "electrifications" of eros. Socrates exemplifies an erotic idea not because of his specific thoughts—not even because eros is the only subject he claimed to know anything about—but because for Carson the act of thinking is erotic. As she says of Socrates, who carried on his incessant questioning in a predominately oral culture and with a personal distrust of writing: "He loved, that is, the process of coming to know."[30] Coming-to-know, as an exploratory process, differs from knowing much as it remains distinct even from the knowledge that it seeks to produce. "In any act of thinking, the mind must reach across this space between known and unknown, linking one to the other but also keeping visible their difference," Carson writes. "It is an erotic space."[31]

The erotic space of coming-to-know is inseparable, in the modern world, from the erotic space of reading, which is also, inescapably for the reader, a space occupied with the process of coming-to-know. What Carson once described as an "erotics of reading," then, does not refer to the subgenre of erotica but rather to the internal process in which coming-to-know makes its crucial appearances. Appearances, for Carson, also hold an erotic power. Her husband, Robert Currie, once gave an interview account of their first meeting and subsequent courtship, but Carson intervened to set the record straight—in her own distinctive style: "There you were, and then you were there more."[32] The there-more-ness, in this strange account, might stand as another version of the erotic thickening of appearances that occur in coming-to-know. Currie appears; he does not dis-appear; then he keeps on appearing. *Nox* mounts an erotic literary resistance to her brother's dis-appearances as Carson pieces together scraps of memory and fragments of ephemerae. Michael is dis-appearing, no question, and he is daily dis-appearing more, but Carson deploys a writer's resources and the power of eros in an effort to find the words that will fend off *nox* and his utter vanishment.

Sisters and brothers possess a unique bond. Unlike husbands and wives, unlike adult partners of any gender, they share a childhood that no one else completely understands or shares. They know each other in ways that no other person alive knows them, in ways that words can't express because much of the experience of children takes place outside language, in the not-known unspoken dimensions of feeling. The death of a brother or the death of a sister takes away this very special part of us—part of our identity, part of our past, no doubt part of our possible futures. When they dis-appear, something has vanished that cannot be replaced, only mourned. The ultimate question for Carson, immersed as a writer in a field of language, is *will her words hold good?* Can eros, with its electrifications and not-knowing, successfully fend off vanishment and oblivion in a scrapbook-style "epitaph" that transforms loss into an intermittent, jagged, epileptic, one-reader-at-a-time, Spinther-like *dis-appearing?*

On Not-Knowing: Flute's Solo

The spark of life for Ruth has gone, even though her body continues to function. Bodily function now is the opposite of health. She is disappearing, slowly but surely, and the spark—once so visible that you could see it in her eyes—has completely vanished. Jean-Do Bauby knew that he was fading away; it added to the terror of locked-in syndrome. I am at least grateful that Ruth is now spared the consciousness of what Alzheimer's disease is relentlessly stripping away. That terror has passed to me. The spark may be what I miss most as Ruth's body—shifted from bed to wheelchair and back to bed—continues to decline. I recall how Michel Foucault identified "thinking" as the distinctive human function and how he celebrated the revolutionary moment (Carson might call it erotic) when we *witness* the birth of new ideas in the bursting outward of their force: "not in books expressing them, but in events manifesting this force, in struggles carried on around ideas, for or against them."[33] Events are appearances—created by individuals caught up within still-unstable ideas and improvised struggles—as impassioned thinking and action begin to break away from the inchoate realm of the not-known. Isn't love, too, in its origins but also in its changes, not just a feeling but an action? A disruptive event, a bursting outward, an impassioned, improvised creation in which bodies and minds, fully present and fully engaged, make their indelible appearances? Love, too, however, can move toward the condition of dis-appearances. I too am resisting a form of vanishment. Husbands and wives (like lovers of every description) may not share a childhood but they have entered together into the unspoken mysteries of eros that always lie somewhere beyond the reach of language.

The spark of life, as I saw it in Ruth's eyes, was wide open to desire. The events she managed to find every day that made her happy found expression in her bodily life as well as in her inner life. Desire adds a brilliance that knowledge and power, for all their social uses, cannot reproduce, and sometimes the disruptive genius of eros proves most revealing in comic moments, as the coming-to-know and the bursting forth of events skids toward sheer chaos and the primal pleasures of not-knowing. *A Midsummer Night's Dream*, in the 1999 film version directed by Michael Hoffman, offers a faithful version of Shakespeare's long night's journey into erotic confusion as all the lovers, including the king and queen of the fairies, experience the power of eros to erode self-knowledge and to loosen rational control. A luminous cinematic moment (unauthorized by Shakespeare's text) occurs, however, in the famous concluding play-within-a-play, as Bottom the Weaver and his Athenian tradesmen accomplices offer a performance of the highbrow Ovidian tragedy *Pyramus and Thisbe*.

Pyramus and Thisbe, before Bottom and his pals reduce it to farce, is a serious play about desire in which tragic events spin out of control, leading to a mistaken suicide. The Ovidian high tragedy spins even further out of control, however, as the amateur, working-class actors (who know next to nothing about the theater) blunder on. Their earnest but laughable performance not only exposes their not-knowing to ridicule but also manages to convey their own endearing ignorance of their not-knowing, as they enter into this alien enterprise of the theater as an expression of their desire to honor the duke's wedding. The clumsiness of the performance continues to spark smug ridicule and unintended merriment among the sophisticated courtiers in audience—until the film takes leave of Shakespeare's text and makes a sudden turn. Bottom as Pyramus has just killed himself, with ham-like dying histrionics, and Flute the Bellows-Mender, wearing a long wig as the romantic heroine Thisbe and mimicking a woman's voice in his squeaky falsetto, bends over the apparently lifeless body. Then it happens. Suddenly the high-flown diction stops. Flute takes off his wig and lowers his register to speak in his natural voice. Why? In his ignorance of theater and its make-believe, Flute seems to believe that the theatrical dead body lying before him (the imitation of a corpse) is not Pyramus but Bottom. Worse, it is not Bottom *playing* dead. ("Asleep, my love?" asks Flute as Thisby. "What, dead, my dove?")[34] It is Flute's bosom friend, Bottom-the-Weaver, *truly* dead.

Flute's blunder and confusion mark a rare moment—amid the pretense and folderol surrounding the duke's marriage ceremony—when eros and not-knowing somehow cross over to make contact with truth or rightness. Flute's knowledge may be flawed or incorrect (it surely is), but his emotion is true. This is, after all, the mystery of the theater. Somehow all the artifice on stage can produce real emotions in the audience. Flute, in his not-knowing, cuts through all the theatrical make-believe; his emotion is real even if it is based on a mistake or not-knowing. In this moment of authentic emotion, he indirectly exposes the falsity of the fawning court-iers and self-satisfied aristocrats in the audience, as they play out their designated social roles, witty, charming, or deferential. Only the women seem to get it. The faces of several brides-to-be, unlike their prospective grooms, register an uneasy sense that something odd is going on. Social actresses almost from birth, bred to play their subordinate roles in the reason-dominated male world, the women perhaps intuitively sense the unexpected arrival of a moment of truth when the masks drop. It is almost as if death—cold as a winter wind slicing through the precoital midsummer hall—has made its appearance, and Flute alone (in his not-knowing) knows.

CONCLUSION

Altered States

Eros—the divine principle of desire and love—surges from our deepest evolutionary roots: the urge to create, to generate new life, to regenerate the species. It is the creative energy immanent in us as living beings.

STEPHEN NACHMANOVITCH, *FREE PLAY* (1990)

*T*HE BIGGEST QUESTION that occupies me in this purposely inconclusive and open-ended conclusion is *So what?* What *good* does it do to explore distinctions between medical eros and medical logos? What real work can medical eros accomplish in the world? How can we turn its advantages—respectfully and without reducing them to a stealth agent of instrumental reason—to practical human *use*? The best way I can address these rude questions is to return to desire. Human health and illness are fundamentally altered by the dynamics of desire, for better or for worse. One touchstone example is the history of tobacco, with its legacy of lung cancer.

The desire for profit as much as the desire for tobacco is what drove the triangular Atlantic slave trade. In a simplified version, European companies traded guns and factory goods in Africa for slaves, then they sold the African slaves in Virginia for tobacco and cotton, and then they sold Virginia tobacco and cotton in Europe, pocketing a large profit at each transaction. Twelve million West African black slaves—and likely more—were brutalized in this triangle of desire, and today big tobacco companies are still in business, after spinning off a few charitable foundations, with continuing damage to global human health. Lung cancer, then, not to mention slavery, has everything to do with desire.

Similar stories could be told about modern industries where desire is not simply a matter of individual psychology—*I want a new car*—but a widespread consumer preference stimulated by well-designed ads, with less than primary concern for the related personal and environmental damage that correlates directly with accidents, disease, debilities, and (in the case of some drugs) birth defects.[1] Medical eros is concerned not only with individual desires, especially because we must accept responsibility for our own desire-driven choices, but also with larger, social, health-related effects of desire as desire is built into late consumer capitalism and the systems of contemporary health care.

Knowledge—the home province of medical logos—is, alone, not enough to change behavior. For over half a century it failed to change medical under-treatment for pain. The U.S. Surgeon General imprints every pack of cigarettes with the warning that cigarette smoke is harmful to your health. Cigarette smoking is now well-documented to cause not only lung cancer but also cancers of the esophagus, larynx, mouth, throat, kidney, bladder, pancreas, stomach, cervix, and blood, in addition to more indirect contributions to heart disease, stroke, aortic aneurysm, chronic obstructive pulmonary disease, asthma, hip fractures, and cataracts.[2] Knowledge alone seems easy to ignore, and reason is not always effective in changing behavior, especially if corporate profits are keyed to sustaining the status quo. Knowledge, as medical eros would claim, is most effective when it engages desire, such as the *desire* for tobacco or the *desire* for clean air, and the goal of enhanced public health offers a powerful incentive for medical logos and medical eros to work together as complements when desire and knowledge can combine forces for better results.

It is important to say here, if it is not already obvious, that medical eros and medical logos are a manner of speaking. They offer unfamiliar terms and broad concepts with which to think about the terrain that moves, sometimes visibly, sometimes invisibly, beneath them. Certain important personal or national conversations do not occur mainly because we lack an enabling vocabulary. Race, for example, never gets the conversation that leaders keep saying needs to happen, partly because Americans are tongue-tied without an enabling vocabulary. The point is not to enshrine a certain manner of speaking. Enabling vocabularies may self-destruct or inspire replacements once the conversation gets under way and generates its own lexicon. What matters most is the conversation.

Medical eros and medical logos are not what philosophers call "natural kinds"—like chemical elements—inscribed in the nature of things. They are also not figures in a grand narrative that seeks to explain the entire field of health and illness. They are, for certain, not boxes into which we can stuff whatever falls out of the medicine cabinet or the bestseller list. The real confinement belongs to a total commitment to the molecular gaze that boxes in our understanding of illness and health so as to neglect their cultural and personal dimensions. Medical eros and medical logos are what icebreakers are to ice. They offer means to unblock stasis and to start the flow of conversations that we urgently need as individuals confronting illness and as cultures dealing with health-care systems and health-care policies. It is a conversation that we can no longer afford to neglect. Nor can we afford to neglect the claims of human desire.

Desire, as we have seen, encompasses serious dilemmas, including some dilemmas that it creates through its tendency toward transgression. Three dilemmas above all seem important to single out. First, desire can be misplaced. Misplaced here doesn't mean lost, as in misplaced car keys, but rather misplacement acknowledges that we can desire persons, objects, or experiences that are directly or indirectly harmful, from cigarette smoke to stony-hearted lovers. Second, desire can be alienated. The alienation of desire occurs by means of a complex psychodynamics through which assertions of desire (*I want to be a doctor*) do not express our own desire but the desire of others, as when it is really the parents who want their son or daughter to enter medicine. Cultures, religions, ideologies, or simply an overbearing individual conscience can encourage us to alienate our own individual desires in preference to the desire of the other. (Certain schools of psychoanalysis would capitalize Other in acknowledgement that *all* desire proceeds from the Unconscious.) Third, and most important here, desire can be hijacked. Hijacked desire is desire put under the control of a usurping power, comparable to terrorists taking over command of a jetliner. Addiction is the most serious individual and social instance of hijacked desire. In addiction, whatever still-unknown neurobiological network it is that underwrites desire gets taken over (or overridden) by the overlapping but separate neurobiology of addiction. The ravaged health and shattered relationships due to addiction are as devastating as bombed-out scenes of a civil war.

"Bring me my Bow of burning gold," wrote William Blake in the voice of a biblical prophet. "Bring me my Arrows of desire."[3] The arrows of desire—not identical with the feathered shafts in Cupid's quiver—are what drove Blake to display his passionate opposition to the then-legal British slave trade. The arrows of desire are what drove his censure of a political status quo in which palace walls were stained with blood and in which churches recoiled from prostitutes created by an unjust social system and by a sanctimonious state religion. They are not merely instruments of protest in bygone times: "the only way to do great work," said Steve Jobs, acclaimed among the most hugely successful, visionary entrepreneurs of the modern era, "is to love what you do."[4] The arrows of desire are certified hazardous, then, but they also can drive personal and cultural change. Nowhere is this double-edged power more evident than in the human impulse to seek various forms of self-transcendence: religious, philosophical, or biochemical. Blake, immersed in his own private mythic cosmos, saw desire as necessary to lead us beyond sensory knowledge and beyond analytical reason to altered and elevated states of consciousness here and now. Liberated desire, for Blake, is what will lead us to grasp the hidden truths accessible only to the expanded mind. "If the doors of perception were cleansed," as he wrote in a famous, much-quoted passage from *The Marriage of Heaven and Hell* (1789), "every thing would appear to man as it is: infinite."[5]

Altered states of consciousness are at times such beneficial, benign, spiritual, erotic, liberating, or simply uncanny conditions—like Joan Didion's year of magical thinking—that they need to be disassociated from statistics on drug addiction. Mike Jay, in *High Society: The Central Role of Mind-Altering Drugs in History, Science and Culture* (2010), provides a fascinating historical account of drug use across cultures and times demonstrating that the desire to alter human consciousness has deep roots, doubtless in the brain as well as in social arrangements.[6] Scientific and social experiments with medical marijuana encourage the need to distinguish between mood-altering substances (with possible therapeutic value) and mind-altering hallucinogens or recreational narcotics. Extreme loneliness, especially among the elderly, might count as an *undesired* state of altered consciousness, which, in its dire effects, may well merit medical or paramedical attention. The crucial point is that a desire for altered states of consciousness does not guarantee liberation—freedom from the mind-forged shackles of our limited, ordinary perception—especially if such desires end in drug addiction and alcoholism.

Desire can surely imprison as well as liberate, and substance abuse has established its position (despite documented historical lulls) as a distinctive contemporary crisis, fueled in part by an unprecedented international traffic in illegal drugs. Emergency rooms, treatment centers, police departments, and prisons absorb much of the trauma and damage. Their stories make for compelling television drama and supply a pipeline of bestselling memoirs about addiction and recovery, but cold numbers describe an equally dramatic calamity. The National Institute on Drug Abuse, an agency within the National Institutes of Health, reports in 2015 that the overall annual cost of illicit drugs—in health-care expenses alone—runs to $11 billion.[7] Other addictive substances run the tab still higher. The annual health-care costs from alcohol are $30 billion, and tobacco tops the list with annual health-care costs of $96 billion. An Internet search of comparative net worth reveals that the combined total cost of $137 billion is enough cash to buy, let's say, Cuba or Morocco.[8]

The personal costs of addictive desire are of course incalculable when we consider lives lost, families destroyed, and children abused or abandoned. Heroin overdoses for the year 2011, according to the National Center on Health Statistics, resulted in 4,397 deaths. Cocaine overdoses resulted in 4,681 deaths, and benzodiazepine overdoses resulted in 6,872 deaths. The largest number of overdose deaths came from opioid pain relievers and synthetic narcotics: 16,917.[9] Is the drug crisis resolving? Not exactly. Deaths from drug overdoses in the decade between 2001 and 2011 increased threefold. Such numbers make melancholy reading, but so do the daily news stories about local drug busts and international drug kingpins. None of this carnage is possible without the arrows of human desire—misplaced, alienated, or outright hijacked—and the neurobiology of addiction. Medical logos has tools to address the neurobiology of addiction. An understanding of eros, it would seem, puts us in a better position to deal with a crisis that owes much of its force and its collateral damage to eros.

One bright California morning in 1953 the distinguished British writer Aldous Huxley dissolved four-tenths of a gram of mescaline in a glass of water, swallowed, and sat down to wait for the results.[10] His wait took place long before epidemiologists began to tote up the disheartening statistics on addiction, before the Haight-Ashbury drug scene, before Harvard professor Timothy Leary's LSD-inspired call to "turn on, tune in, drop out," before even the legendary extravaganzas at Woodstock and Altamont. Numerous modern intellectuals, including a loose confederation of existentialist philosophers, had been trying to lay hands on mescaline; even Jean-Paul Sartre conducted a physician-guided psychedelic experiment, although all he saw on his trip was "a hellish crew of snakes, fish, vultures, toads, beetles and crustaceans," creatures who then followed him around for months.[11] Mescaline is a powerful hallucinogen, and Huxley had long nourished questions about mystics, artists, and visionaries that he felt mescaline might let him address. His brief 1953 encounter with altered consciousness commenced, as he points out, under supervision and in the spirit of a rogue scientific experiment, much like William Morton's self-experiments with the anesthetic properties of ether. Huxley published the results of his May morning research in a fascinating little book that he titled, after William Blake, *The Doors of Perception* (1954).

Huxley's experiment did not go as anticipated. Previous research had led him to believe that mescaline would transport him to an inner world of fantastic visions, something like a Blakean vista of mythic figures striding across star-strewn cosmic landscapes, "But what I had expected," he reports, "did not happen" (*DP* 14–15). Mescaline did not open up an interior realm of subjective vision or of hidden truths. The drug, instead, totally altered his perception of the external environment. The room where he awaited the results of his hallucinogen cocktail, for example, contained a vase with three colorful, oddly matched flowers. "I was not looking now at an unusual flower arrangement," he writes describing his mescaline-inspired response. "I was seeing what Adam had seen on the morning of his creation—the miracle, moment by moment, of naked existence" (*DP* 17). Adam's vision on the morning of creation, as Huxley imagines it, was like experiencing the revelation of a whole new world. Familiar objects shone with a transformed radiance. *Naked existence*, as a description of what mescaline revealed, comes close to what philosophers and theologians mean by *being*: a state stripped bare of all human interpretation and cultural baggage, when existence seems to stand revealed, without mediation, in its basic truth or untouched reality.

His altered state of consciousness led Huxley to surprising intensities and to equally surprising disinterest. Color seemed so fresh, brilliant, and hyperintensified as to feel almost overwhelming. The familiar books in his study took on new life: "Like the flowers, they glowed, when I looked at them, with brighter colors, a profounder significance. Red books, like rubies; emerald books; books bound in white jade; books of agate; of aquamarine, of yellow topaz; lapis lazuli books whose color was so intense, so intrinsically meaningful, that they seemed to be on the point of leaving the shelves to thrust themselves more insistently on my attention" (*DP* 19). Meaningfulness in this altered state is somehow separated from meaning, since the conscious meaning-making processes of reason, logic, and ordinary cognition have lost relevance. Objects simply radiate a mystical significance as self-evident as their colors. What surprised him, however, along with his intensified awareness of external objects, was a simultaneous and profound disinterest in human beings, including himself. "For persons are selves," as he wrote about this odd change in perception, "and, in one respect at least, I was now a Not-self, simultaneously perceiving and being the Not-self of the things around me" (*DP* 35). Language bends nearly to the breaking point of inexpressibility under the burden of this new experience of absent selfhood. As if in a mirror, mescaline reflected his own image as, paradoxically, a "new-born Not-self." This is a very unusual imagery of rebirth in which his new noninterest in human beings extended to a form of self-erasure. His pants commanded more attention than his ego. Fully aware of the Blakean allusions, he describes sitting in his study surrounded by material objects that inspired only a desire for the solitude of selfless and immaterial immensities: "I longed to be left alone with Eternity in a flower, Infinity in four chair legs and the Absolute in the folds of a pair of flannel trousers!" (*DP* 35–36).

We know—from the modern history of substance abuse—where a desire for altered consciousness can take individuals who are less cautious than Huxley and less scientifically inclined, even if some may be equally well-read in Blakean texts and equally well-schooled in Eastern religious traditions. The Not-self for Huxley hadn't completely lost touch with his personal and professional status as a successful writer in his private study wearing flannel pants, and his personal safety net (during what is almost a controlled experiment) certainly sets him apart from people who turn to drugs in a social context of poverty, squalor, racism, and hopelessness. A temporary relaxation of the boundaries of the self—boundaries drawn and policed by outside forces at least as powerful as consciousness in its well-behaved, law-abiding, everyday modes—is for some people an almost necessary escape from utterly oppressive personal experiences and social surroundings. Drugs seem to offer what eros, too, can provide, in its impassioned release from varieties of individual limitation, although the inner life of addiction is—for the long-term drug addict—the direct opposite of liberating.

The desire for an altered consciousness remains, whatever its dangers, an enduring human trait. Huxley describes the "urge" to transcend our ordinary lives, if only for a few moments, as among "the principal appetites of the soul" (*DP* 62). Art, religion, carnivals, dance, saturnalia, and even oratory strike him as means to address this desire for self-transcendence, which tobacco and alcohol also address. If he is right, then the response of governments to ban certain drugs that alter consciousness is like seeking to ban sex. Sex in the age of HIV / AIDS can prove harmful, and there are sex addicts of every gender, but the war on drugs has failed. "If I started a business and it was clearly failing," writes virtuoso British businessman Richard Branson, "I would shut it down. The war on drugs has failed—why isn't it being shut down?"[12] The American habit of declaring war on complex social problems, such as Lyndon Johnson's war on poverty, is only part of the dilemma. Branson urges Americans to heed the Global Commission on Drug Policy and to treat drugs not as a criminal matter but as a health issue. American prisons today are overcrowded—with 1.5 million state and federal inmates in 2014—while 16 percent of state prisoners and 50 percent of federal prisoners are convicted of drug-related offenses.[13] Has failure finally reached a turning point? Might medical eros join with medical logos in addressing the role of desire in drug dependency, especially as desire gets hijacked by addiction and serviced by criminal gangs?

Huxley offers an even more audacious proposal regarding drugs. Because he regards the quest for altered consciousness as an *appetite of the soul*, he believes it is "very likely" that humans will never renounce what Baudelaire called the *artificial paradise* of drugs. Startlingly, he does not advocate fewer drugs but *better* drugs. "What is needed," he argues, "is a new drug which will relieve and console our suffering species without doing more harm in the long run than it does good in the short" (*DP* 64–65). Moralists will seize the opportunity to excoriate Huxley's perhaps poorly phrased concept of "chemical vacations," evoking opium dens and intergalactic drug bars, but a new and ideal drug (potent in minute doses as well as synthesizable) should produce changes in consciousness "more interesting" and "more intrinsically valuable" (*DP* 65), as Huxley puts it, than the narcotic products of sedation or idle dreaminess. Medical logos and the worldwide pharmaceutical industry might take note.

The whole business of eroticism, as Bataille had put it, is to destroy "the self-contained character" of the participators as they are "in their normal lives."[14] Serious disease and disabling conditions of body or mind almost automatically introduce us into a reality so changed that it resembles a foreign land: what Susan Sontag aptly called "the kingdom of the ill."[15] It is not so much a place, of course, as an inner state, an altered state of consciousness. In such a state, as Virginia Woolf described in *On Being Ill*, the self-contained upright character of our normal healthy lives is deeply challenged, and our familiar surroundings come to look as eerily transformed as Huxley's luminous ruby-red books. The medicines prescribed for the treatment of illness or for medical procedures, of course, regularly bring on alterations of consciousness—that is their function—including restful or rejuvenating states such as the pop star Michael Jackson sought from the anesthetic drug propofol, which he used for at least an entire decade in order to help him sleep, before he ultimately died from an overdose of the same medication.[16] Even in a drug-free state we are changed—*translated*—by the experience of serious illness and by our entry, as patients, family, friends, or caregivers, into the uncannily familiar kingdom of the ill.

Illness as an almost involuntary altered state of consciousness runs like a leitmotif through the narratives of medical eros. The "intoxication" that Anatole Broyard experienced, *"as concentrated as a diamond or a micro-chip,"* resembles the experience of British academic Gillian Rose after her diagnosis with advanced ovarian cancer: "What people now seem to find most daunting with me, I discover, is not my illness or possible death, but my accentuated being: not my morbidity, but my renewed vitality."[17] Joan Didion's vortex-punctuated year of "magical thinking" included an altered temporal consciousness: "I had been trying to reverse time, run the film backward."[18] For Virginia Woolf, illness resembled the intoxications of love: "It invests certain faces with divinity, sets us to wait, hour after hour, with pricked ears for the creaking of a stair."[19] The inner life of serious illness, beyond the molecular gaze, is regularly experienced as an altered state of consciousness—and not just among patients. "For the next eight years I would have flashbacks," Dr. H reports after his catastrophic surgical error left a two-year-old boy dead; "I would just be driving down the highway and think about it, or I'd conjure up horrible images. It was like a war scene, so bloody and gross."[20] Medical eros, with its attention to such altered states, offers an important perspective on what happens—on radical changes to our inner lives—not only when we ourselves are seriously ill but also when we enter even the outskirts or environs of illness and its unseen consequences.

The altered states of consciousness typical of illness are often unsought and undesired, but they quickly intersect with desire if only in prayers for a recovery and a return to health. Prayer—from the Latin *precari* (to ask earnestly, to beg, to entreat)—is often an altered state, whether conducted in solemn privacy, or incorporated in dancing, whirling, ecstatic rituals and group joy or *communitas.*[21] Prayer and meditation as everyday altered states, sometimes correlated with alpha brain waves, are important beyond their personal benefits as a reminder that desire leads into regions still poorly understood and perhaps inherently enfolded in states of not-knowing. Does whatever neurobiology correlates with desire somehow intersect with genetic predispositions that, under certain circumstances, lead to alcoholism? What happens if desire veers into the pathological altered state known as obsession? Or when it aligns with the constant craving that Buddhists see as the source of all suffering?

The permutations of desire extend even to efforts to control or eradicate it. Joy E. Corey, in *Divine Eros* (2014), writes about desire as a fundamentalist Christian minister whose point of view marks a 180-degree turn from the eroticism of Audre Lorde. "We guard and watch over our minds," Corey writes, "by being vigilant over our wills and our desires. If these don't conform to God's will and desire, we must struggle to align them with His by turning away from our attachments and carnal passions."[22] *Cultural competence* is the catch-phrase for a valuable new emphasis within medical education on the knowledge and sensitivity needed to practice medicine in an era of increasing national, ethnic, and racial diversity, but such competence needs to extend beyond immigrant populations and religious minorities. Cultural competence—as a measurable, testable, objective knowledge that medical students must master—is perhaps less what doctors need as they confront multiethnic patient populations than an attitude of openness and of respect in the face of human difference. Such otherness will inevitably include the different orientations toward desire that help make every patient unique and that help shape the distinctive individual experience of illness.[23]

Foucault, in his late lecture courses, in both Paris and Berkeley, argues that care of the self—always understood in political and ethical (not strictly medical) contexts—requires, crucially, a relation to others: "one cannot attend to oneself, take care of oneself, without a relationship to another person."[24] We act, ethically and politically, in a landscape of not-knowing where the darkness of the self meets the infinity of the other person. Care of the self, then, is an impossible but necessary task, far beyond the powers of medical logos alone, and medical eros can at least offer as encouragement the recognition that we live surrounded by imperfectly understood, immeasurable forces. Our best scientific instruments detect only a small fragment of the known universe, with dark energy and dark matter (invisible and thus far undetectable) as potent metaphors for what remains both strangely fundamental and nonetheless not-known.[25]

What to do? Ralph Waldo Emerson, whose beloved wife Ellen Louisa Tucker died of tuberculosis at age twenty, viewed eros as the only power that merits our complete allegiance: "Give all to love; / Obey thy heart; / Friends, kindred, days, / Estate, good-frame, / Plans, credit and the Muse,— / Nothing refuse." Eros, despite heartbreak, remains for Emerson, as for Updike a century later, the essential cosmic and spiritual binding force without which everything in human life falls apart: "the glue," as one Emersonian scholar puts it, "that holds the universe and humanity together."[26]

Eros might well stand for the glue-like connections that hold individuals together, and, if so, it could have a surprising role to play in the understanding and treatment of addiction. British journalist Johann Hari recently provided strong arguments for thinking that addiction is best understood not as a disease or as a moral weakness but as a condition that, whatever its direct cause, embodies a profound loss of social connection.[27] Disconnection is the altered state that typifies addicts, according to Hari's extensive research. I was skeptical at first because the genetics and neurobiology of addiction are well established, but Hari changed my mind. His crucial contribution is to emphasize that the psychology of addiction includes an almost pathological absence of social connection. Most drug-dependent patients, for example, easily manage the process of step-by-step withdrawal. Addicts do not. A focus on social disconnection is valuable precisely because it offers an effective means of intervention. Social reconnection, a form of erotic glue-like bonding, both actively assists addicts in the process of recovery and also provides a humane, pragmatic, and economical alternative to high-priced, futile "wars" on drugs.

"If you are loved," Hari concludes of the drug casualties he has interviewed, "you have a chance. For a hundred years we have been singing war songs about addicts. All along, we should have been singing love songs to them."[28] Medical logos is likely to dismiss this claim as sentimental, but significant evidence supports further study into the role of social reconnection.

Portugal at the turn of the twenty-first century, for example, was a gateway for European drug trafficking, and widespread intravenous drug use caused rates of infectious diseases to soar. Facing this dilemma, a government-appointed expert commission proposed a new national policy of decriminalizing personal drug use and introduced a multidimensional drug strategy that included an emphasis on "social reintegration."[29] Portugal adopted this policy in 2001, and the strategy of social reintegration involved taking very practical steps to assist addicts, such as helping underwrite costs of employment. Such moderate costs were more than offset by vastly reduced expenditures in health care, in law enforcement, and in criminal justice. Meanwhile the policy led to major reductions in opiate-related deaths and infections. These measurable benefits to public health parallel transformations in the lives of addicts. Humans, as social animals, run in families, gangs, and tribes; our desire for connection may be what gets lost in addiction. No single policy, of course, can eliminate substance abuse. Social reconnection as a means to help addicts recover, however, suggests that our relations to others—bonds fundamental to eros—also prove basic to human function and to the dynamics of self-care.

Foucauldian care of the self, as the example of addiction suggests, implies far more than good nutrition, a regular gym visit, and vitamin supplements. It is an exercise of desire that leads us, inevitably, into the mind-spinning realm of the not-known, where not-knowing is a condition of inner life that connects us with the lives of others (who are similarly at risk or already at a loss). Care for others, in traditional Christian theology, is an instance of *caritas* or charitable love: the "most excellent" of the virtues, according to Aquinas, and a practice not difficult to imagine at work in secular or nontheological contexts. If care for others is a virtue, self-care too merits a respected place in the system of moral thought known as virtue ethics, since we *are* the other. That is, we are simultaneously self and other, both because our selfhood contains an intrinsic otherness (our own dark or unconscious spaces) and because we already occupy the position of other when viewed by someone else. Care of the self, then, understood as the opposite of solipsistic self-indulgence, is less an issue of personal health than an expression of eros as a binding, connective, even ethical force able to draw us into the gentler registers of human loving-kindness. Self-care matters especially because it is so easy to ignore or to get wrong when—as patients, caregivers, family, friends, doctors, or random others—we enter into the disorienting nightside kingdom of the ill.

It was Susan Sontag who described illness as "the night-side of life."[30] It is reasonable to presume that the metaphor is not false to her experience in 1975 with stage IV metastatic breast cancer. She never mentions her experience with cancer in *Illness as Metaphor* (1978), a brilliant analysis (published several years later) showing how figurative language—such as a metaphoric description of the Watergate scandal as "a cancer on the Presidency"—exposes distinctive individual and cultural beliefs about illness. Such beliefs are largely erroneous and such metaphoric language harmful, in her view, because illness for Sontag is exclusively a biological condition of the body, and the body for Sontag is an organic system known, or in principle always knowable, by medical science. "My mother loved science," writes Sontag's son, David Rieff, "and believed in it (as she believed in reason) with a fierce, unwavering tenacity bordering on religiosity. There was a sense in which reason was her religion."[31] Fierceness suggests passion, and Sontag's passionate belief that medicine and reason hold the answers to illness certainly underlies her own care of the self. A radical mastectomy—removing the breast, the chest-wall muscle, and the lymph nodes in the armpit—left her in an altered state almost the opposite of intoxicated.

"People speak of illness as deepening," Sontag writes in a passage from her journal. "I don't feel deepened. I feel flattened. I've become opaque to myself" (*SSD* 35). What does it mean to become opaque to oneself? Is it like a darkened mirror in which we no longer recognize our own reflection? Rieff believes that this opaqueness extended to "the damage done to her sexuality from which I do not believe she ever fully recovered" (*SSD* 36). For eros, of course, sexuality is a key feature of the inner life, as crucial to our self-understanding as the image in a mirror. Eros matters as much in its failures as in its transcendence. Sontag's fierce religion of cutting-edge medical science saved her life, but it did not offer solace from what Rieff calls "the depth of her despair" (*SSD* 41). Medical logos, outside psychiatry, does not focus closely on such altered states of consciousness.

Sontag's respite lasted until the late 1990s when she was diagnosed with uterine sarcoma. The chemotherapy that she received in treatment precipitated a form of stem-cell disorder known as myelodysplastic syndrome, for which medical science had no effective treatment. The prognosis indicated rapid advance into full-blown acute myeloid leukemia. "When I first met Susan," Rieff quotes her oncologist as saying, "she repeatedly told me that she was 'in freefall'" (*SSD* 116). In free fall, Sontag kept up her determined struggle despite the failure of a bone marrow transplant, as she called upon her prodigious intellect, research skills, and extraordinary will to explore all medical options. Science and reason laid out the steep statistical odds against recovery, and, like Anatole Broyard, she had no patience with optimistic, well-meaning friends who offered consolation. "'Read the statistics,' she'd say, ever factual, 'read the statistics'" (*SSD* 133). When friends continued to express confidence that she would recover, Rieff writes that his mother would explain how bad her chances were "in a pedantic tone that soon spiraled into panic." Medical logos accompanies us as far as reason will extend, but reason, as it encounters the individual mysteries of serious illness and not-knowing, may lead to the edge of an abyss.

David Rieff's memoir *Swimming in a Sea of Death* (2008), in its focus on Sontag's last years, begins with a phone call from his famous mother asking that he accompany her as she met with a specialist to discuss troubling blood tests, and his focus throughout remains on how Sontag deals with illness not as a magnet for false metaphors and erroneous beliefs— as in *Illness as Metaphor*—but as a lived experience. Her lived experience, as Rieff viewed it, took shape from her fierce belief that illness is exclusively a bodily state amenable to scientific, rational, biomedical understanding. There is, amid Rieff's biographical reflections about his mother, another important narrative thread (almost a subtheme) that concerns what he calls "the loved one's dilemma" (*SSD* 21). It is Rieff who swims alongside his mother in a sea of death, and the book also details *his* struggle, which includes continually adjusting *his* responses to what he believes are *his* mother's desires, although he never wholly grasps what her desires *are*. The uncertainties of desire and not-knowing return us, of course, to the native ground of medical eros, and caregivers will doubtless recognize their own anguish in the litany of unanswerable questions that continue, long after Sontag's death, to disturb David Rieff's bittersweet dreams.

Dreams are another common altered state, and for Rieff the incessant questions tumble out, as he says, both in wakefulness and in sleep. For a full two years after his mother's death he continues to replay at night his own tormenting self-indictments. At times he wishes that he had died instead of Sontag—a mental state that he identifies as, in part, *survivor's guilt* (*SSD* 159). The questions are as unresolvable as they are relentless:

"Did I do the right thing? Could I have done more? Or proposed an alternative? Or been more supportive? Or forced the issue of death to the fore? Or concealed it better?" (*SSD* 21). I have asked similar questions, repeatedly, received no answers, and found my altered consciousness reflected in the loved one's dilemma.

Rieff's memoir unfolds as a double narrative, two quite different, parallel accounts, with each matching a prototype described by Arthur W. Frank in *The Wounded Storyteller*. One narrative, a classic *quest narrative*, concerns a famous writer—proud of her "straight-A student" intellect (*SSD* 81)—who remains steadfast in her belief that science and reason hold the ultimate remedy for her condition. Sontag transforms her apartment into an ad hoc research library searching for a cure, while nonetheless caught in the vortex of loss and confusion from which no exertion of intellect could free her. Rieff aptly captures the vicious circle: "But while she knew she had a deadly illness, good student though she undoubtedly was, this did not make her any less lost, as almost all patients are, in the thick fog of the alien language of medicine and biology, and in the thicker fog of passing from being an autonomous adult to an infantilized patient—all need, and fear, and pain" (*SSD* 82).

The second narrative—as if two parallel swimmers told differing adjacent stories—is the lost caregiver's *chaos narrative*. Rieff is caught in currents of unnavigable paradox. Intense loving care of the (unknowable) other, in his case, entails a deferred or misplaced care of the (equally unknowable) self; and even if Rieff guesses right about his mother's concealed desires, he can't know *for sure* that he's right, and meanwhile he blames himself when he responds ineptly to what he imagines her needs are. Their mute exchanges are like the dumb show prelude to a tragedy, in which concealed desires and mounting doubts ultimately take an immense psychic toll. "Inside, I was shutting down," Rieff writes, "almost as if, instinctively, I realized that I could not handle my own emotion as well as hers" (*SSD* 99). In retrospect, he wonders if shutting down was inevitable, or the right choice. ("I am by no means sure.") Occasional doubts happen every day, but unremitting, traumatic uncertainties about the care of a loved one, accompanied by an emotional freeze, soon rise to the level of a pathological altered state. "I was numb for so long," Rieff says ruefully (*SSD* 109). His summary holds no consolation. "I am anything but certain that I did the right thing," he concludes, "and, in my bleaker moments, wonder if in fact I might not have made things worse for her by endlessly refilling that poisoned chalice of hope" (*SSD* 169).

The two parallel narratives—reason and doubt, quest and chaos, mother and son—do not belong to the well-lit world of medical logos. They emerge from the dark side of life: the altered state of not-knowing native to medical eros. Eros may not spring to mind when we think about filial affection, but eros is present, too, in the relations between adult children and declining parents, especially when illness calls them together. David Rieff entered a maze with wrong turns everywhere. "She quickly made it plain," he notes of his mother's less than lucid communication, "though she never came out and said it so bluntly, that there were 'no go' areas on the subject of her illness" (*SSD* 42). Ruth and I also had unspoken "no go" agreements. I feared where the talk might lead. Maybe she did, too, but such speculations simply uncover more not-knowing. My suggestion that we learn sign language was an idiotic proposal, of course, because Ruth wasn't just losing English words but all language facility. Still, caregivers are desperate. Ruth had recently begun to cling ever closer to me. Only after I realized, in my exhaustion, that she might one day wake up beside a corpse did I dare say, as I mentioned earlier, I had visited a residential care facility and (like Rieff, my replays are endless) felt the utter astonishment of hearing Ruth reply, *Can we go see it?*

David Rieff had the grace often to acquiesce in his mother's unspoken desires, even though in silencing his disagreements and his doubts he knowingly betrayed his own code of honesty. "I became her accomplice," he says, "albeit with the guiltiest of consciences" (*SSD* 43). He allows himself in retrospect some critical, personal judgments about his mother—that her faith in reason was "unreasonable" (*SSD* 94), for example—but such opinions are rarely free from the doubt, self-reproach, and guilt that seem the inescapable cost of his caregiver role. As a writer, he could see a value in certain real-life stories or fictions—nontruths or deceptions that we embrace out of care for another person—which nonwriters or truth-squads might call lies. Three times he cites Joan Didion's astute statement (the title of her collected essays) that *we tell ourselves stories in order to live.*[32] The life-sustaining story that Susan Sontag told in the face of illness concerned the power of reason and of science; David Rieff's

companion story is about the limits of reason and about the unreasonable things that we do, for love, in an altered state of doubt, guilt, confusion, fear, and not-knowing what to do.

Hippocrates famously says that the art of healing has three parts: the disease, the patient, and the healer. Medical eros is most Hippocratic, we
might say, in its emphasis on the patient and on the healer. The biology
of disease is the province of medical logos and of the molecular gaze, but
medical logos might reclaim a share of its Asklepian heritage if logos were
permitted to resonate with its pre-Socratic connotations of *word*, *speech*,
discourse, and *meaning*. Joan Didion is right: we tell stories—to ourselves,
to others—in order to live. Such stories, however, do not always resemble
traditional narratives with beginnings, middles, and conclusions. Like
shards or splinters, many stories we tell about illness resemble angular
remnants of a missing and perhaps forever inaccessible plot: true to the
moment, perhaps no more than a random, jotted diary entry, but also at
times almost holographic images in which each fragment recapitulates a
vanished whole. "While I was busy zapping the world with my mind,"
Rieff quotes from Sontag's journal, "my body fell down" (*SSD* 41). This
is the statement of a pubic intellectual who not only "loved reason" and
"loathed appeals to the subjective," as Rieff notes (*SSD* 40), but also
for whom the unreasoning body always took second place. "For my
mother, whose pleasure in her own body—never secure—had been irre-
trievably wrecked by her breast cancer surgery," Rieff concludes, "consciousness was finally all that mattered" (*SSD* 73). Consciousness for
Sontag meant *logos* in its strictest biomedical, scientific meanings as
principle, law, and reason.

Science and fact constitute the only ground on which Sontag would
permit hope—the rationalist story she told herself in order to survive—and
the ground in her final illness was radically unstable. Consciousness
for Rieff holds a different meaning, more consistent with eros and not-
knowing, less wholly aligned with reason and less alienated from the
body. It was only in the last weeks of her life, as he writes, after the bone
marrow transplant in Seattle had failed, that Sontag returned home to
New York and "essentially gave up finding ways to believe there were rational reasons for her to think she would survive. It was an impossible

balancing act" (*SSD* 127). *Rational reasons:* for Rieff, the heart, too, has its reasons, but that is a paradox; it invokes a nonscientific concept of reason. In effect, it belongs to another story.

Illness as Metaphor, despite the skill with which Sontag analyzes the metaphoric language of illness, belongs alongside other 1970s texts of *liberation*. It shares in an antimilitarist spirit typical of the post-Vietnam War era. It also embodies Sontag's desire to free illness from what she regarded as the erroneous, contaminating, metaphoric discourses that prevent us from understanding it as, simply, a biological event. She seeks especially to liberate cancer from the psychoanalytic language of self-denial and repression, implying that patients are responsible for their disease, mainly through forms of erotic refusal. *Illness as Metaphor*, alongside its brilliant analysis of ways in which illness infiltrates literary and nonliterary discourse, is a fierce defense and exposition of the powers of reason, in which reason (employing the analytical tools of biomedicine) identifies the hidden cellular processes that always underlie disease. Her son believes that Sontag never entirely broke free from the suspicion that her own self-denials had caused her illness. What we know for sure is that the network of supra-dyadic erotic relations in which serious illness regularly enfolds us—patient, friends, lovers (past or present), family, and caregivers, in an open-ended series—register in complex biofeedback loops on the organic systems at play in illness, so that (like stories, faiths, and beliefs) they are rarely irrelevant to the truth of an individual malady but rather, like the "nebulous factors" affecting outcomes at the best specialized clinics, contribute to the intricate mind/body interrelations that define illness.

Altered states include the emotional entanglements that come with families and with illness, and David Rieff explains that he preferred to write "as little as possible" about his relations with his mother in the last decade of her life. Their relations, he confesses, were "often strained and at times very difficult" (*SSD* 160). More complications of eros. He describes her dying as "so protracted" that there was "almost too much time" to prepare for her death. Sontag's journey ends, but for Rieff there is no conclusion, no end point, only the continued doubt and not-knowing. Even the nineteenth-century tradition of last words—the closure that comes with whatever concluding statement the dying person utters—in Rieff's case takes a decidedly postmodern turn, as he recalls his final exchange with his mother at her bedside.

> *The day before she died, she asked, "Is David here?"*
> *"Yes, I'm here," I remember hearing myself say.*
> *My mother did not open her eyes, or move her head. For a moment,*
> *I thought that she had fallen back to sleep. But after a pause, she said,*
> *"I want to tell you . . ."*
> *That was all she said. She gestured vaguely with one emaciated*
> *hand and then let it drop onto the coverlet. I think she did fall back to*
> *sleep then. These were the last words my mother spoke to me.*[33]

Eros, amid the transcendence and torment that plays out in the inner life, is the medium of questions to which we cannot find answers; it holds out the promise of an inaccessible but wished-for knowledge that, no matter how hard we reason or try, we will never possess.

Bittersweet. The Greek epithet for eros—*glukopikron*: literally "sweetbitter"—that Sappho invented in fifth-century BCE Lesbos is less a literary figure of speech, an oxymoron (like hot ice), than an accurate description of the contrary states that eros unites or at least brings into alternating contact. The sweet-bitterness of love can range from ecstatic transcendence to abject misery. "Spurn me, strike me," Helena adds to her spaniel-like litany of abjection as she begs her cold lover for attention in *A Midsummer Night's Dream*.[34] Any contact better than no contact. If eros can reduce us to such abject fawning, less an expression of love than of twisted self-contempt, it can also raise us to the stars. The rival who sits face to face with Sappho's beloved—drinking in her "sweet speech and lovely / laughter"—is, as Sappho writes enviously, elevated above mortal status: "peer of the gods" (*theoisin*).[35] Significantly, it is the speech and laughter of the beloved—not her visual beauty—that Sappho extols here. Eros lives through all the senses, even as it lifts the lover at times far beyond the sensual or material world. Still, despite its intoxicating transcendence, the altered states into which eros can draw the lover include jealousy, betrayal, and a lovesickness so extreme that, as Sappho also acknowledges, it approaches the hyperdestructive and ultimate bitter alteration of erotic inner life: "dying."

An account of my own altered states offers at least an inconclusive post-script to the scraps of personal essay scattered throughout. Ruth spends her days now in a conscious but heartbreakingly near-comatose state. She no longer walks, although she once ranged the perimeter of her residential facility in shark-like constant motion. I find her most afternoons lying on her bed, eyes unfocused, lost in space. She takes no notice of me—or anyone. Is her chronic teeth-grinding a sign of anxieties? Does she understand where she is, or who she is? No one can tell me. I arrange for her favorite hairdresser to cut her hair each month, although several years ago we agreed to stop the color treatments. Ruth would have fought grey hair to the bitter end. She would not share my pleasure that her later years promised a gorgeous cascade of silvery-platinum locks. I know that I am losing her. I now rationalize that it is OK to reduce my visits because she doesn't know I'm present or absent. Reasons don't help. Psyche never gave up searching for Cupid. Others—spouses, parents, lovers, kin—have faced harder roads. Like David Rieff, I find no way to step outside this clouded not-knowing state.

Eros, however, is not all bitter. It always holds the promise of an inseparable sweetness. Perhaps eros is with us all along—like an invisible force field we inhabit, or like the (mostly unheard) whisper of being that Levinas imagined surviving even catastrophic extinctions—available to gather suddenly into a *positive* Black Swan event as improbable as Ruth's illness. Well past sixty, I worked up my nerve for some first dates over the Internet. After discovering my complete comic futility on the senior dating scene, I finally met a talented painter, living sixty miles away, who had recently accompanied her husband through an extended, fatal dementia. We don't talk much about brain disease, as you might imagine, but we don't need to. It's in our bones, and luckily eros has given us an unexpected chance to focus, for now, on sweetness.

Medical eros is the power I've relied on when I did not know what to do, but not to the exclusion of medical logos. I think of them working separately as needed, but often in concert, like the right hand and the left hand. Of course, there's no medical diagnosis for getting beaten up, run ragged, and just plain pushed to the limit of your strength, as many caregivers are, and eros then proves indispensable. Sometimes, too, words and images can help more than drugs and surgeries in situations where illness

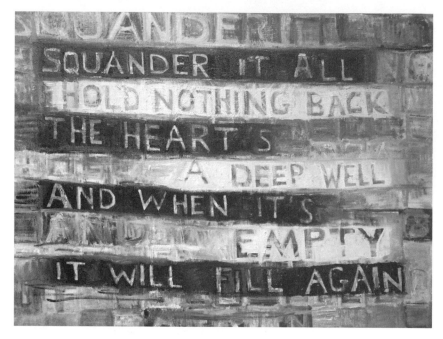

FIGURE 10.1. Trisha Orr. *Squander It All.* Oil on canvas.
Reproduced courtesy of Trisha Orr.

might seem to blot out eros and obliterate an assent to life. Contemporary painter Trisha Orr and her poet-husband, Gregory Orr, joined forces starting in 2006 on a series of *poem-paintings,* as Trisha Orr calls them, in which his words together with her images create a synergy unavailable to either alone. The impact of their collaboration changed in 2009, however, when Trisha was diagnosed with a serious illness. What may have begun, inside a marriage, as an aesthetic engagement with the venerable traditions that combine poetry and painting took on a new, life-sustaining significance. "I came to feel," she writes, "that the poems gave me the courage, faith, and hope necessary to live vitally, not just to survive passively."

"Squander it all / Hold Nothing Back / The Heart's / A Deep Well / And When It's Empty / It Will Fill Again" (Figure 10.1). Like a wall ceaselessly scraped and repainted with graffiti, the canvas in its layered orange and yellow random sprawls of battered color gives the eroded striations of black-and-white linear verse just the right feel of a meaning that survives, absorbs, and transcends whatever powers will continue to resist or oppose it.

I don't know for certain that my heart will always keep refilling—reason says no, wells sometimes run dry, just as language sometimes runs dry, just as Ruth now lives in a nightside world beyond my reach, beyond my touch. But words can also hold good, and a true heart-refilling is what I deeply desire, with no holding back. Call it *survivor's hope*. Not a passive, thin wishful-thinking but instead a sturdy trust in facing the unknown, the not-known, despite the improbabilities ahead, some good, some doubtless not so good. Hope is certainly an inflection of desire. Eros, in its assent to life, is no less than the unofficial guardian of hope and desire: the great god of sprawl, squander, and not-knowing. How will it all end? I don't know. Not-knowing, I continue to relearn, is the one inescapable altered state that eros assures us of.

Notes

INTRODUCTION

Epigraph: John Updike, quoted in Ethan Bronner, "Bethlehem Journal; John Updike Returns to His Source," *New York Times*, November 6, 1998, www.nytimes.com/1998/11/06/us/bethlehem-journal-john-updike-returns-to-his-source.html. Updike was replying to questions from students at Lehigh University, in Bethlehem, Pennsylvania, on November 4, 1998.

1. Hubert Dreyfus and Sean Dorrance Kelly, *All Things Shining: Reading the Western Classics to Find Meaning in a Secular Age* (New York: Simon & Schuster, 2011), 85.

2. For an exemplary collection, see *Erotikon: Essays on Eros, Ancient and Modern*, ed. Shadi Bartsch and Thomas Bartscherer (Chicago: University of Chicago Press, 2005).

3. Georges Bataille, *Erotism: Death and Sensuality*, trans. Mary Dalwood (San Francisco: City Lights Books, 1986), 11. This English translation was first published as *Death and Sensuality: A Study of Eroticism and the Taboo* (New York: Walker, 1962).

4. Georges Bataille, *The Tears of Eros* [1961], trans. Peter Connor (San Francisco: City Lights Books, 1989).

5. Bataille, *Erotism*, 29.

6. Anne Carson, *Eros the Bittersweet* (1986; repr., Normal, Ill.: Dalkey Archive, 1998), 40–41.

7. G. E. Berrios and N. Kennedy, "Erotomania: A Conceptual History," *History of Psychiatry* 13 (2002): 381–400; see also Brendan D. Kelly, "Erotomania," *CNS Drugs* 19 (2005): 657–669.

8. Bataille, *Erotism*, 17 ("une destruction de la structure de l'être fermé qu'est à l'état normal").

9. Kenneth M. Ludmerer, "The Development of American Medical Education from the Turn of the Century to the Era of Managed Care," lecture, Case Western Reserve University, October 12–13, 2001, www.case.edu/artsci/wrss/documents/wrs2001-02ludmerer_000.pdf.

10. Abraham Flexner, *Medical Education in the United States and Canada: A Report to the Carnegie Foundation for the Advancement of Teaching* (1910; repr. New York: Carnegie Foundation for the Advancement of Teaching, 1972), http://archive.carnegiefoundation.org/pdfs/elibrary/Carnegie_Flexner_Report.pdf.

11. See Sander L. Gilman, *Sexuality: An Illustrated History, Representing the Sexual in Medicine and Culture from the Middle Ages to the Age of AIDS* (New York: Wiley, 1989).

12. William Carlos Williams, "The Use of Force" [1938], *The Doctor Stories*, comp. Robert Coles (New York: New Directions, 1984), 59. The subsequent quotations, in order of occurrence, refer to pages 59, 57, 57, and 60.

13. Carson, *Eros the Bittersweet*, 70.

14. Centers for Disease Control and Prevention, "Diphtheria," *Epidemiology and Prevention of Vaccine-Preventable Diseases*, 13th ed. (Atlanta: CDC, 2015), www.cdc.gov /vaccines/pubs/pinkbook/downloads/dip.pdf.

15. Karen Davis, Kristof Stremikis, David Squires, and Cathy Schoen, "Mirror, Mirror on the Wall: How the Performance of the U.S. Health Care System Compares Internationally," *The Commonwealth Fund* (June 2014), publication no. 1755.

16. Martin Makary and Michael Daniel, "Medical Error—The Third Leading Cause of Death in the US," *BMJ*, May 3, 2016, doi: http://dx.doi.org/10.1136/bmj.i2139. For a dissenting voice, see Richard Gunderman and Jae Hyun Kwon, "Deadly Medical Errors Are Less Common Than Headlines Suggest," *The Conversation* (United States edition), accessed August 23, 2016, http://theconversation.com/deadly-medical-errors-are -less-common-than-headlines-suggest-61944. For a wider discussion, see Barbara Starfield, "Is US Health Really the Best in the World?," *JAMA* 248, no. 4 (2000): 483– 485; R. Monina Klevens, Jonathan R. Edwards, Chesley L. Richards Jr., Teresa C. Horan, Robert P. Gaynes, et al., "Estimating Health Care-Associated Infections and Deaths in U.S. Hospitals, 2002," *Public Health Reports* 122 (2007): 160–166; and Institute of Medicine, *Preventing Medication Errors*, ed. Philip Aspden, Julie Wolcott, J. Lyle Bootman, and Linda R. Cronewett (Washington, D.C.: The National Academies Press, 2006).

17. Donna Haraway, *The Companion Species Manifesto: Dogs, People, and Significant Otherness* (Chicago: Prickly Paradigm, 2003), 8; Bruno Latour, *We Have Never Been Modern* [1991], trans. Catherine Porter (Cambridge, Mass.: Harvard University Press, 1993), 41; and Andrew Scholtz, *Concordia discors: Eros and Dialogue in Classical Athenian Literature* (Cambridge, Mass.: Harvard University Press, 2007).

18. Susan Sontag, *Illness as Metaphor* (New York: Farrar, Straus and Giroux, 1978), 3.

19. Jonathan Kipnis, quoted in Josh Barney, "They'll Have to Rewrite the Textbooks," *UVA Today*, March 21, 2016, https://news.virginia.edu/illimitable/discovery/theyll-have -rewrite-textbooks; and Antoine Louveau, Igor Smirnov, Timothy J. Keyes, Jacob D. Eccles, Sherin J. Rouhani, et al. "Structural and Functional Features of Central Nervous System Lymphatics," *Nature* 523 (2015): 337–341.

20. My deepest thanks to Gail Lauzzana for permission to quote from her e-mail.

CHAPTER ONE · THE AMBUSH: AN EROTICS OF ILLNESS

Epigraph: Eugen Herrigel, *Zen in the Art of Archery* [1948], trans. R. F. C. Hull (New York: Pantheon Books, 1953), 51. The Master is the renowned Japanese teacher Awa Kenzō.

1. *A Midsummer Night's Dream*, III.i.18–19, in *The Riverside Shakespeare* (Boston: Houghton Mifflin, 1974).

2. Steven H. Woolf, "The Meaning of Translational Research and Why It Matters," *JAMA* 299, no. 2 (2008): 211–213.

3. Arthur Frank, *At the Will of the Body: Reflections on Illness* (Boston: Houghton Mifflin, 1991), 8.

4. Donald Hall, *Without* (Boston: Houghton Mifflin, 1998), 40.

5. Alzheimer's Association, "2016 Alzheimer's Disease Facts and Figures" www.alz.org /documents_custom/2016-facts-and-figures.pdf.

6. David Rieff, *Swimming in a Sea of Death: A Son's Memoir* (New York: Simon & Schuster, 2008), 28. Rieff observes that Sontag "loathed appeals to the subjective" (40).

7. Susan Sontag, "Directions: Write, Read, Rewrite. Repeat Steps 2 and 3 as Needed" [2000], in *Writers on Writing: Collected Essays from the New York Times*, introduced by John Darnton (New York: Times Books, 2001), 227–228.

8. Ann Jurecic, *Illness as Narrative* (Pittsburgh: University of Pittsburgh Press, 2012), 18. See also Anne Hunsaker Hawkins, *Reconstructing Illness: Studies in Pathography*, 2nd ed. (Lafayette, Ind.: Purdue University Press, 1999).

9. Among relevant accounts, see Rachel Hadas, *Strange Relation: A Memoir of Marriage, Dementia, and Poetry* (Philadelphia: Paul Dry, 2011); Edward Bliss Jr., *For Love of Lois* (New York: Fordham University Press, 2003); Michael S. Pritchard, *Moments with Millie: A Memory Walk* (Haslett, Mich.: Buttonwood Press, 2007); and Lisa Genova, *Still Alice: A Novel* (New York: Pocket Books, 2009).

10. Alzheimer's Association, "2016 Alzheimer's Disease Facts and Figures," *Alzheimer's & Dementia* 12, no. 4 (2016), www.alz.org/documents_custom/2016-facts-and-figures .pdf.

11. Kirsten P. Smith and Nicholas A. Christakis, "Social Networks and Health," *Annual Review of Sociology* 34 (2008): 405–429.

12. Anne E. Becker, "New Global Perspectives on Eating Disorders," *Culture, Medicine and Psychiatry* 28 (2004): 433–437; and "Television, Disordered Eating, and Young Women in Fiji: Negotiating Body Image and Identity during Rapid Social Change," *Culture, Medicine and Psychiatry* 28 (2004): 533–559.

13. Rose McDermott, James H. Fowler, and Nicholas A. Christakis, "Breaking Up Is Hard to Do, Unless Everyone Else Is Doing It Too: Social Network Effects on Divorce in a Longitudinal Sample," *Social Forces* 92 (2013): 491–519.

14. Susan Sontag, "The Way We Live Now" [1986], in *The Way We Write Now: Short Stories from the AIDS Crisis*, ed. Sharon Oard Warner (New York: Citadel Press, 1995), 9.

15. Richard Schulz and Scott R. Beach, "Caregiving as a Risk Factor for Mortality: The Caregiver Health Effects Study," *JAMA* 282 (1999): 2215–2219.

16. Connie Matthiessen, "Caregiving: Does It Have to Be This Hard?" *Caring.com*, April 3, 2008, www.caring.com/blogs/caring-currents/caregiving-are-you-getting-the -support-you-need.

17. Oliver Sacks, *The Man Who Mistook His Wife for a Hat and Other Clinical Tales* (New York: Simon & Schuster, 1985), 81.

18. For two basic texts, see Nancy L. Mace and Peter V. Rabins, *The 36-Hour Day: A Family Guide to Caring for People Who Have Alzheimer's Disease, Related Dementias, and Memory Loss*, 5th ed. (Baltimore: Johns Hopkins University Press, 2011), and *Always on Call: When Illness Turns Families into Caregivers*, rev. ed., ed. Carol Levine (Nashville: Vanderbilt University Press, 2004).

19. Rebecca Garden, "The Problem of Empathy: Medicine and the Humanities," *New Literary History* 38 (2007): 551–567.

20. Danielle Ofri, *What Doctors Feel: How Emotions Affect the Practice of Medicine* (Boston: Beacon, 2013), 3.

21. Reynolds Price, *A Whole New Life: An Illness and a Healing* (New York: Atheneum, 1994), 184 (italics added).

22. *King Lear*, V.iii.307–308, in *The Riverside Shakespeare*.

23. See Victor Strandberg, "The Religious / Erotic Poetry of Reynolds Price," *Studies in the Literary Imagination* 35 (2002): 85.

24. Helen Fisher, *Why We Love: The Nature and Chemistry of Romantic Love* (New York: Henry Holt, 2004), 77–98. For a sociological account, see Eva Illouz, *Why Love Hurts* (Malden, Mass.: Polity, 2012).

25. Price, *Whole New Life*, 183.

26. Carol Levine, "One Loss May Hide Another," *Hastings Center Report* 34, no. 6 (2004): 19.

27. Arthur Kleinman, "Caregiving: The Odyssey of Becoming More Human," *The Lancet* 373 (2009): 293; and "Catastrophe and Caregiving: The Failure of Medicine as an Art," *The Lancet* 371 (2008): 22–23.

28. John Bayley, *Elegy for Iris* (New York: St. Martin's Press, 1999), 76.

29. See E. P. Thompson, "The Moral Economy of the English Crowd in the Eighteenth Century," *Past & Present*, 50 (1971): 76–136.

30. Georges Bataille, "The Notion of Expenditure" [1933], in *The Bataille Reader*, ed. Fred Botting and Scott Wilson (Oxford: Blackwell, 1997), 169.

31. Lore K. Wright, "The Impact of Alzheimer's Disease on the Marital Relationship," *The Gerontologist* 31 (1991): 224–237. For contrast, see Stacy Tessler Lindau, L. Phillip Schumm, Edward O. Laumann, Wendy Levinson, Colm A. O'Muircheartaigh, and Linda J. Waite, "A Study of Sexuality and Health among Older Adults in the United States," *New England Journal of Medicine* 357 (2007): 762–774.

32. William Carlos Williams, "The Use of Force" [1938], *The Doctor Stories*, comp. Robert Coles (New York: New Directions, 1984), 60.

33. Jean Baudrillard, *Seduction*, trans. Brian Singer (New York: St. Martin's Press, 1990; published in French in 1979), 34.

34. See Harold Schweizer, *On Waiting* (New York: Routledge, 2008).

35. W. H. Vanstone, *The Stature of Waiting* (London: Darton, Longman and Todd, 1982); and Henri J. M. Nouwen, *Adam: God's Beloved* (Maryknoll, N.Y.: Orbis, 1997).

36. For a values-based ethics, see Mark D. Bennett and Joan McIver Gibson, *A Field Guide to Good Decisions: Values in Action* (Westport, Conn.: Praeger, 2006).

37. Lisa Diedrich, "Conclusion: Toward an Ethics of Failure," in *Treatments: Language, Politics, and the Culture of Illness* (Minneapolis: University of Minnesota Press, 2007), 148–166.

38. Donnie McClurkin, "Stand," released September 25, 2007, under the Verity Label.

39. John Milton, Sonnet XVI ("When I consider how my light is spent"), in *The Shorter Poems*, ed. Barbara Kiefer Lewalski and Estelle Haan (Oxford: Oxford University Press, 2012), 245 (spelling normalized).

40. Aaron Alterra, *The Caregiver: A Life with Alzheimer's* (1999; repr., New York: Cornell University Press, 2007), 17. Aaron Alterra is the pen name for fiction writer E. S. Goldman.

41. Alterra, *The Caregiver*, 188. On presence, see Hans Ulrich Gumbrecht, *Production of Presence: What Meaning Cannot Convey* (Stanford, Calif.: Stanford University Press, 2004); on testimony, see Arthur W. Frank, *The Wounded Storyteller: Body, Illness, and Ethics*, 2nd ed. (Chicago: University of Chicago Press, 2013).

42. *World Alzheimer Report 2015: The Global Impact of Dementia* (London: Alzheimer's Disease International, 2015), 71. The figure includes aggregated direct and indirect "societal costs."

CHAPTER TWO · UNFORGETTING ASKLEPIOS: MEDICAL EROS AND ITS LINEAGE

Epigraph: William Blake, *The Marriage of Heaven and Hell* [1789-1790], in *The Complete Poetry and Prose of William Blake*, rev. ed., ed. David V. Erdman, commentary by Harold Bloom (Berkeley: University of California Press, 1982), 34 (plate three).

1. Euripides, "Hippolytus," in *Euripides II*, rev. ed., ed. and trans. David Kovacs (Cambridge, Mass.: Harvard University Press, 2005), ll. 540–542.

2. Apuleius, *The Golden Ass*, trans. P. G. Walsh (Oxford: Oxford University Press, 2008), 76 (IV.30).

3. Anne Carson, *Eros the Bittersweet* (1986; repr., Normal, Ill.: Dalkey Archive, 1998), 32.

4. *A Midsummer Night's Dream*, III.ii.115, in *The Riverside Shakespeare* (Boston: Houghton Mifflin Company, 1974). Subsequent quotations will be indicated in the text by act, scene, and line number (in parentheses).

5. See Ralph Jackson, *Doctors and Diseases in the Roman Empire* (Norman: University of Oklahoma Press, 1988), 142.

6. Darrell W. Amundsen, *Medicine, Society, and Faith in the Ancient and Medieval Worlds* (Baltimore: Johns Hopkins University Press, 1996), 146.

7. On Socrates' last words, see Glenn W. Most, "'A Cock for Asklepios,'" *Classical Quarterly* 43 (1993): 96–111.

8. P. Aelius Aristides, "An Address Regarding Asclepius," in *The Complete Works*, trans. Charles A. Behr, 2 vols. (Leiden: Brill, 1981), 2:247.

9. For the description of Anatole Broyard as a "fabled libertine," see Henry Louis Gates Jr., *Thirteen Ways of Looking at a Black Man* (New York: Random House, 1997), 196. Broyard insists—awkwardly—that "it was ultimately with girls' souls that I grappled"; see Anatole Broyard, *Kafka Was the Rage: A Greenwich Village Memoir* (New York: Carol Southern, 1993), 146.

10. Anatole Broyard, "Intoxicated by My Illness," in *Intoxicated by My Illness and Other Writings on Life and Death*, ed. Alexandra Broyard (New York: Clarkson Potter, 1992), 4. Subsequent quotations will be indicated in the text as *IMI*. The essay "Intoxicated by My Illness" first appeared in the *New York Times* in 1982.

11. On desire as discussed by classical thinkers who held the purpose of philosophy to be medicinal and therapeutic, see Martha C. Nussbaum, *The Therapy of Desire: Theory and Practice in Hellenistic Ethics* (Princeton, N.J.: Princeton University Press, 1994).

12. Carson, *Eros the Bittersweet*, 10, 37.

13. Chris Kraus, *I Love Dick* (1997; repr. Los Angeles: Semiotext[e]: 2006), 239.

14. Anatole Broyard, *Aroused by Books* (New York: Random House, 1974).

15. See John Hoberman, *Black and Blue: The Origins and Consequences of Medical Racism* (Berkeley: University of California Press, 2013).

16. Vivian Nutton, *Ancient Medicine*, 2nd ed. (New York: Routledge, 2013), 104. *Asklepios* is the Greek spelling; the Latin spelling *Asculapius* is regularly anglicized to *Asklepius*. All are in common usage. I follow the Greek spelling in my text, but retain each author's original usage in endnotes. See, above all, Emma J. Edelstein and Ludwig Edelstein in their monumental *Asclepius: Collection and Interpretation of the Testimonies* (1945; repr., Baltimore: Johns Hopkins University Press, 1998). I am also indebted to Gerald D. Hart, *Asclepius: The God of Medicine* (London: Royal Society of Medicine Press, 2000); and Sara B. Aleshire, *The Athenian Asklepieion: The People, Their Dedications, and The Inventories* (Amsterdam: Gieben, 1989).

17. Bronwen L. Wickkiser, *Asklepios, Medicine, and the Politics of Healing in Fifth-Century Greece: Between Craft and Cult* (Baltimore: Johns Hopkins University Press, 2008), 1.

18. Gary B. Ferngren, "Introduction," in Emma J. Edelstein and Ludwig Edelstein, *Asclepius: Collection and Interpretation of the Testimonies* (Baltimore: Johns Hopkins University Press, 1998), xviii. This book reprints the famous two-volume study by the Edelsteins published in 1945. Ferngren is summarizing claims argued by the Edelsteins.

19. James Longrigg, *Greek Medicine from the Heroic to the Hellenistic Age: A Source Book* (1998; repr., New York: Routledge, 2012), 1.

20. Roy Porter, *The Greatest Benefit to Mankind: A Medical History of Humanity* (New York: W. W. Norton, 1997), 7.

21. See Sarah Cant and Ursula Sharma, *A New Medical Pluralism?: Alternative Medicine, Doctors, Patients, and the State* (1999; repr., New York: Routledge, 2014); Ted J. Kaptchuk and David M. Eisenberg, "Varieties of Healing. 1: Medical Pluralism in the United States," *Annals of Internal Medicine* 135, no. 3 (2001): 189–195; and Charles Leslie, "Medical Pluralism in World Perspective," *Social Science & Medicine* 14B, no. 4 (1980): 191–195.

22. On ancient theories of dreaming, see Patricia Cox Miller, *Dreams in Late Antiquity: Studies in the Imagination of a Culture* (Princeton, N.J.: Princeton University Press, 1994). Wickkiser discusses the two-tier system of medicine in *Asklepios, Medicine, and the Politics of Healing*, 42–61.

23. Nutton, *Ancient Medicine*, 104 and 115.

24. See Hart, *Asclepius*, 12–15.

25. On representations of Hippocrates, see Jacques Jouanna, *Hippocrates*, trans. M. B. DeBevoise (1992; repr., Baltimore: Johns Hopkins University Press, 1999), 38–39.

26. "The Oath," in *Hippocratic Writings*, ed. G. E. R. Lloyd, trans. J. Chadwick and W. N. Mann (1978; repr., New York: Penguin, 1983), 67.

27. C. Kerényi, *Asklepios: Archetypal Image of the Physician's Existence*, trans. Ralph Mannheim (1947; repr., New York: Pantheon, 1959), 41.

28. Mabel L. Lang, *Cure and Cult in Ancient Corinth: A Guide to the Asklepieion* (Princeton, N.J.: American School of Classical Studies at Athens, 1977), 15, 22.

29. Rachel Naomi Remen, *Kitchen Table Wisdom: Stories That Heal* (New York: Riverhead, 1994), 164; and Pausanias, *Guide to Greece*, trans. Peter Levi, 2 vols. (New York: Penguin Books, 1971), 1:194 (ii.27.3). I am unable to identify Remen's source in Cicero.

30. Plato, *The Symposium*, trans. Christopher Gill (New York: Penguin Books, 1999), 18–19. Significantly, Gill cites as parallels two tracts from the Hippocratic corpus.

31. Rafael Campo, *The Desire to Heal: A Doctor's Education in Empathy, Identity, and Poetry* (New York: W. W. Norton, 1997), 13. Subsequent citations will be indicated in the text as *DH*.

32. Ariel Roguin, "Rene Theophile Hyacinthe Laënnec (1781–1826): The Man behind the Stethoscope," *Clinical Medicine and Research* 4, no. 3 (2008): 230–235.

33. Audre Lorde, *The Cancer Journals*, 2nd ed. (San Francisco: Aunt Lute, 1980). Subsequent citations will be indicated in the text as *CJ*. See also Audre Lorde, "Uses of the Erotic: The Erotic as Power" (1978), *Sister Outsider: Essays and Speeches* (1984; repr., Berkeley: Crossing Press, 2007), 53–59.

34. Virginia Woolf, *On Being Ill*, introduction by Hermione Lee (Ashfield, Mass.: Paris Press, 2002), 6–7. Subsequent citations will be indicated in the text as *OBI*. *On Being Ill* first appeared in 1926 as an essay in the journal *New Criterion*, edited by T. S. Eliot, and it went through minor revisions thereafter. The Paris Press edition closely replicates the 1930 Hogarth Press edition.

35. Martin Cutts, *Oxford Guide to Plain English*, 2nd ed. (New York: Oxford University Press, 2004), 19.

36. Richard Horton, *Health Wars: On the Global Front Lines of Modern Medicine* (New York: New York Review of Books, 2003), 58.

37. Aristotle in *Categories* 10 discusses the varieties of opposition, including the relation of contraries. See *The Complete Works of Aristotle: The Revised Oxford Translation*, ed. Jonathan Barnes, 2 vols. (Princeton, N.J.: Princeton University Press, 1984), 1:18–21.

38. In *The Complete Poems of D. H. Lawrence*, ed. Vivian de Sola Pinto and Warren Roberts (New York: Penguin Books, 1964), 620 (spelling normalized).

39. Richard Selzer, "The Exact Location of the Soul," in *Mortal Lessons: Notes on the Art of Surgery* (New York: Simon & Schuster, 1976), 18.

40. *The Oxford Illustrated Companion to Medicine*, 3rd ed., ed. Stephen Lock, John M. Last, and George Dunea (Oxford: Oxford University Press, 2001), 262.

41. American Medical Association, "The Symbol for a New AMA: Medicine for the 21st Century," *AMA News*, June 20, 2005, www.amednews.com/article/20050620/opinion/306209958/4/.

42. Jennifer Glaser, "Mortality Can Be a Powerful Aphrodisiac," *New York Times*, August 13, 2006, www.nytimes.com/2006/08/13/fashion/13love.html.

CHAPTER THREE · NOT-KNOWING: MEDICINE IN THE DARK

Epigraph: John Berryman, *77 Dream Songs* (New York: Farrar, Straus, 1964), 74 (no. 67).

1. Florida Scott-Maxwell, *The Measure of My Days* (1968; repr., New York: Penguin, 1979), 69–70. I am grateful to Professor Margaret A. Miller for this reference.

2. Centers for Disease Control and Prevention, "HIV among Older Americans," November 2013, www.cdc.gov/hiv/pdf/library_factsheet_HIV_%20AmongOlder Americans.pdf.

3. Larry J. Young and Zuoxin Wang, "The Neurobiology of Pair Bonding," *Nature Neuroscience* 7 (2004): 1048–1054.

4. Larry J. Young, "Love: Neuroscience Reveals All," *Nature* 457 (2009): 148; and Jarred Younger, Arthur Aron, Sara Parke, Neil Chatterjee, and Sean Mackey, "Viewing Pictures of a Romantic Partner Reduces Experimental Pain: Involvement of Neural Reward Systems," *PLoS One* 5 (2010), doi: 10.1371/journal.pone.0013309.

5. Slavoj Zizek, "The Swerve of the Real," in *Erotikon: Essays on Eros, Ancient and Modern*, ed. Shadi Bartsch and Thomas Bartscherer (Chicago: University of Chicago Press, 2005), 215.

6. William Carlos Williams, *Sappho: A Translation by William Carlos Williams* (San Francisco: Grabhorn, 1957). This single poem was printed separately as a broadside.

7. Williams, *Sappho*.

8. Kathryn Montgomery, *How Doctors Think: Clinical Judgment and the Practice of Medicine* (New York: Oxford University Press, 2006), 4–5, 49–51, and 86–90.

9. Atul Gawande, *Complications: A Surgeon's Notes on an Imperfect Science* (New York: Picador, 2003), 109, 110.

10. See Montgomery, *How Doctors Think*, and Jerome Groopman, *How Doctors Think* (Boston: Houghton Mifflin, 2007).

11. Don DeLillo, *Zero K* (New York: Scribner, 2016), 131.

12. In *The Letters of John Keats 1814–1821*, ed. Hyder Edward Rollins, 2 vols. (Cambridge, Mass.: Harvard University Press, 1958), 1:193 (21, 27 [?] December 1817).

13. Donald Barthelme, "Not-Knowing," in *Not-Knowing: The Essays and Interviews of Donald Barthleme*, ed. Kim Herzinger (New York: Random House, 1997), 11.

14. Paul Kalanithi, *When Breath Becomes Air* (New York: Random House, 2016), 170.

15. Nikolas Rose, *The Politics of Life Itself: Biomedicine, Power, and Subjectivity in the Twenty-First Century* (Princeton, N.J.: Princeton University Press, 2007), 7, 4.

16. See Tamar Sharon, *Human Nature in an Age of Biotechnology: The Case for Mediated Posthumanism* (New York: Springer, 2014).

17. Lori Arviso Alvord and Elizabeth Cohen Van Pelt, *The Scalpel and the Silver Bear* (New York: Bantam, 1999), 190.

18. Meghan O'Rourke, "Doctors Tell All and It's Far Worse Than You Think," *The Atlantic*, November 2014, www.theatlantic.com/magazine/archive/2014/11/doctors-tell -all-and-its-bad/380785/.

19. Eva S. Schernhammer and Graham A. Colditz, "Suicide Rates among Physicians: A Quantitative and Gender Assessment (Meta-Analysis)," *American Journal of Psychiatry* 161 (2004): 2295–2302. See also Niku K. Thomas, "Resident Burnout," *JAMA* 292 (2004): 2880–2889; and Elizabeth J. D'Amico, Susan M. Paddock, Audrey Burnam, and Fuan-Yue Kung, "Identification of and Guidance for Problem Drinking by General Medical Providers: Results from a National Survey," *Medical Care* 43 (2005): 229–236.

20. Alvord and Van Pelt, *Scalpel and the Silver Bear*, 190–191.

21. See, for example, Antonio R. Damasio, *Descartes' Error: Emotion, Reason, and the Human Brain* (New York: G. P. Putnam's Sons, 1994); Norman Doidge, *The Brain That Changes Itself: Stories of Personal Triumph from the Frontiers of Brain Science* (New York: Penguin, 2007); Jonah Lehrer, *How We Decide* (Boston: Houghton Mifflin Harcourt, 2009); and Sara Algoe and Jonathan Haidt, "Witnessing Excellence in Action: The 'Other-Praising' Emotions of Elevation, Gratitude, and Admiration," *Journal of Positive Psychology* 4 (2009): 105-127. On the neurobiology of moral action and decisions, see also Michael S. Gazzaniga, *The Ethical Brain* (New York: Dana Press, 2005).

22. See Joseph LeDoux, *The Emotional Brain: The Mysterious Underpinnings of Emotional Life* (New York: Simon & Schuster, 1996); and Daniel Goleman, *Emotional Intelligence* (New York: Bantam, 1995).

23. John Milton, *Paradise Lost* [1667], 2nd ed., rev. ed., ed. Alistair Fowler (London: Pearson Longman, 2007), I.250-251. See A. Roger Ekirch, *At Day's Close: Night in Time Past* (New York: W. W. Norton, 2006).

24. William Kentridge, *Six Drawing Lessons* (Cambridge, Mass.: Harvard University Press, 2014), 80.

25. Anna Steidle and Lioba Werth, "Freedom from Constraints: Darkness and Dim Illumination Promote Creativity," *Journal of Environmental Psychology* 35 (2013): 67-80.

26. Perri Klass, "When Doctors and Patients Speak a Different Language," in *A Not Entirely Benign Procedure: Four Years as a Medical Student* (New York: G. P. Putnam's Sons, 1987), 183.

27. Klass, "Baby Poop," in *A Not Entirely Benign Procedure*, 161.

28. E. L. Doctorow, "False Documents" [1977], in *E. L. Doctorow: Essays and Conversations*, ed. Richard Trenner (Princeton, N.J.: Ontario Review Press, 1983), 25, 26.

29. Tod Chambers, "From the Ethicist's Point of View: The Literary Nature of Ethical Inquiry," *Hastings Center Report* 26, no. 1 (1996): 25.

30. Didier Eribon, *Insult and the Making of the Gay Self*, trans. Michael Lucey, ed. Michèle Aina Barale, Jonathan Goldberg, Michael Moon, and Eve Kosofsky Sedgwick (1999; repr., Durham, N.C.: Duke University Press, 2004), 264, 265.

31. Michel Foucault, "Les Reportages d'idées," *Corriere della sera*, November 12, 1978, in Didier Eribon, *Michel Foucault*, trans. Betsy Wing (1989; repr., Cambridge, Mass.: Harvard University Press, 1991), 282. Eribon describes Foucault as a "militant intellectual" (210).

32. Quoted in Rux Martin, "Truth, Power, Self: An Interview with Michel Foucault," *Technologies of the Self*, ed. Luther H. Martin, Huck Gutman, and Patrick H. Hutton (Amherst: University of Massachusetts Press, 1988), 9.

33. John Cage, quoted in John Ashbery, "Cheering Up Our Knowing," *New York*, April 10, 1978, 69.

34. Richard Kearney, *On Stories* (New York: Routledge, 2002), 83.

35. David M. Eddy, "Variations in Physician Practice: The Role of Uncertainty" [1984], in *Professional Judgment: A Reader in Clinical Decision Making*, ed. Jack Dowie and Arthur Elstein (Cambridge: Cambridge University Press, 1988), 45. I owe this reference to Groopman, *How Doctors Think*.

36. Wendy Steiner, *The Scandal of Pleasure: Art in an Age of Fundamentalism* (Chicago: University of Chicago Press, 1995).

37. Oliver Sacks, *Musicophilia: Tales of Music and the Brain* (New York: Alfred A. Knopf, 2007). As Michiko Kakutani puts it, "In Dr. Sacks' view, music can aid aphasics and patients with parkinsonism, and it can help orient and anchor patients with advanced dementia because 'musical perception, musical sensibility, musical emotion and musical memory can survive long after other forms of memory have disappeared'" ("Power to Soothe the Savage Breast and Animate the Hemispheres," review of *Musicophilia: Tales of Music and the Brain*, by Oliver Sacks, *New York Times*, November 20, 2007, www.nytimes.com/2007/11/20/books/20kaku.html).

38. Stephen Nachmanovitch, *Free Play: Improvisation in Life and Art* (New York: Tarcher/Putnam, 1990), 43.

39. See Robin Wright, "Theatre of War: Sophocles' Message for American Veterans," *The New Yorker*, September 12, 2016, www.newyorker.com/culture/culture-desk/theatre-of-war-sophocles-message-for-american-veterans. I am grateful to Professor Marcia Childress for first calling my attention to Theater of War performances.

40. "Overview," Theater of War, *Outside the Wire*, www.outsidethewirellc.com/projects/theater-of-war/overview. For interpretations of *catharsis*, see *Aristotle's Poetics: A Translation and Commentary for Students of Literature*, trans. Leon Golden, commentary O. B. Hardison Jr. (Tallahassee: University of Florida Press, 1981), 114–120.

41. *A Midsummer Night's Dream*, IV.i.204–206, in *The Riverside Shakespeare* (Boston: Houghton Mifflin, 1974).

42. See the chapter entitled "Records and Progress Notes," in Brian N. Baird, *The Internship, Practicum, and Field Placement Handbook: A Guide for the Helping Professions*, 7th ed. (New York: Routledge, 2013). Baird includes the subsequent passage on prosecuting attorneys.

43. Wislawa Szymborska, "A Note," in *Monologue of a Dog: New Poems*, trans. Clare Cavanagh and Stanislaw Baranczak (New York: Harcourt, 2006), 79–81.

44. Wislawa Szymborska, "Nobel Lecture," December 7, 1996, in *Poems New and Collected 1957–1997*, trans. Stanislaw Baranczak and Clare Cavanagh (New York: Harcourt, 1998), xv, xvi.

45. Scott Fishman, M.D., quoted in Claudia Wallis, "The Right (and Wrong) Way to Treat Pain," *Time*, February 20, 2005, http://content.time.com/time/magazine/article/0,9171,1029836,00.html.

CHAPTER FOUR · VARIETIES OF EROTIC EXPERIENCE: FIVE ILLNESS NARRATIVES

Epigraph: William James, "Conclusions," in *The Varieties of Religious Experience: A Study in Human Nature* (New York: Random House, 1902), 492.

1. Arthur W. Frank, *The Wounded Storyteller: Body Illness, and Ethics*, 2nd ed. (Chicago: University of Chicago Press, 2013).

2. Anne Hunsaker Hawkins, *Reconstructing Illness: Studies in Pathography*, 2nd ed. (Lafayette, Ind.: Purdue University Press, 1999), 3.

3. Anonymous, "Our Family Secrets," *Annals of Internal Medicine* 163 (2015): 321. See also the accompanying editorial regarding the decision to publish (p. 320).

4. Abraham Verghese, "Medicine and Writing," in *Abraham Verghese: FAQ*, no date, http://abrahamverghese.mc2beta.com/home/faq/#Medicine%20and%20Writing.

5. See Arthur Kleinman, *The Illness Narratives: Suffering, Healing, and the Human Condition*, 2nd ed. (New York: Basic Books, 1992); Rita Charon, *Narrative Medicine: Honoring the Stories of Illness* (New York: Oxford University Press, 2006); Arthur W. Frank, *Letting Stories Breathe: A Socio-Narratology* (Chicago: University of Chicago Press, 2010); James W. Pennebaker, *Opening Up: The Healing Power of Expressing Emotions*, rev. ed. (1990; New York: Guilford, 1997); Richard G. Tedeschi and Lawrence G. Calhoun, "Posttraumatic Growth: Conceptual Foundations and Empirical Evidence," *Psychological Inquiry* 15, no. 1 (2004): 1–18. The second edition (2013) of Frank's *Wounded Storyteller* contains a valuable new preface that surveys work on illness and narrative over the preceding decade.

6. William Styron, *Darkness Visible: A Memoir of Madness* (New York: Random House, 1990), 64. Subsequent citations will be indicated in the text as *DV*.

7. Georges Bataille, *Erotism: Death and Sensuality*, trans. Mary Dalwood (San Francisco: City Lights Books, 1986), 11.

8. See National Institute of Mental Health, "Major Depression among Adults," no date, www.nimh.nih.gov/health/statistics/prevalence/major-depression-among-adults.html.

9. See Rita Charon, "Narrative Medicine: A Model for Empathy, Reflection, Profession, and Trust," *JAMA* 286, no. 15 (2001): 1897, 1898.

10. Rose Styron, "Strands," in *Unholy Ghost: Writers on Depression*, ed. Nell Casey (New York: HarperCollins, 2001), 133. Subsequent quotations will be indicated in the text as *S*.

11. Alexandra Styron, *Reading My Father: A Memoir* (New York: Scribner, 2011), 3. Subsequent quotations will be indicated in the text by *RMF*.

12. Sandra Butler and Barbara Rosenblum, *Cancer in Two Voices* (San Francisco: Spinsters Book Company, 1991), i. Subsequent citations will be indicated in the text as *CTV*.

13. Richard Kearney, *On Stories* (New York: Routledge, 2002), 5.

14. National Cancer Institute, "SEER Stat Fact Sheets: Female Breast Cancer" (Bethesda, Md.: National Cancer Institute), no date, http://seer.cancer.gov/statfacts/html/breast.html.

15. Stephanie Nolen, *28: Stories of AIDS in Africa* (New York: Walker & Company, 2007), 5. Subsequent quotations will be indicated in the text by *AA*. I am indebted to Nolen for facts and figures cited in my discussion.

16. See Desmond Tutu HIV Foundation, "Background," http://desmondtutuhivfoundation.org.za/about/background/.

17. For additional discussion, see Michael Battle, *Reconciliation: The Ubuntu Theology of Desmond Tutu*, rev. ed. (Cleveland: Pilgrim Press, 2009); and Christian B. N. Gade, "What Is Ubuntu? Different Interpretations among South Africans of African Descent," *South African Journal of Philosophy* 31 (2012): 484–503.

18. Desmond Tutu, "The Politics of Ubuntu," *Huffington Post*, June 10, 2014, www.huffingtonpost.com/desmond-tutu/the-politics-of-ubuntu_b_5125854.html.

19. See Kathryn Montgomery Hunter, *Doctors' Stories: The Narrative Structure of Medical Knowledge* (Princeton, N.J.: Princeton University Press, 1991).

20. Jean-Dominique Bauby, *The Diving Bell and the Butterfly: A Memoir of Life in Death*, trans. Jeremy Leggatt (1997; repr., New York: Random House, 1997), 9. Subsequent citations will be indicated in the text as *DB*.

21. William James, "Conclusions," in *Varieties of Religious Experience*, 492.

22. Eric J. Leed, *The Mind of the Traveler: From Gilgamesh to Global Tourism* (New York: Basic Books, 1991), 276.

23. Bill T. Jones, with Peggy Gillespie, *Last Night on Earth* (New York: Pantheon, 1995), 246. Subsequent citations will be indicated in the text as *LN*.

24. Judith Mackrell quoted in John O'Mahony, "Body Artist," *The Guardian*, June 11, 2004, www.theguardian.com/stage/2004/jun/12/dance.

25. Arlene Croce, "Discussing the Undiscussable" [1994], in *Writing in the Dark, Dancing in the New Yorker* (New York: Farrar, Straus and Giroux, 2000), 708. Croce's objections to (what she calls) "victim art" are badly outdated. See Tobin Siebers, *Disability Aesthetics* (Ann Arbor: University of Michigan Press, 2010).

26. In *Bill T. Jones: Still/Here* (1997), prod. Bill Moyers (New York: Films Media Group, 2006).

27. World Health Organization, "WHO Definition of Palliative Care," May 26, 2014, www.who.int/cancer/palliative/definition/en/.

28. David B. Morris, "Palliation: Shielding the Patient from the Assault of Symptoms," *Academy Update* 7, no. 3 (1997): 1ff; reprinted as "The Cloak and the Shield: A Thumbnail History of Palliation," in *Illness, Crisis, & Loss* 6, no. 2 (1998): 229–232.

29. Butler and Rosenblum, *Cancer in Two Voices*, 162.

30. Ezekiel J. Emanuel, "Cost Savings at the End of Life: What Do the Data Show?" *JAMA* 275 (1996): 1907–1914. See also Baohui Zhang, Alexi A. Wright, Haiden A. Huskamp, Matthew E. Nilsson, Matthew L. Maciejewski, et al., "Health Care Costs in the Last Week of Life: Associations with End-of-Life Conversations," *Archives of Internal Medicine* 169 (2009): 480–488.

31. See the essays collected in *Dying Well: The Prospect for Growth at the End of Life*, ed. Ira Byock (New York: Riverhead, 1997). For a general introduction to palliative care, see *Hospice and Palliative Care: Concepts and Practice*, ed. Denice C. Sheehan and Walter B. Forman (Sudbury, Mass.: Jones and Bartlett, 1996).

32. David Barnard, Anna Towers, Patricia Boston, and Yanna Lambrinidou, *Crossing Over: Narratives of Palliative Care* (New York: Oxford University Press, 2000), 14. On the need for new options, see Angelo E. Volandes, *The Conversation: A Revolutionary Plan for End-of-Life Care* (New York: Bloomsbury, 2015).

33. Oliver Sacks, *Gratitude* (New York: Alfred A. Knopf, 2016). Sacks's medical circumstances, during the period of composition, are described in a foreword to *Gratitude* by Kate Edgar and Bill Hayes.

CHAPTER FIVE · EROS MODIGLIANI: ASSENTING TO LIFE

Epigraph: Georges Bataille, *Erotism: Death and Sensuality*, trans. Mary Dalwood (San Francisco: City Lights Books, 1986), 17: "*L'action décisive est la mise à nu.*"

1. Jacques Lipchitz, "Amedeo Modigliani," in *Modigliani* (New York: Harry N. Abrams, 1953), 5.

2. Jean Cocteau, *My Contemporaries*, ed. and trans. Margaret Crosland (1935; repr., Philadelphia: Chilton, 1968), 69.

3. Jean Cocteau, "Preface," in Franco Russoli, *Modigliani* (New York: Harry N. Abrams, 1959), 9.

4. Lipchitz, "Amedeo Modigliani," 6 ("une vie brève mais intense").

5. Another version reads "Cover him with flowers"; see Charles Douglas, *Artist Quarter: Reminiscences of Montmartre and Montparnasse in the First Two Decades of the Twentieth Century* (London: Faber and Faber, 1941), 300. "Charles Douglas" is the pen name for coauthors Charles Beadle and Douglas Goldring.

6. Douglas, *Artist Quarter*, 301.

7. Robert Hughes, "And Now the Nudes," *The Guardian*, June 10, 2004, www.theguardian.com/artanddesign/2004/jun/10/art.

8. Aaron Smith, "Modigliani's 'Reclining Nude' Sells for $170 Million at Christie's," *CNN Money*, November 10, 2015, http://money.cnn.com/2015/11/09/luxury/reclining-nude-modigliani-christies/index.html?iid=ob_article_footer.

9. Quoted in Douglas, *Artist Quarter*, 112. On Picasso's changing costumes, see Dan Franck, *Bohemian Paris: Picasso, Modigliani, Matisse, and the Birth of Modern Art*, trans. Cynthia Hope Liebow (1998; repr., New York: Grove, 2001), 72.

10. Ilya Ehrenburg, *People and Life 1891–1921*, trans. Anna Bostock and Yvonne Kapp (New York: Alfred A. Knopf, 1962), 152.

11. Gertrude Stein, *Paris France* (New York: Charles Scribner's Sons, 1940), 11.

12. Marevna Vorobëv, *Life in Two Worlds*, trans. Benet Nash (New York: Abelard-Schuman, 1962), 157. See also Douglas, *Artist Quarter*, 98; and Nina Hamnett, *Laughing Torso: Reminiscences of Nina Hamnett* (1932; repr., London: Virago, 1984), 54.

13. Herbert Lottman, *Man Ray's Montparnasse* (New York: Harry N. Abrams, 2001), 33.

14. Cocteau, "Preface," in Russoli, *Modigliani*, 10.

15. "*Je suis Modigliani. Juif*" (quoted in Douglas, *Artist Quarter*, 211).

16. Ehrenburg, *People and Life*, 154–155.

17. Quoted in Meryle Secrest, *Modigliani: A Life* (New York: Alfred A. Knopf, 2011), 165. Survage (1879–1968) is of complicated Russian-Danish-Finnish descent, and his surname has numerous ethnic spellings.

18. In Douglas, *Artist Quarter*, 87, 201.

19. Douglas, *Artist Quarter*, 203.

20. Cocteau, "Preface," in Russoli, *Modigliani*, 10.

21. Quoted in Pierre Sichel, *Modigliani: A Biography of Amedeo Modigliani* (New York: Dutton, 1967), 295.

22. Kenneth Clark, *The Nude: A Study in Ideal Form* (Princeton, N.J.: Princeton University Press, 1956); see chapter 1 ("The Naked and the Nude").

23. Lynda Nead, *The Female Nude: Art, Obscenity and Sexuality* (New York: Routledge, 1992), 16.

24. Giorgio Agamben, "Nudity," in *Nudities*, trans. David Kishik and Stefan Pedatella (Stanford, Calif.: Stanford University Press, 2011), 55–90.

25. Francis Carco, *The Last Bohemia, from Montmartre to the Quartier Latin*, trans. Madeleine Elise Reynier Boyd (New York: H. Holt, 1928), 237.

26. Meryle Secrest identifies this passage—inscribed on the back of a painting—as from Italian novelist Gabriele D'Annunzio (1863–1938), a Modigliani favorite (*Modigliani: A Life*, 167).

27. Douglas, *Artist Quarter*, 227. The unnamed speaker—a "poet friend"—is likely Max Jacob.

28. In Douglas, *Artist Quarter*, 194.

29. Lipchitz, "Amedeo Modigliani," 2.

30. Umberto Boccioni, Carlo Carrá, Luigi Russolo, Giacomo Ball, and Gino Severini, "Futurist Painting: Technical Manifesto 1910," in *Futurist Manifestos*, ed. Umbro Apollonio, trans. Robert Brain, R. W. Flint, J. C. Higgitt, and Caroline Tisdall (1970; repr., New York: Viking, 1973), 30–31. See also, F. T. Marinetti, "The Founding and Manifesto of Futurism 1909," in *Futurist Manifestos*, 19–24.

31. André Salmon, quoted in Douglas, *Artist Quarter*, 202.

32. Picasso, quoted in Jean Clair, "The School of Darkness," in *Picasso Érotique*, ed. Jean Clair (New York: Prestel, 2001), 14.

33. Douglas, *Artist Quarter*, 107–108.

34. Tsuguharu Foujita, quoted in Sichel, *Modigliani*, 407.

35. *The Education of a French Model: Kiki's Memoirs*, trans. Samuel Putnam, introduced by Ernest Hemingway (1930; repr., New York: Belmont, 1962), 36. First published in English as *The Education of a French Model: The Loves, Cares, Cartoons and Caricatures of Alice Prin*, trans. Samuel Putnam (New York: Boar's Head Books, 1950); and in French as *Les souvenirs de Kiki* (Paris: H. Broca, 1929).

36. Anne Carson, *Eros the Bittersweet* (1986; repr., Normal, Ill.: Dalkey Archive, 1998), 12–17.

37. Bataille, *Erotism*, 17.

38. In Douglas, *Artist Quarter*, 260.

39. Franck, *Bohemian Paris*, 23.

40. Archibald MacLeish, "Ars Poetica," in *Collected Poems 1917–1982* (Boston: Houghton Mifflin, 1985).

41. Philip Roth, *The Dying Animal* (Boston: Houghton Mifflin, 2001), 98.

42. Ehrenburg, *People and Life*, 154–155.

43. Franck, *Bohemian Paris*, 181.

44. See Holger Afflerback, "The Topos of Improbable War in Europe before 1914," in *An Improbable War?: The Outbreak of World War I and European Culture before 1914*, ed. Holger Afflerback and David Stevenson (Oxford: Oxford University Press, 2007), 161–182; and Christopher Clark, *The Sleepwalkers: How Europe Went to War in 1914* (New York: Harper, 2012), 562.

45. On socialists as "bald-headed parrots," see Ehrenburg, *People and Life*, 199; on Modigliani as a "violent pacifist," see Douglas, *Artist Quarter*, 268–269.

46. Modris Eksteins, *Rites of Spring: The Great War and the Birth of the Modern Age* (Boston: Houghton Mifflin, 1989), 144.

47. Quoted in Secrest, *Modigliani: A Life*, 166–167.

48. Charles Baudelaire, *Artificial Paradises*, trans. Stacy Diamond (1860; repr., New York: Citadel Press, 1996), 29.

49. Jean Cocteau, *Opium: The Diary of a Cure*, trans. Margaret Crosland and Sinclair Road, rev. ed. (1930; repr., London: Peter Owen, 1968), 66.

50. *The Education of a French Model: Kiki's Memoirs*, 41.

51. Secrest, *Modigliani: A Life*, 184.

52. Douglas, *Artist Quarter*, 123.

53. Secrest, *Modigliani: A Life*, 298.

54. Douglas, *Artist Quarter*, 258, 122.

55. Ehrenburg, *People and Life*, 156–157.

56. Cocteau, *My Contemporaries*, 56.

57. See Wassily Kandinsky, *Concerning the Spiritual in Art*, trans. M. T. H. Sadler (1911; repr., New York: Dover, 1977), 38.

58. Philip Ball, *Bright Earth: Art and the Invention of Color* (New York: Farrar, Straus and Giroux, 2002), 176.

59. Quoted by Russoli, *Modigliani*, 33 ("Mais, monsieur, je n'aime pas les fesses").

60. Cocteau, *My Contemporaries*, 57.

61. Ehrenburg, *People and Life*, 157–158.

CHAPTER SIX · THE INFINITE FACES OF PAIN: EROS AND ETHICS

Epigraph: "Grace and Clarity" [1944], in *Silence: Lectures and Writings by John Cage* (Middleton, Conn.: Wesleyan University Press, 1961), 93.

1. See Kay L. Larson, *Where the Heart Beats: John Cage, Zen Buddhism, and the Inner Life of Artists* (New York: Penguin, 2012); and John Russon, "Self and Suffering in Buddhism and Phenomenology: Existential Pain, Compassion and the Problems of Institutional Healthcare," *Cultural Ontology of the Self in Pain*, ed. Siby K. George and P. G. Jung (New York: Springer, 2016), 181–195.

2. Cage, "Grace and Clarity," 95.

3. Institute of Medicine, *Relieving Pain in America: A Blueprint for Transforming Prevention, Care, Education, and Research* (Washington, D.C.: National Academies Press, 2011), 1.

4. Richard L. Nahin, "Estimates of Pain Prevalence and Severity in Adults: United States, 2012," *Journal of Pain* 16, no. 8 (2015): 769–780.

5. Institute of Medicine, *Relieving Pain in America*, 1.

6. See David B. Morris, *The Culture of Pain* (Berkeley: University of California Press, 1991); and "Sociocultural Dimensions of Pain Management," in *Bonica's Management of Pain*, 4th ed., ed. Jane C. Ballantyne, James P. Rathmell, and Scott M. Fishman (New York: Lippincott Williams & Wilkins, 2010), 133–145; also *Pain and its Transformations: The Interface of Biology and Culture*, ed. Sarah Coakley and Kay Kaufman Shelemay (Cambridge, Mass.: Harvard University Press, 2008).

7. David Mikics, *A New Handbook of Literary Terms* (New Haven, Conn.: Yale University Press, 2010), 156.

8. Elaine Scarry, *The Body in Pain: The Making and Unmaking of the World* (New York: Oxford University Press, 1985), 11; quotations that follow refer to the introduction (pp. 3–23).

9. See Ronald Melzack, "The McGill Pain Questionnaire: Major Properties and Scoring Methods," *Pain* 1, no. 3 (1975): 277–299.

10. Virginia Woolf, *On Being Ill*, introduction by Hermione Lee (Ashfield, Mass.: Paris Press, 2002), 6–7. As noted previously, *On Being Ill* first appeared as an essay in 1926.

11. David Biro, *The Language of Pain: Finding Words, Compassion, and Relief* (New York: W. W. Norton, 2010), 12, 20. See also David Biro, *One Hundred Days: My Unexpected Journey from Doctor to Patient* (New York: Pantheon, 2000).

12. SUPPORT Principal Investigators, "A Controlled Trial to Improve Care for Seriously Ill Hospitalized Patients," *JAMA* 274 (1995): 1591–1598.

13. John D. Loeser, "What Is Chronic Pain?," *Theoretical Medicine* 12 (1991): 215, 216.

14. *Classification of Chronic Pain*, 2nd ed., ed. Harold Merskey and Nikolai Bogduk (1994; repr., Seattle: IASP Press, 2002), 210.

15. Timothy L. Bayer, Paul E. Baer, and Charles Early, "Situational and Psychophysiological Factors in Psychologically Induced Pain," *Pain* 44 (1991): 45–50.

16. See, in order of reference, David A. Williams and Beverly E. Thorn, "An Empirical Assessment of Pain Beliefs," *Pain* 36 (1989): 351–358; David A. Williams, "Acute Pain Management," in *Psychological Approaches to Pain Management: A Practitioner's Handbook*, ed. Robert J. Gatchel and Dennis C. Turk (New York: Guilford, 1996), 55–77; David A. Williams and Francis J. Keefe, "Pain Beliefs and the Use of Cognitive-Behavioral Coping Strategies, *Pain* 46 (1991): 185–190; Mark P. Jensen and Paul Karoly, "Pain-Specific Beliefs, Perceived Symptom Severity, and Adjustment to Chronic Pain," *Clinical Journal of Pain* 8 (1992): 123–130; Michael S. Shutty Jr., Douglas E. DeGood, and Diane H. Tuttle, "Chronic Pain Patients' Beliefs about their Pain and Treatment Outcomes," *Archives of Physical Medicine and Rehabilitation* 71 (1990): 128–132.

17. Lous Heshusius, *Inside Chronic Pain: An Intimate and Critical Account* (Ithaca, N.Y.: Cornell University Press, 2009). Subsequent citations will be indicated in the text as *ICP*.

18. R. H. Gracely, M. E. Geisser, T. Giesecke, M. A. B. Grant, F. Petzke, et al., "Pain Catastrophizing and Neural Responses to Pain among Persons with Fibromyalgia," *Brain* 127, no. 4 (2004): 835–843.

19. Timothy D. Wilson, *Redirect: The Surprising New Science of Psychological Change* (New York: Little, Brown, 2011).

20. Daniel B. Carr and Ylisabyth S. Bradshaw, "Time to Flip the Pain Curriculum?" *Anesthesiology* 120 (2014): 1–3.

21. See, in order of reference, Henriët van Middendorp, Mark A. Lumley, Johannes W. G. Jacobs, Johannes W. J. Bijlsma, and Rinie Greenen, "The Effects of Anger and Sadness on Clinical Pain Reports and Experimentally-Induced Pain Thresholds in Women with and without Fibromyalgia," *Arthritis Care & Research* 62 (2010): 1370–1376; William Breitbart, Barry D. Rosenfeld, Steven D. Passik, Margaret V. McDonald, Howard Thaler, and Russell K. Portenoy, "The Undertreatment of Pain in Ambulatory AIDS Patients," *Pain* 65 (1996): 243–249; Roger B. Fillingim, Christopher D. King, Margarete C. Ribeiro-Dasilva, Bridgett Rahim-Williams, and Joseph L. Riley III, "Sex, Gender, and Pain: A Review of Recent Clinical and Experimental Findings," *Journal of Pain* 10 (2009): 447–485; Anita M. Unruh, "Gender Variations in Clinical Pain Ex-

perience," *Pain* 65 (1996): 123–167; Maryann S. Bates, W. Thomas Edwards, and Karen O. Anderson, "Ethnocultural Influences on Variation in Chronic Pain Perception," *Pain* 52 (1993): 101–112; and Steven F. Brena, Steven H. Sanders, and Hiroshi Motoyama, "American and Japanese Chronic Low Back Pain Patients: Cross-Cultural Similarities and Differences," *Clinical Journal of Pain* 6 (1990): 118–124.

22. Sean Mackey, quoted in Tara Parker-Pope, "Love and Pain Relief," *New York Times*, October 13, 2010.

23. Jill Bolte Taylor, *My Stroke of Insight: A Brain Scientist's Personal Journey* (New York: Viking, 2006), 151.

24. See William Hirstein, *Brain Fiction: Self-Deception and the Riddle of Confabulation* (Cambridge, Mass.: MIT Press, 2005), 5: "There is also a clear connection here to the human gift for storytelling."

25. Roland Barthes, *The Pleasure of the Text*, trans. Richard Miller (1973; repr., New York: Hill and Wang, 1975).

26. Arthur W. Frank, *The Wounded Storyteller: Body, Illness, and Ethics*, 2nd ed. (Chicago: University of Chicago Press, 2013), 23–25.

27. Quoted in Keith H. Basso, *Wisdom Sits in Places: Landscape and Language among the Western Apache* (Albuquerque: University of New Mexico Press, 1996), 59.

28. Jean-François Lyotard and Jean-Loup Thébaud, *Just Gaming*, trans. Wlad Godzich (Minneapolis: University of Minnesota Press, 1985), 32–35.

29. Robert Coles, *The Call of Stories: Teaching and the Moral Imagination* (Boston: Houghton Mifflin, 1989).

30. Mark Johnson, *Moral Imagination: Implications of Cognitive Science for Ethics* (Chicago: University of Chicago Press, 1993), 11.

31. See, for example, *Narrative Ethics: The Role of Stories in Bioethics*, ed. Martha Montello, *Hastings Center Report* 44, no. 1 (2014): S2–S44; *Stories Matter: The Role of Narrative in Medical Ethics*, ed. Rita Charon and Martha Montello (New York: Routledge, 2002); Tod Chambers, *The Fiction of Bioethics: Cases as Literary Texts* (New York: Routledge, 1999); *Stories and Their Limits: Narrative Approaches to Bioethics*, ed. Hilde Lindemann Nelson (New York: Routledge, 1997); Sally Gaddow, "Relational Narrative: The Postmodern Turn in Nursing Ethics," *Scholarly Inquiry for Nursing Practice* 13, no. 1 (1999): 57–69; Adam Zachary Newton, *Narrative Ethics* (Cambridge, Mass.: Harvard University Press, 1995); and William J. Ellos, *Narrative Ethics* (Avebury, UK: Ashgate, 1994).

32. Emily Dickinson, *The Complete Poems of Emily Dickinson*, ed. Thomas H. Johnson (Boston: Little, Brown, 1960), no. 650.

33. My account is based on Robert Pear, "Mothers on Medicaid Overcharged for Pain Relief," *New York Times*, March 8, 1999, www.nytimes.com/1999/03/08/us/mothers-on -medicaid-overcharged-for-pain-relief.html.

34. Harald Schrader and Diana Obelieniene, "Natural Evolution of Late Whiplash Syndrome outside the Medicolegal Context," *The Lancet* 347 (1996): 1207–1211.

35. George Mendelson, "Compensation and Chronic Pain," *Pain* 48 (1992): 121–123; and Robert W. Teasell, "Compensation and Chronic Pain," *Clinical Journal of Pain* 17 (2001): S46–S51.

36. *Back Pain in the Workplace: Management of Disability in Nonspecific Conditions: A Report of the Task Force on Pain in the Workplace of the International Association for the Study of Pain*, ed. Wilbert E. Fordyce (Seattle: IASP Press, 1995), xiii.

37. Ben A. Rich, "A Legacy of Silence: Bioethics and the Culture of Pain," *Journal of Medical Humanities* 18 (1997): 233–259.

38. Fiona Stockard, "Painkiller Addiction Facts and Statistics," Lighthouse Recovery Institute, http://lighthouserecoveryinstitute.com/painkiller-addiction-facts/.

39. Centers for Disease Control and Prevention, "Today's Heroin Epidemic," July 7, 2015, www.cdc.gov/vitalsigns/heroin/.

40. Peter M. Grace, Keith A. Strand, Erika L. Galer, Daniel J. Urban, Xiaohui Wang, et al., "Morphine Paradoxically Prolongs Neuropathic Pain in Rats by Amplifying Spinal NLRP3 Inflammasome Activation," *Proceedings of the National Academy of Sciences of the United States of America* 113, no. 24 (2016): E3441–E3450.

41. Art Van Zee, "The Promotion and Marketing of OxyContin: Commercial Triumph, Public Health Tragedy," *American Journal of Public Health* 99, no. 2 (2009): 221–222.

42. Richard Kearney, *On Stories* (New York: Routledge, 2002), 91–117.

43. Carmen R. Green, Karen O. Anderson, Tamara A. Baker, Lisa C. Campbell, Sheila Decker, et al., "The Unequal Burden of Pain: Confronting Racial and Ethnic Disparities in Pain," *Pain Medicine* 4, no. 3 (2003): 277–294; and Sophie Trawalter, Kelly M. Hoffman, and Adam Waytz, "Racial Bias in Perceptions of Others' Pain," PLoS ONE 7, no. 11 (2012), http://journals.plos.org/plosone/article?id=10.1371/journal.pone.0048546.

44. Joan Stephenson, "Experts Say AIDS Pain 'Dramatically Undertreated,'" *JAMA* 276 (1996): 1369–1370.

45. Raymond Tait, quoted in Abby Goodnough, "Minorities Seeking Pain Relief Are Shortchanged in Treatment," *New York Times*, August 10, 2016. See Raymond C. Tait, John T. Chibnall, Elena M. Anderson, and Nortin M. Hadler, "Management of Occupational Back Injuries: Differences among African Americans and Caucasians," *Pain* 112 (2004): 389–396; and Raymond C. Tait and John T. Chibnall, "Racial/Ethnic Disparities in the Assessment and Treatment of Pain," *American Psychologist* 69 (2014): 131–141.

46. Knox H. Todd, "Influence of Ethnicity on Emergency Department Pain Management," *Emergency Medicine* 13 (2001): 274–278; Salimah H. Meghani, Eeeseung Byun, and Rollin M. Gallagher, "Time to Take Stock: A Meta-Analysis and Systematic Review of Analgesic Treatment Disparities for Pain in the United States," *Pain Medicine* 13 (2012): 150–174.

47. R. Sean Morrison, Sylvan Wallenstein, Dana K. Natale, Richard S. Senzel, and Lo-Li Huang, "'We Don't Carry That'—Failure of Pharmacies in Predominantly Nonwhite Neighborhoods to Stock Opioid Analgesics," *New England Journal of Medicine* 342 (2000): 1023–1026; and Anthony DePalma, "In Mexico, Pain Relief Is a Medical and Political Issue," *New York Times*, June 19, 1996, www.nytimes.com/1996/06/19/world/in-mexico-pain-relief-is-a-medical-and-political-issue.html.

48. Roger B. Fillingim, "Individual Differences in Pain Responses," *Current Rheumatology Reports* 7, no. 5 (2005): 342–347; Zsuzsanna Wiesenfeld-Hallin, "Sex Differences in Pain Perception," *Gender Medicine* 2, no. 3 (2005): 137–145; and Catherine J. Binkley,

Abbie Beacham, William Neace, Ronald G. Gregg, Edwin B. Liem, and Daniel I. Sessler, "Genetic Variations Associated with Red Hair Color and Fear of Dental Pain, Anxiety Regarding Dental Care and Avoidance of Dental Care," *Journal of the American Dental Association* 140 (2009): 896–905.

49. *The Great Moment*, dir. Preston Sturges (1944; repr., Universal City, Calif.: Universal, 2006), DVD. The screenplay (entitled *Triumph over Pain*) is available in *Four More Screenplays by Preston Sturges*, introduction by Brian Henderson (Berkeley: University of California Press, 1995). Paramount edited Sturges's film before its release. See René Fülöp-Miller, *Triumph over Pain*, trans. Eden and Cedar Paul (New York: The Literary Guild of America, 1938); and Susan Sontag, *Regarding the Pain of Others* (New York: Farrar, Straus and Giroux, 2003).

50. Edmund D. Pellegrino, "Emerging Ethical Issues in Palliative Care," *JAMA* 279 (1998): 1521.

51. Antonio R. Damasio, *Descartes' Error: Emotion, Reason, and the Human Brain* (New York: G. P. Putnam's Sons, 1994), 34–51.

52. Rafael Campo, *The Desire to Heal: A Doctor's Education in Empathy, Identity, and Poetry* (New York: W. W. Norton, 1997), 132.

53. Emanuel Levinas, *Ethics and Infinity: Conversations with Philippe Nemo*, trans. Richard A. Cohen (1982; repr., Pittsburgh: Duquesne University Press, 1985), 87.

54. Levinas, *Ethics and Infinity*, 87; and Emmanuel Levinas, *Totality and Infinity: An Essay on Exteriority*, trans. Alphonso Lingis (1961; repr., Pittsburgh: Duquesne University Press, 1969), 201, containing a section titled "Ethics and the Face" (pp. 194–219).

CHAPTER SEVEN · BLACK SWAN SYNDROME: PROBABLE IMPROBABILITIES

Epigraph: Richard Dawkins, *The Blind Watchmaker: Why the Evidence of Evolution Reveals a Universe without Design* (New York: W. W. Norton, 1986), 317.

1. "The Oath of Maimonides," in S. Y. Tan and M. E. Yeow, "Moses Maimonides (1135–1204): Rabbi, Philosopher, Physician," *Singapore Medical Journal* 43, no. 11 (2002): 551–553.

2. Guy B. Faquet, *The War on Cancer: An Anatomy of Failure, A Blueprint for the Future* (New York: Springer, 2008), 109.

3. Ian Hacking, *The Emergence of Probability: A Philosophical Study of Early Ideas about Probability, Induction and Statistical Inference* (1975; repr., Cambridge: Cambridge University Press, 1978), 11.

4. "Angelina Jolie Cancer Surgery: Actress to Have Another Procedure to Prevent Disease," *Huffington Post*, March 13, 2014, www.huffingtonpost.com/2014/03/13/angelina -jolie-cancer-surgery_n_4954496.html.

5. Angelina Jolie Pitt, "Angelina Jolie Pitt: Diary of a Surgery," *New York Times*, March 24, 2015, www.nytimes.com/2015/03/24/opinion/angelina-jolie-pitt-diary-of-a-surgery.html.

6. Elizabeth Wurtzel, "The Breast Cancer Gene and Me," *New York Times*, September 27, 2015, www.nytimes.com/2015/09/27/opinion/sunday/elizabeth-wurtzel-the-breast -cancer-gene-and-me.html.

7. Nassim Nicholas Taleb, *The Black Swan: The Impact of the Highly Improbable*, 2nd ed. (New York: Random House, 2010); see also *Fooled by Randomness: The Hidden Role of Chance in Life and in the Markets*, 2nd ed. (New York: Random House, 2005).

8. Taleb, *Black Swan*, 7.

9. See Leo Hickman, "How Algorithms Rule the World," *The Guardian*, July 1, 2013, www.theguardian.com/science/2013/jul01/how-algorithms-rule-the-world-nsa; and Thomas E. Kottke and Courtney Jordan Baechler, "An Algorithm that Identifies Coronary and Heart Failure Events in the Electronic Health Record," *Preventing Chronic Disease*, February 28, 2013, doi: http://dx.doi.org/10.5888/pcd10.120097.

10. See Alan Hájek, "Interpretations of Probability," in *The Stanford Encyclopedia of Philosophy*, ed. Edward N. Zalta (Stanford, Calif.: Metaphysics Research Lab, Center for the Study of Language and Information, December 19, 2011, revision), http://plato.stanford.edu/entries/probability-interpret/.

11. Joan Didion, *The Year of Magical Thinking* (New York: Alfred A. Knopf, 2005), 3 (italics in the original).

12. Didion, *Year of Magical Thinking*, 27.

13. David Lewis-Williams, *The Mind in the Cave: Consciousness and the Origins of Art* (London: Thames & Hudson, 2002), 124–126.

14. William James, "Mysticism," in *The Varieties of Religious Experience: A Study in Human Nature* (New York: Random House, 1902), 378–379.

15. Didion, *Year of Magical Thinking*, 42.

16. Leslie Jamison, *The Empathy Exams: Essays* (Minneapolis: Greywolf, 2014), 1.

17. Cristian Tomasetti and Bert Vogelstein, "Variations in Cancer Risk among Tissues Can Be Explained by the Number of Cell Divisions," *Science*, 347, no. 6217 (2015): 78–81. See "Most Types of Cancer Largely Down to Bad Luck Rather Than Lifestyle or Genes," *The Guardian*, January 1, 2015, www.theguardian.com/society/2015/jan/01/two-thirds-cancer-cases-caused-bad-luck-lifestyle-genes.

18. Taleb, *Black Swan*, xxiii.

19. Quoted in Margaret Plews-Ogan, Justine E. Owens, and Natalie May, *Choosing Wisdom: Strategies and Inspiration for Growing through Life-Changing Difficulties* (Philadelphia: Templeton, 2012), 45.

20. Institute of Medicine, *To Err Is Human: Building a Safer Health System* (Washington, D.C.: National Academy Press, 1999); Jawahar Kalra, Natasha Kalra, and Nick Baniak, "Medical Error, Disclosure and Patient Safety: A Global View of Quality Care," *Clinical Biochemistry* 46, nos. 13–14 (2013): 1161–1169; and Martin Makary and Michael Daniel, "Medical Error—The Third Leading Cause of Death in the US," *BMJ*, May 3, 2016, doi: http://dx.doi.org/10.1136/bmj.i2139.

21. Plews-Ogan, Owens, and May, *Choosing Wisdom*, 45.

22. Danielle Ofri, *What Doctors Feel: How Emotions Affect the Practice of Medicine* (Boston: Beacon, 2013), 131.

23. Stephen Jay Gould, "The Median Isn't the Message," *Discover Magazine* 6 (June 1985): 40–42.

24. Alex Cipriano, "The 7 Most Bizarrely Unlucky People Who Ever Lived," *Cracked*, June 1, 2009, www.cracked.com/article_17416_the-7-most-bizarrely-unlucky-people-who-ever-lived.html.

25. Centers for Disease Control and Prevention, "Heart Disease Facts," August 10, 2015, www.cdc.gov/HeartDisease/facts.htm.

26. V. S. Ramachandran, *The Tell-Tale Brain: Unlocking the Mystery of Human Nature* (New York: Windmill, 2011), 232.

27. Rachel Naomi Remen, *Kitchen Table Wisdom: Stories That Heal* (New York: Riverhead, 1996), 247.

28. See Guy Lyon Playfair, *Twin Telepathy*, 2nd ed. (Gloucestershire, UK: History Press, 2008), xiv.

29. Nate Silver, *The Signal and the Noise: Why So Many Predictions Fail—But Some Don't* (New York: Penguin, 2012).

30. David M. Eisenberg, Roger B. Davis, Susan L. Ettner, Scott Appel, Sonja Wilkey, et al., "Trends in Alternative Medicine Use in the United States, 1990–1997: Results of a Follow-up National Survey," *JAMA* 280 (1998): 1569–1575; David Eisenberg and Catherine Woteki, *Exploring Complementary and Alternative Medicine* (Washington, D.C.: National Academies Press, 2003); and Hilary A. Tindle, Roger B. Davis, Russell S. Phillips, and David M. Eisenberg, "Trends in Use of Complementary and Alternative Medicine by US Adults: 1997–2002," *Alternative Therapies in Health and Medicine* 11 (2005): 42–49.

31. Francis S. Collins, "NIH Complementary and Integrative Health Agency Gets New Name," *NIH News & Events*, December 17, 2014, www.nih.gov/news-events/news -releases/nih-complementary-integrative-health-agency-gets-new-name.

32. National Center for Complementary and Integrative Health, "The Use of Complementary and Alternative Medicine in the United States: Cost Data," January 4, 2016, https://nccih.nih.gov/news/camstats/costs/costdatafs.htm.

33. Bernard D. Beitman, *Connecting with Coincidence: The New Science for Using Synchronicity and Serendipity in Your Life* (Deerfield Beach, Fla.: Health Communications, 2016).

34. Jean-Dominique Bauby, *The Diving Bell and the Butterfly: A Memoir of Life in Death*, trans. Jeremy Leggatt (New York: Random House, 1997), 17.

35. Anne Louise Germaine de Staël, Letter to Juliette Récamier (1810), in J. Christopher Herold, *Mistress to an Age: A Life of Madame de Staël* (Indianapolis: Bobbs-Merrill, 1958), 401.

36. Charles Perrow, *Normal Accidents: Living with High-Risk Technologies* (New York: Basic Books, 1984), 11.

37. Erik B. Schelbert, Jie J. Cao, Sigurdur Sigurdsson, Thor Aspelund, Peter Kellman, et al., "Prevalence and Prognosis of Unrecognized Myocardial Infarction Determined by Cardiac Magnetic Resonance in Older Adults," *JAMA* 308 (2012): 890–897.

38. Centers for Disease Control and Prevention, "Ehrlichiosis: Statistics and Epidemiology," September 5, 2013, www.cdc.gov/Ehrlichiosis/stats/. See also, Barbara Fouts Flicek, "Rickettsial and Other Tick-Borne Infections," *Critical Care Nursing Clinics of North America* 19 (2007): 27–38.

39. Warren H. Cole, "Efforts to Explain Spontaneous Regression of Cancer," *Journal of Surgical Oncology* 17, no. 3 (1981): 201–209.

40. Andrew Weil, *Spontaneous Healing: How to Discover and Enhance Your Body's Natural Ability to Maintain and Heal Itself* (New York: Alfred A. Knopf, 1995); and Jacalyn

Duffin, *Medical Miracles: Doctors, Saints, and Healing in the Modern World* (Oxford: Oxford University Press, 2009).

41. Atul Gawande, "The Bell Curve: What Happens When Patients Find Out How Good Their Doctors Really Are?," *The New Yorker*, December 6, 2004, www.newyorker .com/magazine/2004/12/06/the-bell-curve.

42. Milton DeLugg and Willie Stein, "Orange Colored Sky" (New York: Frank Music Corp., 1950). It was first recorded in 1950 with Janet Brace singing; in 1950 it also became a *Billboard* hit song when recorded by Nat "King" Cole.

CHAPTER EIGHT · LIGHT AS ENVIRONMENT: HOW *NOT* TO LOVE NATURE

Epigraph: Joseph Warton, "The Enthusiast, Or The Lover of Nature" [1744], in *English Poetry of the Mid and Late Eighteenth Century*, ed. Ricardo Quintana and Alvin Whitley (New York: Alfred A. Knopf, 1963). Warton's reference to *enthusiasm* still carried its earlier religious connotation as "possession by a god" (Greek *en=within* and *theos=god*).

1. Cheryl Keenan, "Thousands Affected by 'Once-in-a-Millennium' Flooding," *The Lafayette Tribune*, June 27, 2016, www.fayettetribune.com/news/thousands-affected-by -once-in-a-millennium-flooding/article_c5d3d3ce-3c1d-11e6-bcbe-ef7611dd6cfd.html.

2. René Descartes, *Discourse on the Method of Rightly Conducting One's Reason and of Seeking Truth in the Sciences* [1637], ed. and trans. Charles W. Eliot, Harvard Classics (New York: Collier, 1909–1914), part vi (*"maîtres et possesseurs de la nature"*). On the gendering of the natural world, a persistent theme in ecofeminism, see Carolyn Merchant, *The Death of Nature: Women, Ecology, and the Scientific Revolution* (New York: Harper & Row, 1980).

3. Terry Tempest Williams and Mary Frank, *Desert Quartet: An Erotic Landscape* (New York: Pantheon, 1995), 3. Frank provides illustrations.

4. Terry Tempest Williams, "The Erotics of Place," *Whole Earth* 91 (Winter 1997), 53–54, reprinted from *An Unspoken Hunger: Stories from the Field* (New York: Pantheon, 1994). See also Sarah McFarland Taylor, "Land as Lover: Mormon Eco-Eroticism and Planetary Plural Marriage in the Work of Terry Tempest Williams," *Nova Religio: The Journal of Alternative Religions* 8, no. 1 (2004): 39–56.

5. Williams and Frank, *Desert Quartet*, 10.

6. Kim Levin, "The Eye of Ra," *Light in Art*, ed. Thomas B. Hess and John Ashbery (New York: Collier, 1969), 21–36. See also Erik Hornung, *Akhenaten and the Religion of Light* [1995], trans. David Lorton (Ithaca, N.Y.: Cornell University Press, 1999).

7. See Patrik Reuterswärd, "What Color Is Divine Light?" in *Light in Art*, ed. Hess and Ashbery, 101–124.

8. Albert Einstein, quoted in Emil Wolf, "Einstein's Researches on the Nature of Light," *Optics News* 5 (1979): 24.

9. Ralph Baierlein, *Newton to Einstein: The Trail of Light: An Excursion to the Wave-Particle Duality and the Special Theory of Relativity* (Cambridge: Cambridge University Press, 1992), 170.

10. See Sidney Perkowitz, *Empire of Light: A History of Discovery in Science and Art* (Washington, D.C.: Joseph Henry, 1996), 19–39; Arthur Zajonic, *Catching the Light: The*

Entwined History of Light and Mind (New York: Bantam, 1993); and David Park, *The Fire within the Eye: A Historical Essay on the Nature and Meaning of Light* (Princeton, N.J.: Princeton University Press, 1997).

11. Quoted in Elaine Pagels, *The Gnostic Gospels* (New York: Random House, 1979), 120.

12. Jodi Magness, "Illuminating Byzantine Jerusalem: Oil Lamps Shed Light on Early Christian Worship," *Biblical Archaeology Review* 24, no. 2 (1998): 42.

13. Wolfgang Schivelbusch, *Disenchanted Night: The Industrialization of Light in the Nineteenth Century* [1983], trans. Angela Davies (1988; repr., Berkeley: University of California Press, 1995), 124–126. Also see Ruth G. Sikes, "The History of Suntanning: A Love/Hate Affair," *Journal of Aesthetic Science* 1, no. 2 (1998): 1–7; and Ferenc Morton Szasz, *The Day the Sun Rose Twice: The Story of the Trinity Site Nuclear Explosion, July 16, 1945* (Albuquerque: University of New Mexico Press, 1984).

14. Eviatar Nevo, *Mosaic Evolution of Subterranean Mammals: Regression, Progression, and Global Convergence* (New York: Oxford University Press, 1999); and, in a review of Nevo, Hynek Burda, "Light from Underground," *Nature* 402 (1999): 725.

15. J. Lawson Dick, *Rickets: A Study of Economic Conditions and Their Effects on the Health of the Nation* (London: Heinemann, 1922), 3, 91.

16. See, for example, Michael J. Lillyquist, *Sunlight and Health* (New York: Dodd, Mead, 1985).

17. J. A. Parrish, "The Scope of Photomedicine," *The Science of Photomedicine*, ed. James D. Regan and John A. Parrish (New York: Plenum, 1982), 6.

18. Natalie Angier, "Do Races Differ? Not Really, Genes Show," *New York Times*, August 22, 2000, www.nytimes.com/2000/08/22/science/do-races-differ-not-really -genes-show.html. See also Alan H. Goodman, "Why Genes Don't Count (for Racial Differences in Health)," *American Journal of Public Health* 90, no. 11 (2000): 1699–1702.

19. See *Physiology and Pharmacology of Biological Rhythms*, ed. Peter H. Redfern and Björn Lemmer (New York: Springer-Verlag, 1997); *Biological Clocks: Mechanisms and Applications*, ed. Yvan Touitou (New York: Elsevier, 1998); and *Biologic Effects of Light 2001: Proceedings of a Symposium*, ed. Michael F. Holick (Boston: Kluwer Academic, 2002).

20. Robert Y. Moore, "The Organization of the Human Circadian Timing System," *The Human Hypothalamus in Health and Disease*, ed. D. F. Swaab, M. A. Hofman, M. Mirmiran, et al. (New York: Elsevier, 1992), 101–115.

21. *Biological Rhythms in Clinical and Laboratory Medicine*, ed. Y. Touitou and E. Haus (New York: Springer-Verlag, 1992).

22. H. J. Lynch, M. H. Deng, and R. J. Wurtman, "Indirect Effects of Light: Ecological and Ethological Considerations," *Annals of the New York Academy of Sciences* 453 (1985), 231–241.

23. Gregory M. Brown, "Light, Melatonin and the Sleep-Wake Cycle," *Journal of Psychiatry and Neuroscience* 19 (1994): 345–353.

24. Karen T. Stewart, Benita C. Hayes, and Charmane I. Eastman, "Light Treatment for NASA Shiftworkers," *Chronobiology International* 12 (1995): 141–151.

25. Norman E. Rosenthal, David A. Sack, J. Christian Gillin, Alfred J. Lewy, Frederick K. Goodwin, et al., "Seasonal Affective Disorder: A Description of the Syndrome and

Preliminary Findings with Light Therapy," *Archives of General Psychiatry* 41 (1984): 72–80.

26. Dan G. Blazer, Ronald C. Kessler, and Marvin S. Swartz, "Epidemiology of Recurrent Major and Minor Depression with a Seasonal Pattern: The National Comorbidity Survey," *British Journal of Psychiatry* 172 (1998): 164–167; C. I. Eastman, M. A. Young, and L. F. Fogg, "A Comparison of Two Different Placebo-Controlled SAD Light Treatment Studies," *Light and Biological Rhythms in Man*, ed. L. Wetterberg (New York: Pergamon, 1993), 371–383; and Michael Terman, Jiuan Su Terman, and Donald C. Ross, "A Controlled Trial of Timed Bright Light and Negative Air Ionization for Treatment of Winter Depression," *Archives of General Psychiatry* 55 (1998): 875–882. See also *Seasonal Affective Disorder and Beyond: Light Treatment for SAD and Non-SAD Conditions*, ed. Raymond W. Lam (Washington, D.C.: American Psychiatric Press, 1998).

27. Dan A. Oren, Marek Koziorowski, and Paul H. Desan, "SAD and the Not-So-Single Photoreceptors," *American Journal of Psychiatry* 170 (2013): 1403. See also Melissa Lee Phillips, "Of Owls, Larks and Alarm Clocks," *Nature* 458 (2009): 142–145.

28. Kathleen M. Beauchemin and Peter Hays, "Sunny Hospital Rooms Expedite Recovery from Severe and Refractory Depressions," *Journal of Affective Disorders* 40 (1996): 49–51.

29. Jeff Hecht and Dick Teresi, *Laser: Light of a Million Uses* (1982; repr., Mineola, N.Y.: Dover, 1998), 6. My account of lasers is indebted to Hecht and Teresi.

30. Gero Miesenböck, "The Optogenetic Catechism," *Science* 326 (2009): 395. For the use of optogenetics in research on pain, see Shrivats Mohan Iyer, Kate L. Montgomery, Chris Towne, Soo Yeun Lee, Charu Ramakrishnan, et al., "Virally Mediated Optogenetic Excitation and Inhibition of Pain in Freely Moving Nontransgenic Mice," *Nature Biotechnology* 32 (2014): 274–278. On optogenetics and memory, see Ewen Callaway, "Flashes of Light Show How Memories Are Made," *Nature.com*, June 2, 2014, www.nature.com/news/flashes-of-light-show-how-memories-are-made-1.15330.

31. Eliane A. Lucassen, Claudia P. Coomans, Maaike van Putten, Suzanne R. de Kreij, Jasper H. L. T. van Genugten, et al., "Environmental 24-hr Cycles Are Essential for Health," *Current Biology* 26 (2016): 1843–1853.

32. Marion Kuhn, Elias Wolf, Jonathan G. Maier, Florian Mainberger, Bernd Feige, et al., "Sleep Recalibrates Homeostatic and Associative Synaptic Plasticity in the Human Cortex," *Nature Communications*, August 23, 2016, doi: 10.1038/ncomms12455.

33. I closely follow John J. DiGiovanna, "Xeroderma Pigmentosum: A Model of Accelerated Photodamage," *Photodamage*, ed. Barbara A. Gilchrest (Cambridge, Mass.: Blackwell Science, 1995), 157–167.

34. National Institutes of Health, "Xeroderma pigmentosum," June 7, 2016, https://ghr.nlm.nih.gov/condition/xeroderma-pigmentosum; and "What Really Has a 1 in a Million Chance?," www.stat.berkeley.edu/~aldous/Real-World/million.html.

35. Quoted in Eraldo Peres, "Rare Disease Afflicts Brazilian Village," May 6, 2014, http://medicalxpress.com/news/2014-05-rare-disease-afflicts-brazilian-village.html.

36. Anne B. Britt, "Plant Biology: An Unbearable Beating by Light?," *Nature* 406 (2000): 30–31; and Paul R. Bergstresser, "Immediate and Delayed Effects of UVR on Immune Responses in Skin," in *Photodamage*, 81–99.

37. Susan Solomon, Diane J. Ivy, Doug Kinnison, Michael J. Mills, Ryan R. Neely III, and Anja Schmidt, "Emergence of Healing in the Antarctic Ozone Layer," *Science*, June 30, 2016, doi: 10.1126/science.aae0061.

38. Shannon C. Harrison and Wilma F. Bergfeld, "Ultraviolet Light and Skin Cancer in Athletes," *Sports Health* 1 (2009): 335–340. See also Dallas R. English, Bruce K. Armstrong, Anne Kricker, and Claire Fleming, "Sunlight and Cancer," *Cancer Causes and Control* 8 (1997): 271–283; Avril D. Woodhead, Richard B. Setlow, and Michiko Tanaka, "Environmental Factors in Nonmelanoma and Melanoma Skin Cancer," *Journal of Epidemiology* 9 (1999): S102–S114; and Frederick Urbach, "Ultraviolet Radiation and Skin Cancer," *Topics in Photomedicine*, ed. Kendric C. Smith (New York: Plenum, 1984), 39–142.

39. See Allen Guttmann, *The Erotic in Sports* (New York: Columbia University Press, 1996); Thomas F. Scanlon, *Eros and Greek Athletics* (New York: Oxford University Press, 2002); and Alain Fleischer, *Éros / Hercule: Pour une érotique du sport* (Paris: La Musardine / l'Attrape-corps, 2005).

40. World Wildlife Fund, *Living Blue Planet Report: Species, Habitats, and Human Well-Being* (Gland, Switzerland: WWF International, 2015), 2.

41. Steven C. Sherwood, Sandrine Bony, and Jean-Louis Dufresne, "Spread in Model Climate Sensitivity Traced to Atmospheric Convective Mixing," *Nature* 505 (2014): 376–343; Benjamin H. Strauss, Scott Kulp, and Anders Levermann, "Carbon Choices Determine US Cities Committed to Futures Below Sea Level," *Proceedings of the National Academy of Sciences* 112 (2015): 13508–13513.

42. James Lovelock, *The Ages of Gaia: A Biography of Our Living Earth*, rev. ed. (New York: W. W. Norton, 1995). The Gaia Hypothesis, in Lovelock's *Gaia: A New Look at Life on Earth* (New York: Oxford University Press, 1982), postulated that biota "regulate" the surface of the earth. *The Ages of Gaia* adds a description of the earth as a "*self-regulating* super-organism": "I now see the system of the material Earth and the living organisms on it, evolving so that self-regulation is an emergent property" (pp. 19–20).

43. Lovelock, *Ages of Gaia*, 30.

44. U.S. Environmental Protection Agency, "Climate Impacts on Human Health," www3 .epa.gov/climatechange/impacts/health.html. See also the National Center for Environmental Assessment, *Review of the Impacts of Climate Variability and Change on Aeroallergens and Their Associated Effects*, EPA / 600 / R-06/164F (Washington, D.C.: Office of Research and Development, EPA, August 2008).

45. Ralph Waldo Emerson, "Nature," in *Essays and Lectures*, ed. Joel Porte (New York: Library of America, 1983), 28 (chapter 5). On an ethics of biocentrism, see Paul W. Taylor, *Respect for Nature: A Theory of Environmental Ethics* (Princeton, N.J.: Princeton University Press, 1986).

46. International Energy Agency, "Solar Energy Perspectives: Executive Summary," 2011, www.iea.org/Textbase/npsum/solar2011SUM.pdf.

47. Maria Neira, "Climate Change: An Opportunity for Public Health," *Specimen News*, September 14, 2014, https://web.archive.org/web/20151007195114/http://specimennews .com/2015/10/07/climate-change-an-opportunity-for-public-health/. Dr. Neira is director of the Department of Public Health, Environmental and Social Determinants of Health—at the World Health Organization.

48. *Explaining Ocean Warming: Causes, Scale, Effects and Consequences*, ed. J. M. Baxter and Daniel D'A. Laffoley (Gland, Switzerland: IUCN, 2016); "Soaring Ocean Temperature is 'Greatest Hidden Challenge of our Generation,'" *The Guardian*, September 5, 2016, www.theguardian.com/environment/2016/sep/05/soaring-ocean-temperature -is-greatest-hidden-challenge-of-our-generation; and Paul Watson, "If the Oceans Die, We All Die!," September 29, 2015, www.seashepherd.org/commentary-and-editorials /2015/09/29/if-the-ocean-dies-we-all-die-741.

49. Quoted in "James Turrell: Interview by Esa Laaksonen," *Architectural Design* 68, nos. 7–8 (1997): 77. See also the interview with Turrell by Martin Gayford, "Seeing the Light," *Modern Painters* 13, no. 4 (2000): 26–30.

50. Ezra Pound, *ABC of Reading* (New York: New Directions, 1960), 73.

51. See Amanda Petrusich, "Fear of the Light: Why We Need Darkness," *The Guardian*, August 23, 2016, www.theguardian.com/environment/2016/aug/23/why-we-need -darkness-light-pollution-stars.

52. Quoted in "Turrell: Interview by Esa Laaksonen," 78.

53. James Turrell, quoted in Alison de Lima Greene, "As It Is, Infinite: *The Work of James Turrell,*" *James Turrell: A Retrospective*, ed. Michael Govan and Christine Y. Kim (Los Angeles: Los Angeles County Museum of Art, 2013), 127.

54. Turrell, quoted in Michael Govan, "Inner Light: The Radical Reality of James Turrell," *Turrell: A Retrospective*, 13.

55. Mark C. Taylor, *Refiguring the Spiritual: Beuys, Barney, Turrell, Goldsworthy* (New York: Columbia University Press, 2012), 117; and Stuart A. Kauffman, *Reinventing the Sacred: A New View of Science, Reason, and Religion* (New York: Basic Books, 2008).

56. *Oxford Textbook of Spirituality in Healthcare*, ed. Mark Cobb, Christina M. Puchlaski, and Bruce Rumbold (Oxford: Oxford University Press, 2012).

57. Thomas Nashe, "A Litany in Time of Plague," www.poets.org/poetsorg/poem/litany -time-plague. The lyric first appeared in Nashe's play *Summer's Last Will and Testament*, performed in the autumn of 1592. "The Choice of Valentines" circulated in manuscript.

58. Gowri Anandarajah and Ellen Hight, "Spirituality and Medical Practice: Using the HOPE Questions as a Practical Tool for Spiritual Assessment," *American Family Physician* 63 (2001): 81–89.

59. Peter Speck, Irene Higginson, and Julia Addington-Hall, "Spiritual Needs in Health Care: May Be Distinct from Religious Ones and Are Integral to Palliative Care," *BMJ* 329 (2004): 123.

60. Rachel Naomi Remen, *Kitchen Table Wisdom: Stories That Heal* (New York: Riverhead Books, 1996), 164.

61. Cynthia A. Moe-Lobeda, *Resisting Structural Evil: Love as Ecological-Economic Vocation* (Minneapolis: Fortress, 2013), 165–299. On social power as it affects health, see Paul Farmer, *Pathologies of Power: Health, Human Rights, and the New War on the Poor* (Berkeley: University of California Press, 2003).

62. Matilda Coxe Stevenson, *The Zuñi Indians: Their Mythology, Esoteric Fraternities, and Ceremonies*, 23rd Annual Report of the Bureau of American Ethnology (Washington, D.C.: U.S. Government Printing Office, 1904), 293.

63. Ruth L. Bunzel, *Zuñi Ceremonialism* (1932; repr., Albuquerque: University of New Mexico Press, 1992), 635. See also M. W. Stirling, "Concepts of the Sun among Amer-

ican Indians," *Smithsonian Report for 1945* (Washington, D.C.: Smithsonian Institution, 1945), 387–400.

64. Peter Schulte, Laia Alegret, Ignacio Arenillas, José A. Arz, Penny J. Barton, et al., "The Chicxulub Asteroid Impact and Mass Extinction at the Cretaceous-Paleogene Boundary," *Science* 327 (2010): 214–218. (Note that this article has forty international coauthors.) See also N. R. Longrich, J. Scriberas, and M. A. Wills, "Severe Extinction and Rapid Recovery of Mammals across the Cretaceous-Palaeogene Boundary, and the Effects of Rarity on Patterns of Extinction and Recovery," *Journal of Evolutionary Biology* 29, no. 8 (2016): 1495–1512.

65. Jean-Dominique Bauby, *The Diving Bell and the Butterfly*, trans. Jeremy Leggatt (New York: Knopf, 1997), 28–29.

CHAPTER NINE · THE SPARK OF LIFE: APPEARANCES/DISAPPEARANCES

Epigraph: Walt Whitman, *Leaves of Grass* (Brooklyn, N.Y., 1855), 17. In Whitman's many revisions, this long poem is retitled "Song of Myself." This passage too is later revised, very slightly.

1. See Alice Munro, "The Bear Came over the Mountain," in *Hateship, Friendship, Courtship, Loveship, Marriage* (New York: Alfred A. Knopf, 2001), 276.

2. Hans-Georg Gadamer, *The Enigma of Health: The Art of Healing in a Scientific Age*, trans. Jason Gaiger and Nicholas Walker (Stanford, Calif.: Stanford University Press, 1996), 96. *Verborgenheit* is a key term in the philosophy of Martin Heidegger, with whom Gadamer studied, and refers to *concealment* or *hiddenness*, which Heidegger associates with the concept of Being.

3. See, for example, Bindu Kalesan, Clare French, Jeffrey A. Fagan, Dennis L. Fowler, and Sandro Galea, "Firearm-Related Hospitalizations and In-Hospital Mortality in the United States, 2000–2010," *American Journal of Epidemiology* 179 (2014): 303–312; Carl E. Fisher and Jeffrey A. Lieberman, "Getting the Facts Straight about Gun Violence and Mental Illness: Putting Compassion before Fear," *Annals of Internal Medicine* 159 (2013): 423–424; and Mike Mitka, "Firearm-Related Hospitalizations: 20 US Children, Teens Daily," *JAMA* 311 (2014): 664. For a comprehensive view, see the American Psychological Association, *Gun Violence: Prediction, Prevention, and Policy* (2013), www.apa.org/pubs/info/reports/gun-violence-prevention.aspx.

4. Alice W. Flaherty, *The Midnight Disease: The Drive to Write, Writer's Block, and the Creative Brain* (New York: Houghton Mifflin, 2004), 2.

5. Quoted by Teresa Wiltz, "The Operating Room Is Her Studio," *Chicago Tribune*, December 4, 1998, http://articles.chicagotribune.com/1998-12-04/features/9812040380 _1_plastic-surgeon-french-orlan.

6. See Carl Elliott and Peter D. Kramer, *Better Than Well: American Medicine Meets the American Dream* (New York: W. W. Norton, 2003).

7. See David Hilfiker, *Not All of Us Are Saints: A Doctor's Journey with the Poor* (New York: Ballantine, 1996).

8. Wallace Stevens, "The Poems of Our Climate" [1938], in *The Palm at the End of the Mind: Selected Poems and a Play*, ed. Holly Stevens (New York: Alfred A. Knopf, 1971).

9. See Tobin Siebers, *Disability Aesthetics* (Ann Arbor: University of Michigan Press, 2010); and, for its indispensable overview, *The Disability Studies Reader*, 4th ed., ed. Lennard J. Davis (New York: Routledge, 2013)—with a fifth edition on the horizon.

10. Jo Spence, *Putting Myself in the Picture: A Political, Personal and Photographic Autobiography* (London: Camden, 1986), 83. See Terry Dennett, "The Wounded Photographer: The Genesis of Jo Spence's Camera Therapy," *Afterimage* 29, no. 3 (2001): 26–27; and Susan E. Bell, "Photo Images: Jo Spence's Narratives of Living with Illness," *Health: An Interdisciplinary Journal for the Social Study of Health, Illness and Medicine* 6, no. 1 (2002): 5–30.

11. World Health Organization, *Constitution of the World Health Organization*, 45th ed., supplement (October 2006), www.who.int/governance/eb/who_constitution_en.pdf.

12. Global Burden of Disease Study 2013 Collaborators, "Global, Regional, and National Incidence, Prevalence, and Years Lived with Disability for 301 Acute and Chronic Diseases and Injuries in 188 Countries, 1990–2013: A Systematic Analysis for the *Global Burden of Disease Study 2013*," *The Lancet* 386: 743–800. See also *Against Health: How Health Became the New Morality*, ed. Jonathan M. Metzl and Anna Kirkland (New York: New York University Press, 2010).

13. Metzl and Kirkland, eds., *Against Health*.

14. René Girard, *Violence and the Sacred*, trans. Patrick Gregory (1972; repr., Baltimore: Johns Hopkins University Press, 1977), 262.

15. Eric Trump, "My Illness, the Third Partner in Our Relationship," *New York Times*, April 24, 2014, www.nytimes.com/2014/04/27/fashion/Modern-Love-My-Illness-the -Third-Partner-in-Our-Relationship.html.

16. Girard, *Violence and the Sacred*, 37.

17. Gadamer, *Enigma of Health*, 164.

18. Gadamer, *Enigma of Health*, 164.

19. Perri Klass, *Love and Modern Medicine* (Boston: Houghton Mifflin, 2001). Subsequent citations will be indicated in the text as *LMM*.

20. Centers for Disease Control and Prevention, "About SUID and SIDS," June 8, 2016, www.cdc.gov/sids/aboutsuidandsids.htm.

21. Terry Tempest Williams, *Finding Beauty in a Broken World* (New York: Pantheon, 2008), 29.

22. Anne Carson, *Nox* (New York: New Directions, 2009).

23. Ben Ratliff, "Lamentation," review of *Nox*, by Anne Carson, *New York Times*, June 11, 2010, www.nytimes.com/2010/06/13/books/review/Ratliff-t.html.

24. Rachel Deahl, "How E-book Sales Compare to Print . . . So Far," *Publishers Weekly*, November 1, 2010, www.publishersweekly.com/pw/by-topic/digital/content-and -e-books/article/45015-how-e-book-sales-compare-to-print-so-far.html.

25. Anne Carson, *Economy of the Unlost (Reading Simonides of Keos with Paul Celan)* (Princeton, N.J.: Princeton University Press, 1999), 82.

26. Carson, *Economy of the Unlost*, 121.

27. David Rieff, *Swimming in a Sea of Death: A Son's Memoir* (New York: Simon & Schuster, 2008), 5.

28. Paul Virilio, *The Aesthetics of Disappearance*, trans. Philip Beitchman (Los Angeles: Semiotext[e], 2009), 19.

29. Anne Carson, *Eros the Bittersweet* (1986; repr., Normal, Ill.: Dalkey Archive, 1998), 109.

30. Carson, *Eros the Bittersweet*, 171.

31. Carson, *Eros the Bittersweet*, 171.

32. Anne Carson, quoted in Sam Anderson, "The Inscrutable Brilliance of Anne Carson," *New York Times Magazine*, March 14, 2013, www.nytimes.com/2013/03/17/magazine/the -inscrutable-brilliance-of-anne-carson.html.

33. Michel Foucault, "Les Reportages d'idées," *Corriere della sera*, November 12, 1978, in Didier Eribon, *Michel Foucault*, trans. Betsy Wing (1989; repr., Cambridge, Mass.: Harvard University Press, 1991), 282.

34. *A Midsummer Night's Dream*, V.i.324–325, in *The Riverside Shakespeare* (Boston: Houghton Mifflin, 1974).

CONCLUSION: ALTERED STATES

Epigraph: Stephen Nachmanovitch, *Free Play: Improvisation in Life and Art* (New York: Tarcher/Putnam, 1990), 163.

1. See Anne Nadakavukaren, *Our Global Environment: A Health Perspective*, 7th ed. (Long Grove, Ill.: Waveland, 2011); *Illness and the Environment: A Reader in Contested Medicine*, ed. Steve Kroll-Smith, Phil Brown, and Valerie J. Gunter (New York: New York University Press, 2000); and *Critical Condition: Human Health and the Environment*, ed. Eric Chivian, Michael McCally, Howard Hu, and Andrew Haines (Cambridge, Mass.: MIT Press, 1993).

2. National Cancer Institute, "Harms of Smoking and Health Benefits of Quitting," December 3, 2014, www.cancer.gov/about-cancer/causes-prevention/risk/tobacco /cessation-fact-sheet.

3. William Blake, Preface to *Milton: A Poem in 2 Books* [ca. 1804–1810], in *The Complete Poetry and Prose of William Blake*, rev. ed., ed. David V. Erdman, commentary by Harold Bloom (Berkeley: University of California Press, 1982), 95.

4. Steve Jobs, "'You've Got to Find What You Love,' Jobs Says," Stanford University Commencement Address on June 12, 2005, *Stanford News*, June 14, 2005, http://news .stanford.edu/2005/06/14/jobs-061505/.

5. Blake, "The Marriage of Heaven and Hell" [1789–1790], in *Complete Poetry and Prose*, 39 (plate 14).

6. Mike Jay, *High Society: The Central Role of Mind-Altering Drugs in History, Science and Culture* (Rochester, Vt.: Park Street, 2010).

7. National Institute on Drug Abuse, "Trends and Statistics," August 2015, www .drugabuse.gov/related-topics/trends-statistics.

8. "15 Things Apple Could Buy with Its $137B Cash Reserve," *ZD Net*, February 10, 2013, www.zdnet.com/pictures/15-things-apple-could-buy-with-its-137b-cash-reserve/.

9. National Institute on Drug Abuse, "Overdose Death Rates," December 2015, www .drugabuse.gov/related-topics/trends-statistics/overdose-death-rates.

10. Aldous Huxley, *The Doors of Perception*, in *The Doors of Perception and Heaven and Hell* (1954; repr., New York: Harper Colophon, 1963), 12. Subsequent citations will be indicated in the text as *DP*.

11. Sarah Bakewell, *At the Existentialist Café: Freedom, Being, and Apricot Cocktails* (New York: Other Press, 2016), 99.

12. Richard Branson, "The War on Drugs Has Failed, So Let's Shut It Down," *Huffington Post*, August 3, 2014, www.huffingtonpost.com/richard-branson/the-war-on-drugs-has -fail_1_b_5439312.html.

13. "U.S. Prison Population Declined One Percent in 2014," Bureau of Justice Statistics, September 17, 2015, www.bjs.gov/content/pub/press/p14pr.cfm.

14. Georges Bataille, *Erotism: Death and Sensuality*, trans. Mary Dalwood (1957; repr., San Francisco: City Lights Books, 1986), 17 (*la structure de l'être fermé*).

15. Susan Sontag, *Illness as Metaphor* (New York: Farrar, Straus and Giroux, 1978), 3.

16. "Michael Jackson Requested Propofol Long before Death, Says Doctor," *CBS News*, August 29, 2013, www.cbsnews.com/news/michael-jackson-requested-propofol-long -before-death-says-doctor/.

17. Gillian Rose, *Love's Work* (London: Chatto & Windus, 1995), 72.

18. Joan Didion, *The Year of Magical Thinking* (New York: Alfred A. Knopf, 2005), 107, 183–184.

19. Virginia Woolf, *On Being Ill* (1926), introduction by Hermione Lee (Ashfield, Mass.: Paris Press, 2002), 6.

20. Quoted in Margaret Plews-Ogan, Justine E. Owens, and Natalie May, *Choosing Wisdom: Strategies and Inspiration for Growing Through Life-Changing Difficulties* (Philadelphia: Templeton Press, 2012), 46.

21. Edith Turner, *Communitas: The Anthropology of Collective Joy* (New York: Palgrave Macmillan, 2011).

22. Joy E. Corey with Mark Sanford, *Divine Eros: A Timeless Perspective on Homosexuality* (La Vergne, Tenn.: Lightning Source, 2014), 113.

23. See Sunil Kripalani, Jada Bussey-Jones, Mara G. Katz, and Inginia Genao, "A Prescription for Cultural Competence in Medicine," *Journal of General Internal Medicine* 21, no. 10 (2006): 1116–1120.

24. Michel Foucault, *The Government of Self and Others*, ed. Frédéric Gros, trans. Graham Burchell (New York: Palgrave Macmillan, 2010), 43.

25. National Aeronautics and Space Administration, "Dark Energy, Dark Matter," *NASA Science: Astrophysics*, updated June 5, 2015, http://science.nasa.gov/astrophysics/focus -areas/what-is-dark-energy/.

26. Ralph Waldo Emerson, "Give All to Love," in *Essays and Poems*, ed. Joel Porte, Harold Bloom, and Paul Kane (New York: Library of America, 1996); and Len Gougeon, *Emerson and Eros: The Making of a Cultural Hero* (Albany: State University of New York Press, 2007), 7.

27. Johann Hari, *Chasing the Scream: The First and Last Days of the War on Drugs* (2015; repr. New York: Bloomsbury, 2016). See also Robert Weiss, "The Opposite of Addiction is Connection," *Psychology Today*, September 30, 2015, www.psychologytoday.com /blog/love-and-sex-in-the-digital-age/201509/the-opposite-addiction-is-connection.

28. Hari, *Chasing the Scream*, 293.

29. Caitlin Elizabeth Hughes and Alex Stevens, "What Can We Learn from the Portuguese Decriminalization of Illicit Drugs?," *British Journal of Criminology* 50 (2010): 999–1022.

30. Sontag, *Illness as Metaphor*, 3.

31. David Rieff, *Swimming in a Sea of Death: A Son's Memoir* (New York: Simon & Schuster, 2008), 31. Subsequent citations will be indicated in the text as *SSD*.

32. Rieff, *Swimming in a Sea of Death*, 38, 43, 121.

33. Rieff, *Swimming in a Sea of Death*, 162–163. I have omitted several sentences (which I believe do not alter the sense of the passage) in order to convey the gist of the deathbed encounter, and I have italicized the text *in order to indicate* my editorial intrusion.

34. *A Midsummer Night's Dream*, II.i.205, in *The Riverside Shakespeare* (Boston: Houghton Mifflin, 1974).

35. William Carlos Williams, *Sappho: A Translation by William Carlos Williams* (San Francisco: Grabhorn Press, 1957). Williams's translation of Sappho's famous ode 31 was printed separately as a broadside.

Acknowledgments

WRITING FOR ME is so tangled up in incessant rewriting and rethinking that it is at best a continuous stop-and-go process (prolonged over many years and many revisions) that only gradually discovers the shape and substance of what emerges as a book. Here, as usual, I call upon fragmentary materials lodged in previous essays as I come to recognize where earlier tryouts might have led, but nothing here merely reproduces previous essays or articles. Everything stands under correction—revised, turned, expanded, cut, plundered, redirected, and substantially altered—as it meets with new thinking, new purposes, and (a gift from the anonymous readers at Harvard University Press) invaluable new critiques. A full acknowledgment is impossible—it would resemble a prose *curriculum vitae* over the last ten years—but I want to extend grateful thanks to the editors, journals, and presses whose support stands behind the fragments and chunks of previous work that I have, inescapably, rethought and substantially reworked here. I owe ongoing thanks for their vision to five gifted scholars who have worked at the crossroads where medicine and the humanities intersect: Arthur Kleinman, Joanne Trautmann Banks, Arthur Frank, Rita Charon, and Kathryn Montgomery. My particular household pantheon has a permanent niche as well for Michel Foucault and Mikhail Bakhtin.

No road this long and winding is traveled alone. I want to express deepest gratitude to Joan Gaustad for her generous spirit, loving heart, invaluable insight, and saving encouragement. My incomparable brothers—Christopher, Michael, and Jess—again proved how much I need them. Heartfelt thanks for improving several preliminary versions go to Julie Sando—astute reader, fine critic, and fast friend. Gerald Bruns, Christopher Morris, Danny Becker, Peg Miller, and Larry Zaroff all helped in ways that they might not recognize or agree on, while Lindsay Waters, Al Zuckerman, and Joy Deng contributed crucial support. No one could wish for a finer editor than Amanda Peery. Her deft guidance was invaluable. Meanwhile, I take steady inspiration, on all roads, from my family trio of writers, scholars, and intrepid explorers: Ellen Morris, Severin Fowles, and Julia Fowles Morris. Ruth Morris, my wife, despite the illness that separates us, inhabits whatever I feel, think, do, and write. I dedicate this book to Ruth, but, in so many ways, it is really her book.

Index